Global Health Governance and Policy

Global Health Governance and Policy outlines the fundamentals of global health, a key element of sustainable development. Taking an interdisciplinary approach, it explores the relationship between the globalization process and global health's social, political, economic and environmental determinants. It points the attention to the actors and forces that shape global policies and actions with an impact on peoples' health in an increasingly complex global governance context. Topics discussed include:

- The relationship between globalization and the determinants of health
- The essentials of global health measurements
- The evolution of public health strategies in the context of the global development agenda
- The actors and influencers of global health governance
- The role of health systems
- The dynamics and mechanisms of global health financing and Development Assistance for Health
- Career opportunities in global health governance, management and policy

Looking in depth at some of the more significant links between neoliberal globalization, global policies and health, *Global Health Governance and Policy: An Introduction* discusses some specific health issues of global relevance such as changes in the ecosystem, epidemics and the spread of infectious diseases, the global transformation of the food system, the tobacco epidemic, human migration, macroeconomic processes and global financial crisis, trade and access to health services, drugs and vaccines, and eHealth and the global "health 4.0" challenge.

Written by a team of experienced practitioners, scientists and teachers, this textbook is ideal for students of all levels and professionals in a variety of disciplines with an interest in global health.

Eduardo Missoni has decades-long experience in international development cooperation, and is currently adjunct professor at the Bocconi University and SDA-Bocconi School of Management, at the Milano-Bicocca University, and at the Medical School of the University of Pavia, Italy. He is also a member of the Faculty of the Geneva School of Diplomacy, and has teaching duties at the Instituto Nacional de Salud Pública in Cuernavaca, Mexico.

Guglielmo Pacileo is a senior physician at the Management Directorate of the Alessandria Local Health Authority, and an adjunct professor at SDA-Bocconi School of Management, Italy. He also holds teaching duties at the Medical School of the University of Pavia, Italy.

Fabrizio Tediosi is Group Leader for Health Policy and System Research at the Department of Epidemiology and Public Health of the Swiss Tropical and Public Health Institute, and Privat Dozent (Associate Professor) at the University of Basel.

Global Health Governance and Policy

An Introduction

Eduardo Missoni, Guglielmo Pacileo and Fabrizio Tediosi

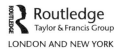

LONDON AND NEW YORK

First published 2019
by Routledge
2 Park Square, Milton Park, Abingdon, Oxon OX14 4RN

and by Routledge
52 Vanderbilt Avenue, New York, NY 10017

Routledge is an imprint of the Taylor & Francis Group, an informa business

© 2019 Eduardo Missoni, Guglielmo Pacileo and Fabrizio Tediosi

The right of Eduardo Missoni, Guglielmo Pacileo and Fabrizio Tediosi to be identified as authors of this work has been asserted by them in accordance with sections 77 and 78 of the Copyright, Designs and Patents Act 1988.

All rights reserved. No part of this book may be reprinted or reproduced or utilised in any form or by any electronic, mechanical, or other means, now known or hereafter invented, including photocopying and recording, or in any information storage or retrieval system, without permission in writing from the publishers.

Trademark notice: Product or corporate names may be trademarks or registered trademarks, and are used only for identification and explanation without intent to infringe.

British Library Cataloguing-in-Publication Data
A catalogue record for this book is available from the British Library

Library of Congress Cataloging-in-Publication Data
Names: Missoni, Eduardo, author. |
Pacileo, Guglielmo, author. | Tediosi, Fabrizio, author.
Title: Global health governance and policy / Eduardo Missoni,
Guglielmo Pacileo, Fabrizio Tediosi.
Description: Abingdon, Oxon ; New York, NY : Routledge, 2019. |
Includes bibliographical references and index.
Identifiers: LCCN 2018051589 | ISBN 9780815393283 (hardback) |
ISBN 9780815393290 (pbk.) | ISBN 9781351188999 (e-book)
Subjects: | MESH: Global Health | Health Policy
Classification: LCC RA418 | NLM WA 530.1 | DDC 362.1–dc23
LC record available at https://lccn.loc.gov/2018051589

ISBN: 978-0-8153-9328-3 (hbk)
ISBN: 978-0-8153-9329-0 (pbk)
ISBN: 978-1-351-18899-9 (ebk)

Typeset in Times New Roman
by Newgen Publishing UK

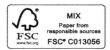

Printed and bound in Great Britain by
TJ International Ltd, Padstow, Cornwall

Contents

List of illustrations ix
Acknowledgements xi
List of abbreviations xii

1 Introduction 1

SECTION 1
Globalization, development and health 9

2 Development, globalization and health 11
   2.1 *The idea of development 11*
      2.1.1 The attributes of development 18
      2.1.2 Overturning the paradigm 19
   2.2 *What is globalization? 21*
      2.2.1 The three dimensions of the globalization process 22
   2.3 *The impact of globalization on human health 24*
      2.3.1 Looking for a methodological framing 24
      2.3.2 Is globalization good for your health? 27

3 Global estimates of health indicators 33
   3.1 *Need and use of global health estimates 33*
   3.2 *The Global Burden of Disease Study 38*
   3.3 *Global health estimate challenges 38*

4 The right to health and the evolution of public health strategies in the context of global development policies 44
   4.1 *The global right to health 44*
   4.2 *From disease eradication programs to health for all and primary health care 45*
   4.3 *The international financial institutions and health systems reform 48*
      4.3.1 From the debt crisis to structural adjustment plans 49
      4.3.2 Structural adjustment and health sector reform 50
   4.4 *Local health systems and health promotion 52*
   4.5 *Sectorial programs and poverty reduction strategies 53*

4.6 Health returns to the center of the global debate 54
4.7 The right to health and commercial interests 61
4.8 The renewed interest in a systemic vision 63

SECTION 2
Global governance and health

5 Global governance in health
   5.1 Introduction 77
   5.2 From international to global health governance, and global governance for health 77
   5.3 Global health governance map 80

6 International institutions: the United Nations system
   6.1 Introduction 83
   6.2 The United Nations Organization 83
      6.2.1 The origins 83
      6.2.2 Structure and functions 84
      6.2.3 Subsidiary organs and other entities 87
      6.2.4 The specialized institutions 88
   6.3 The World Health Organization 89
      6.3.1 The origins 89
      6.3.2 Functions and structure 89
      6.3.3 The evolution of WHO's role as the directing and coordinating authority in global health 94
   6.4 The Bretton Woods institutions: the International Monetary Fund and the World Bank 105
      6.4.1 The origins 105
      6.4.2 Structure and functions of the International Monetary Fund 106
      6.4.3 Structure and functions of the World Bank 107
   6.5 UNAIDS 112
      6.5.1 Origins 112
      6.5.2 Structure and functions 112
   6.6 The World Trade Organization and other free trade regimes 113
      6.6.1 The origins 113
      6.6.2 Structure and functions 114
      6.6.3 The WTO system of multilateral trade agreements: main health-related aspects 115
      6.6.4 Interagency collaboration on intellectual property rights and health 118
      6.6.5 Free trade agreements negotiated outside the WTO 119

7 Governments and their groupings
   7.1 Introduction 127
   7.2 Groups of most influential countries: G8, G20 and BRICS 128
      7.2.1 The G7/G8 129
      7.2.2 The G20 135
      7.2.3 The BRICS 136

Contents vii

8 Non-state actors 140
   8.1 The origins *140*
   8.2 Transnational private business sector entities and their relevance in influencing policies affecting global health *141*
   8.3 Civil society organizations and their relevance in influencing policies affecting global health *145*
   8.4 Global philanthropy and its relevance in influencing policies affecting global health *153*

9 Global action networks and transnational hybrid organizations 160
   9.1 The origins *160*
   9.2 Definition, functions and structure *163*
      9.2.1 Governance *165*
      9.2.2 Management and strategy *166*
      9.2.3 Financing *167*
   9.3 Global public-private partnerships' influence on global policies for health *167*
   9.4 The GAVI Alliance *170*
   9.5 The Global Fund to Fight AIDS, Tuberculosis and Malaria *172*

10 Future challenges toward global governance for health 180
   10.1 Introduction *180*
   10.2 The "chaotic" nature of global health governance and its "narrative" *181*
   10.3 Leadership for *health 183*
   10.4 Facing the challenge: which instruments? *184*

SECTION 3
Global policies and issues 187

11 Neoliberal globalization, global policies and health 189
   11.1 Introduction *189*
   11.2 Changes in the ecosystem *191*
   11.3 Epidemics and the global spread of infectious diseases *197*
   11.4 The transformation of the global food system *202*
      11.4.1 The impact on nutritional status and health *203*
      11.4.2 Food security, food safety and food sovereignty *204*
      11.4.3 The global framework of policies and response *208*
   11.5 The tobacco epidemic *210*
   11.6 Human migration *213*
   11.7 Macroeconomic processes and global financial crises *217*
   11.8 Trade, intellectual property rights and access to drugs *220*
   11.9 eHealth and the global "health 4.0" challenge *229*
      11.9.1 Internet-related health risks *229*
      11.9.2 eHealth potential and challenges *230*
      11.9.3 eHealth policy and governance *233*

12 Health systems in the global health landscape — 246
- *12.1 Introduction 246*
- *12.2 The Universal Health Coverage movement 248*
  - 12.2.1 Policies towards Universal Health Coverage 249
- *12.3 Global challenges to health system sustainability 251*
  - 12.3.1 The epidemiological transition and the challenge of noncommunicable diseases (NCDs) 258
- *12.4 System approaches to address contemporary global health complexity 259*
  - 12.4.1 A fragmented global health governance 260
  - 12.4.2 Social determinants of health, demographic and epidemiological transitions 261
  - 12.4.3 The specialization of health care and health professionals 262
  - 12.4.4 The pluralistic nature of health systems 263

13 Global health financing and Development Assistance for Health — 268
- *13.1 Introduction 268*
- *13.2 Development Assistance for Health and global financing instruments 272*
  - 13.2.1 Global Innovative Financing Instruments (GIFIs) 274
- *13.3 DAH modalities and health systems 277*
  - 13.3.1 Project aid 277
  - 13.3.2 Program assistance 278
  - 13.3.3 From International Health Partnership to UHC2030 281
- *13.4 Main issues and challenges 282*
  - 13.4.1 DAH resources 282
  - 13.4.2 Fragmentation 284
  - 13.4.3 Verticalization 285
  - 13.4.4 Geographical allocation 286

14 Career opportunities in global health — 292
- *14.1 Global health trends and education 292*
- *14.2 "Hands-on" training: internships and first steps in the "career" 294*
- *14.3 Working in global health 296*
- *14.4 The ethical global health professional 299*

Index 304

Illustrations

Figures

2.1	The determinants of health	25
2.2	Framework for globalization and health	26
2.3	Influence on human health of changes related to globalization	27
5.1	Global health governance	81
7.1	WHO Member States with the highest representation in the professional and higher categories	129
9.1	Classification of THOs, GPPPs and other global networks	165
9.2	Contributors to the GFTAM – 2001–2016	175
11.1	Migrant population between 1995 and 2015	214
11.2	Migration phases framework	215
11.3	Migrant health and SDGs	216
12.1	Health systems' building blocks and goals	247
12.2	The dynamic architecture and interconnectedness of health system building blocks	248
12.3	Global determinants of health system sustainability	257
13.1	DAH sources, channels, implementing organizations and flows (a simplified representation)	270
13.2	Development Assistance for Health 1990–2017 (US$ millions)	271
13.3	Global Innovative Financing Instruments (GIFIs): cumulative revenue by instrument (2002–2015)	277
13.4	Program assistance financing	280

Tables

11.1	The direct and indirect pathways from climate change to NCDs	195
11.2	Food security: risks and opportunities linked to global trade liberalization	206
11.3	Guiding principles and priorities to promote the health of refugees and migrants	218
11.4	World Trade Organization (WTO) measures taken in response to the TRIPS agreement	225
13.1	Global Innovative Financing Instruments (GIFIs)	275
13.2	Comparing project assistance and sector-wide approach	280
14.1	List of areas and institutions interested in global health recruitment	298

Boxes

3.1	DHS and MICS programs	34
3.2	Child Health Epidemiology Reference Group (CHERG)	36
3.3	The Health Data Collaborative (HDC)	37
3.4	The National Evaluation Platform (NEP)	41
3.5	The Data for Health initiative	41
4.1	The Alma-Ata Declaration – excerpts	46
4.2	Millennium Development Goals	56
4.3	Case study: politics-based evidence – the creation of the Global Fund to Fight HIV/AIDS, Tuberculosis and Malaria	57
4.4	Sustainable Development Goals	67
4.5	Health targets and actions for Sustainable Development Goal 3	68
6.1	The International Health Regulations	91
6.2	The Framework Convention on Tobacco Control (FCTC)	97
6.3	WHO priorities for the period 2014–2019	102
8.1	Non-state actors	141
8.2	The Red Cross and Red Crescent Movement: governance and membership	147
8.3	The Bill & Melinda Gates Foundation	154
11.1	CIPIH report: main recommendations	226
11.2	The Global Strategy and Plan of Action on Public Health, Innovation and Intellectual Property	228
12.1	Case study: health systems and Ebola	252
13.1	Sources of DAH data	271

Acknowledgements

We would express our gratitude to the many people who encouraged us to pursue this endeavor; to all those who provided support, discussed, read our work and offered their comments.

We owe our deepest thanks to over fifteen cohorts of undergraduate, graduate and post-graduate students that since 2001 have made our didactic effort meaningful with their encouraging feedback and have been the real inspiration of our work.

A heartful thank you to those that allowed us to share our experience with future generations of professionals in different disciplines, offering us individually or as a team the possibility to further explore and teach what we had learnt through both research and experience in the field, at local, national and global levels. A special thanks goes to Alberto Giasanti, who allowed us to pioneer in global health education in Italy, at the Department of Sociology and Social Research, University of Milano-Bicocca; to Elio Borgonovi, who opened for us the doors of the Bocconi University and the SDA Bocconi Management School, entrusting us with the then innovative area of teaching and research in global health and development, at the Center for Research in Health and Social Care of the Bocconi University; to Colum Murphy, who enthusiastically received our proposal to introduce global health governance teaching at the Geneva School of Diplomacy; to the colleagues of the Swiss Tropical and Public Health Institute, Marcel Tanner and Don de Savigny for their inspiring guidance and passion for global health research; and to Nelly Salgado de Sneyder, who prompted the collaboration with the Mexican Instituto Nacional de Salud Pùblica in Cuernavaca.

Thanks to Francesco Cicogna for his valuable comments on the chapter on the World Health Organization, to Lodovica Longinotti for her suggestions regarding development theories and UN-related issues, and to Serafino Marchese for his inputs on the World Trade Organization chapter.

Among the many good friends and colleagues with whom we shared passion and initiatives to advocate for global health, we cannot avoid remembering Giovanni Berlinguer, who in Italy paved the way for the debate on the relations between globalization and human health.

Last but not least, a sincere thanks to Maitreyi Sahu for her generous help with excellent proof-reading, to Afua Asante-Poku for her immediate availability to help and Benedetta Armocida for her assistance with indexing.

Finally, we thank our loved ones, who supported and encouraged us selflessly, despite the many hours that we took from them during this endeavor.

Abbreviations

ACT	Artemisin-based Combination Therapy
ACTA	Anti-counterfeiting Trade Agreement
AFRO	African Regional Office (of the World Health Organization)
AMC	Advance Market Commitment
AMFm	Affordable Medicines Facility for Malaria
AMR	Anti-Microbial Resistance
AMRO	American Regional Office (of the World Health Organization)
BCG	Boston Consulting Group
BRICS	Brazil Russia India China South Africa
CCM	Chronic Care Model
CCM	Country Coordination Mechanism (GFATM)
CEB	Chief Executives Board
CETA	Canada Europe Trade Agreement
CHERG	Child Health Epidemiology Reference Group
CIFF	Child Investment Facility Foundation
COP	Conference of the Parties
CSDH	Commission on Social Determinants of Health
CSO	Civil Society Organizations
CSR	Corporate Social Responsibility
DAC	Development Assistance Committee
DAH	Development Assistance in Health
DFID	UK Department for International Development
DHS	Demographic and Health Surveys Program
DPHAC	Diet, Physical Activity and Health (Global Strategy)
EBF	Extra-Budgetary Funds
ECOSOC	Economic and Social Council
EU	European Union
EURO	European Regional Office (of the World Health Organization)
FAO	Food and Agriculture Organization
FCTC	Framework Convention on Tobacco Control
FENSA	Framework of Engagement with Non-State Actors
GATS	General Agreement on Trade in Services
GAVI	Global Alliance on Vaccines and Immunization
GBS	General Budget Support
GDP	Gross Development Product
GFATM	Global Fund to fight Aids Tuberculosis and Malaria

GHD	Global Health Diplomacy
GHG	Global Health Governance
GIFI	Global Innovative Financing Instruments
GNI	Gross National Income
GOe	Global Observatory on eHealth
GPEDC	Global Partnership for Effective Development Cooperation
GPF	Global Financial Facility
GPPP	Global Public-Private Partnership
HAART	Highly Active Antiretroviral Therapy
HDC	The Health Data Collaborative
HDI	Human Development Index
HER	Health Electronic Records
HIA	Health Impact Assessment
HLCM	High-Level Committee on Management – CEB
HLCP	High-Level Committee on Programme – CEB
HLPF	High-Level Political Forum
HNP	Health Nutrition and Population
IBRD	International Bank for Reconstruction and Development
ICC	Interagency Coordination Committee (GAVI)
ICJ	International Court of Justice
ICRC	International Committee of the Red Cross
ICS	Investor Court System
ICSID	International Centre for Settlement of Investment Disputes
ICT	Information and Communication Technology
IDA	International Development Agency (World Bank Group)
IFC	International Finance Corporation
IFFIm	International Finance Facility for Immunizations
IFI	International Financial Institutions
IFRC	International Federation of the Red Cross and Red Crescent Societies
IHDI	Inequality-adjusted Human Development Index
IHME	Institute for Health Metrics and Evaluation
IHR	International Health Regulations
IIs	International Institutions
ILO	International Labour Organization
IOM	International Organization for Migrations
IPPC	International Plant Protection Convention
ISDS	Investor-State Dispute Settlement
JICA	Japan International Cooperation Agency
LDC	Least Developed Countries
LHS	Local Health Systems
LICs	Low-Income Countries
LMICs	Low-Middle-Income Countries
MNCH&N	Maternal, Newborn and Child Health and Nutrition
MDG	Millennium Development Goals
MICS	Multiple Indicator Cluster Surveys Program
MIGA	Multilateral Investment Guarantee Agency
MPI	Multidimensional Poverty Index

MTEF	Medium-Term Expenditure Framework
NAFTA	North Atlantic Free Trade Agreement
NCD	Non-Communicable Diseases
NEE	Newly Emerging Economies
NEP	The National Evaluation Platform
NGO	Non-Governmental Organization
NIEO	New International Economic Order
NRCMS	New Rural Cooperative Medical System
NT	National Treatment
OCHA	Office for the Coordination of Humanitarian Affairs
OCP	Onchocerciasis Control Programme
ODA	Official Development Aid
ODAH	Official Development Aid in Health
OECD	Organization for Economic Cooperation and Development
OoP	Out of Pocket
OPEC	Organization of Petroleum Exporting Countries
PAHO	Pan American Health Organization
PASB	Pan American Sanitary Bureau
PCB	Programme Coordinating Board
PEPFAR	President's Emergency Plan for AIDS Relief
PHC	Primary Health Care
PHEIC	Public Health Emergency of International Concern
PoW	Plan of Work
PRSP	Poverty Reduction Strategy Papers
PWC	PricewaterhouseCoopers
QoC	Quality of Care
RBF	Regular Budget Funds
RoI	Return on Investment
RTA	Regional Trade Agreements
SAP	Structural Adjustment Program
SBS	Budget Support
SC	Security Council
SEARO	South-East Asia Regional Office (World Health Organization)
SPS	Agreement on the Application of Sanitary and Phytosanitary Measures
SWAp	Sector Wide Approach
TA	Technical Assistance
TBT	Technical Barriers to Trade
THO	Transnational Hybrid Organization
TNC	Transnational Company
TPP	Trans-Pacific Partnership
TRIPS	Trade-Related Intellectual Property Rights
TTIP	Transatlantic Trade and Investment Partnership
UBRAF	Unified Budget, Results and Accountability Framework (UNAIDS)
UHC	Universal Health Coverage
UIA	Union of International Associations
UN	United Nations
UNAIDS	United Nations Programme on HIV/AIDS

UNCTC	United Nations Centre on Transnational Corporations
UNDESA	United Nations Department for Social Affairs
UNDG	United Nations Development Group
UNDP	United Nations Development Programme
UNESCO	United Nations Educational Scientific and Cultural Organization
UNFPA	United Nations Fund for Population Activities
UNGA	United Nations General Assembly
UNHRC	United Nations Human Rights Council
UNICEF	United Nations Children's Fund
UNO	United Nations Organization
UNODC	United Nations Office on Drugs and Crime
U5MR	Under-Five Mortality Rate
WEF	World Economic Forum
WFP	World Food Programme
WHA	World Health Assembly
WHO	World Health Organization
WHR	World Health Report
WIPO	World Intellectual Property Organization
WMO	World Meteorological Organization
WTO	World Trade Organization

1 Introduction

A search made in 2018 on the most popular internet search engine using the keyword "globalization"[1] generates approximately 52,400,000 hits; the same search gave 35,800,000 hits only two years earlier and in 2005 there were only 7,000,000 results. Despite being increasingly and widely used, there is no agreement about the meaning of this term, which describes an essential characteristic of the contemporary era. Some consider globalization as just a new, captivating term to rename the expansion of the neo-liberal development model (which we prefer to define as "neoliberal globalization"), while others see in it a century-old process of integration which has seen an impressive acceleration since the second half of the last century. Whatever the interpretation, due to the technological advances in communications and transport and the ever-growing level of world interconnectedness, people, goods and diseases are moving fast across borders. World citizens and governments have to increasingly deal with these issues which have transnational dimensions and that require equally transnational responses. Also, the temporal dimension of globalization is modified with ever-faster technological, but also environmental and microbiological, changes. Additionally, cognitive changes have facilitated knowledge-sharing but also impacted the traditional cultures and behaviors, including production, distribution and consumption patterns. These have impacted health directly as have changes in the ecosystem. Humanity today faces unprecedented social, economic and environmental global, i.e. planetary, challenges.

The consequences are particularly significant in terms of human health: new infectious diseases are emerging and spreading; the prevalence of chronic, degenerative and socio-behavioral pathologies is increasing; the right to health is often questioned or denied; utilitarian approaches consider human health as a factor of economic growth, rather than a right in itself; access to care is often limited as part of macroeconomic interventions which include public expenditure reduction policies; and avoidable and unfair disparities in health outcomes, i.e. inequities,[2] are increasing. More in general, inequities between the North and the South of the world are increasing, whereby "North" and "South" have lost any geographical connotation. Instead, this represents the distance between the few in the various Norths in whose hands wealth and opportunities are concentrated, and the multitudes of the many Souths who are excluded from the benefits of modernity and suffer from poverty and marginalization. These inequities also exacerbate health risks and threats, with critical implications for sustainable development.

Health has been increasingly recognized as a key element of sustainable economic development, global security, effective governance and human rights promotion (Frenk

2010). Since the late 1990s, the role of health in global development policies has become more relevant, as shown by the fact that three out of the eight Millennium Development Goals (MDGs) set forth in the year 2000 by United Nations Millennium Declaration – "the blueprint agreed to by all the world's countries and all the world's leading development institutions" – were related to health targets (MDG 4: Reduce child mortality; MDG 5: Improve maternal health; MDG 6: Combat HIV/AIDS, malaria and other diseases).

The Sustainable Development Goals (SDGs) approved in 2015 confirmed the central role of global health in the much broader agenda for global development as defined by the Agenda 2030 and its universal and indivisible 17 SDGs.[3]

This shift in attention to health has also resulted in an unprecedented growth of financial resources at a global level destined for the development of the health sector, a trend that has been partially reversed since 2013, with 2017 levels comparable to those of 2012.[4]

Over the last few decades, the number of global health initiatives as well as both public and private actors involved in the global health governance increased substantially, leading to a highly complex scenario. This has even challenged the World Health Organization's (WHO) mandate as the "directing and coordinating authority" in international health. Indeed, the relative weight of the actors traditionally active in the health sector is changing. Economic forces strongly influence national and international public policies that tend to benefit the creation of favorable environments for economic investments, over health promotion and control of the determinants negatively impacting on the living conditions and health of the populations.

However, a parallel increased focus on the importance of the social, economic, political and environmental determinants of health that are influenced by decisions made in other global policy-making arenas (such as those governing international trade, environment, migration) has prompted the debate on the need to protect and promote health in global governance processes outside the global health system. This approach has been conceptualized as "global governance *for* health" (Frenk and Moon 2013).

Judging by the scope of topics covered by existing resources on global health, almost everything has been thrown into the "global" pot, often re-labeling as "global" issues and modalities defined by terms (such as international) that have proven perfectly adequate in the past. "The health field has been equally guilty of this tendency which, in turn, has led to conceptual and empirical imprecision" (Lee 2004).

According to the same trend, teaching "Global Health" also became fashionable. In 2009, Richard Horton, chief editor of *The Lancet*, highlighted that global health was becoming a critical aspect of the educational, scientific and moral mission of universities (Horton 2009). Beyond the academic sector, the media are increasingly referring to the idea of global health. International and bilateral institutions as well as private organizations are also putting increasing emphasis on it. The subject attracts new generations of students and scholars, new journals are dedicated to this field of studies, and the offer of courses in this new area has been booming over the last decade or so.

However, there is still wide discrepancy about what global health stands for and about the content of global health courses offered around the world, whereby sometimes the denomination global health is arguably used to refurbish pre-existing courses in "international health", "tropical medicine" and others in a mere response to marketing needs (Koplan *et al.* 2009). This presents an interesting conundrum because, as pointed out by Bozorgmehr (2010), "Social innovations are unlikely to evolve if 'Global Health' becomes or remains a cosmetic re-labeling of old patterns, objects, and interests".

Thus, the question arises "what should be taught when we teach global health?" (Missoni and Martino 2011), and by extension what is the scope of global health governance and policies?

Regarding the definition, there has been some debate over the past years. The term global health was, and still is, applied liberally and with little attempt to fully explain the true definition and contents of the terminology (Bozorgmehr 2010). Clearly, once the global health community examines how health determinants and policies range beyond the interactions between nation states, the inadequacy of the "international" attribute becomes evident (Missoni and Martino 2011). Similarly, the need to include multiple consolidated disciplines (sociology, political sciences, economics, anthropology, environmental sciences and others) allows the understanding of global health as more than simply the global dimension of public health (Fried *et al.* 2010). Also, what is meant with global health policies and projects and how they are implemented are deeply discordant (Rieder 2016).

Bozorgmehr (2010) identifies four ways in which the term "global" is understood in the health literature. The first meaning for global is: "worldwide" or "everywhere". The second criterion refers to health issues that are not limited by national boundaries (e.g. pandemics and the spread of infectious disease). According to the third criterion, the term global refers to a broad-spectrum approach that is multidisciplinary in character. Thus, the study of global health is the study of social, political, economic, biological and technological relationships that impact health in diverse means. Highlighting the diversity and complexity of those relations in the global space, Rieder (2016) synthesizes global health as "a set of processes that occur at the intersections of transnational networks". Finally, the term "global" refers to what Scholte (2002) coined "supra-territoriality", or social connections that move beyond simple territorial geography, a phenomenon which has increased exponentially through both the number of social media tools as well as the number of users. According to Bozorgmeher (2010), it is the fourth interpretation – supra-territoriality – that allows global health to focus "on the globality of the social determinants of health and the power relations in global social space" (Bozorgmeher 2010). However, it is important to note that underlying these four interpretations of the terminology "global" is one unifying ideal: equity. Addressing the current inequities in health status worldwide has become one of the primary goals in all global health studies (CSDH 2008).

Lack of agreement on the definition of global health and a general discord regarding theories that can generalize findings do not yet allow the classification of global health as a self-standing discipline. Indeed, as pointed out above, an interdisciplinary approach is essential to understand this new area of studies and the complexity of this approach may have limited the education of practitioners and the emergence of an intellectually robust field (Kleinmann 2010).

More recently, the concept of "planetary health" was launched by *The Lancet* (Horton *et al.* 2014) and supported by the Rockefeller Foundation, with a scope supposedly going beyond the boundaries of "the existing global health framework to take into consideration the natural systems upon which human health depends". It was nevertheless presented as "A New Discipline in Global Health" (Rodin 2015), thus part of this interdisciplinary area of studies. In the original "Manifesto", planetary health is presented as "an attitude towards life and a philosophy for living" (Horton *et al.* 2014). The emphasis on people and equity, the recognition of the impact of neoliberal globalizations on health and the sustainability of human development, as well as the focus on equity and on "interdependence and the interconnectedness of the risks we face" (Horton *et al.* 2014), all belong to a comprehensive understanding of global health. The ecosystem is undoubtedly one of the most important determinants of human health and in that sense the emphasis that planetary health places on the link between human health and a healthy planet is highly welcome.

In Italy, global health as a field of studies, research and practice was identified from the very beginning of the debate at the end of the 1990s, with the interaction between globalization and health. This would include the planetary dimension of the issues at stake; a people-centered, human right and health determinants approach; ethically minded and focused on equity. Thus, the global health goal would require global responses with solid roots in local awareness and action, and moral responsibility toward future generations (Berlinguer 1999).[5]

Since 2008, we have adopted a definition that encompasses most of the elements discussed above, such as interdisciplinarity, focus on equity, people-centered and health determinants approach, the worldwide transnational dimension of both determinants and solutions:

> Global health is an emerging area for interdisciplinary studies, research and practice that considers the effects of globalization on health – understood as a complete state of physical, mental and social well-being – and the achievement of equity in health for all people worldwide, emphasizing transnational health issues, determinants and solutions, and their interactions with national and local systems.
> (CERGAS 2011)

The development and implementation of transnational, i.e. global, solutions imply global governance and policies, a dimension of global health that, in our opinion, is still lacking an introductory, but comprehensive textbook in the English language.

To this end, we use an interdisciplinary approach, combining health sciences with economic, social and management sciences, in exploring global health, social, political, economic and environmental determinants, and the role of both State and non-State actors in an increasingly complex global governance scenario.

The book is divided into three sections: the first provides an overview on the links between globalization, development and health; the central section focuses on global governance and health; and the third offers an insight on most relevant global issues and related policies.

In the first section, an introductory chapter (Chapter 2) sets the theoretical bases that connect development, globalization and health. It first briefly and critically illustrates how the concept of development was generated, and how it evolved in the context of the international agenda, situating health in that context. The chapter then explains the acceleration of the globalization process and uses its three dimensions (temporal, spatial and cognitive) (Lee 2000) to illustrate how it relates to health. Finally, the chapter provides the reader with a framework linking globalization and societal determinants of health.

The following chapter (Chapter 3) analyzes how the rise in the importance of global health has been accompanied by the increasing need for global estimates of health indicators. It describes the need for global health estimates based on statistical modeling that has evolved in a new field referred to as "science of global health estimates". It then reviews the sources of data and the main challenges of health information metrics and systems, showing how global health estimates are produced. Finally, Chapter 3 discusses the institutions involved and their funding, and reflects some of the contemporary challenges in global health governance.

The next chapter (Chapter 4) in the section uses a "right to health" approach in historically describing the evolution of health policies, priorities and practices in the context of the global development agenda, from the establishment of the World Health Organization and the Universal Declaration of Human Rights to the Agenda 2030 for sustainable development. It highlights most significant passages, such as: the Alma Ata Declaration, the Primary Health Care strategy and counteractive emergence of selective approaches; the Structural Adjustment Programs and Health Systems Reforms; health promotion and health in the context of integrated poverty reduction programs; the emergence of the Global Public-Private Partnership model, and the emphasis put on the potential role of market and finance for health; the renewed commitment for a systemic approach to health; and most recent changes and trends in the sustainable development global platform.

In the second section, a short chapter (Chapter 5) introduces, and differentiates between, the concepts of global health governance and global governance *for* health, i.e. prioritizing and promoting health through policies and processes in non-health sectors, and maps the main actors in today's global scene.

The following chapters look into the organizational governance and role in influencing health policies of the main actors in global health. First intergovernmental organizations (Chapter 6) are described, including the UN, and its funds and programs (e.g. UNICEF and UNFPA), its specialized agencies and specifically the World Health Organization, and the Bretton Wood Institutions (IMF and World Bank), UNAIDS and UN-related organizations, and specifically the World Trade Organization.

Then in Chapter 7 the reader is introduced to the role of "donor" countries especially in the context of development assistance (developed separately in Section 3), but also in the multiple international forums where they exercise their influence. It also describes the origins, structure, functions and influence of some specific "groupings" of countries, such as the G7/G8, the G20 and the BRICS in orienting global health policies.

A following chapter (Chapter 8) analyzes the evolution of the participation and role of non-State actors in health, as well as their relevance in influencing policies affecting global health. Transnational companies, civil society organizations and global philanthropy are separately analyzed.

The notion and classification of global action networks and transnational hybrids and their relevance in global health are dealt with in Chapter 9, which also describes their origins, the way they are structured and function, and their influence on global health policies.

The concluding chapter (Chapter 10) of the second section traces the most important challenges in health-related global governance and possible future scenarios.

In the third section, a wide chapter (Chapter 11) explores the impact of consumerist neoliberal globalization on the population's health and the relevant global policy and action responses. Specific phenomena and health issues are used as examples, such as the changes in the ecosystem, epidemics and the spread of infectious diseases, the global transformation of the food system, the tobacco epidemic, human migration, the macro-economic processes and global financial crisis, intellectual property rights and access to drugs, and the challenges of eHealth.

6 *Introduction*

The next chapter (Chapter 12) analyzes the concept, objectives, functions and actors of health systems as proximal health determinants. It focuses on investing in health systems and the challenge of building health-care systems that can sustainably attain the Universal Health Coverage (UHC) global target, vis-á-vis the impact of the global epidemic of noncommunicable diseases (NCDs) and pervasive health consumerism. The chapter concludes by highlighting the need for a system thinking to address contemporary global health complexities.

A chapter (Chapter 13) is then dedicated to development assistance in health, providing the reader with an overview of current issues, mechanisms and flows in global health financing. It also illustrates the basic concepts, goals and mechanisms of development cooperation in health; it describes how they have evolved according to the changing nature and influence of international and transnational actors, and explores future scenarios and challenges.

Finally, the last chapter (Chapter 14) of the book provides a synthetic overview of education and career opportunities in global health governance, management and policy. We conclude that chapter by focusing attention on the moral commitment of the ethical global health professional.

It is our hope that this book, besides providing the theoretical and knowledge bases to engage in global health and to face the complex and challenging dynamics of its governance and policy-making, may contribute to the creation of new generations of people acting *for* health regardless of their discipline, sector of involvement, or position. These will be people who are willing to dedicate their personal and professional long-term commitment to their community and to the whole planet, sharing the goal of health and wellbeing everywhere and for every human being, including future generations.

Notes

1 We used the American English spelling for the purpose.
2 Health inequities are systematic, unnecessary, avoidable, unfair and unjust differences in health outcomes and their determinants between segments of the population (Whitehead 1990).
3 https://sustainabledevelopment.un.org/post2015/transformingourworld.
4 https://vizhub.healthdata.org/fgh/.
5 A small group of experienced researchers and practitioners joined forces in 2002 and established the Italian Global Health Watch (OISG) to advocate global health concepts, research, policies and action among Italian institutions and public. This led, among other things, to nationwide initiatives for the teaching of global health including the creation of a specific network linking all those experiences and providing a forum to identify a common understanding and methodological approach to global health (Missoni 2013). The authors of this book were part of those experiences and in 2001 pioneered the introduction of global health in non-health disciplines and contexts, such as the Faculty of Sociology at the Milano-Bicocca University (Missoni *et al.* 2013) and the SDA Bocconi Management School (Missoni *et al.* 2013a), and later (in 2008) the Geneva School of Diplomacy; as well as the publication of the first Global health textbook in Italian (Missoni and Pacileo 2005).

References

Berlinguer, G., 1999. Globalization and global health. *International Journal of Health Services*, 29(3), 579–595.
Bozorgmehr, K., 2010. Rethinking the 'global' in global health: a dialectic approach. *Global Health*, 6, 19.

CERGAS, 2011. *Area Global Health and Development. Activity Report 2008–2010*. Center for Research on Health and Social Care Management, Area Global Health and Development. Milano: Bocconi University, 3.

CSDH, 2008. *Closing the gap in a generation: Health equity through action on the social determinants of health*. Commission on the Social Determinants of Health. Geneva: World Health Organization.

Frenk, J., 2010. The global health system: strengthening national health systems as the next step for global progress. *PLoS Medicine*, 7(1), e1000089.

Frenk, J., Moon, S., 2013. Governance challenges in global health. *New England Journal of Medicine*, 368(10), 936–942.

Fried, L.P., et al., 2010. Global health is public health. *The Lancet*, 375, 535–537.

Horton, R., 2009. Global science and social movements: toward a rational politics of global health. *International Health*, 1, 26–30.

Horton, R., et al., 2014. From public to planetary health: a manifesto. *The Lancet*, 383, 847.

Kleinman, A., 2010. The art of medicine. Four social theories for global health. *The Lancet*, 7(375), 1518–9.

Koplan, J.P., et al., 2009. Towards a common definition of global health. *The Lancet*, 373, 1993–1995.

Lee, K. 2000. Global dimensions of health. In Parsons, L., Lister, G. (Eds.), *Global Health: A Local Issue*. London: The Nuffield Trust.

Lee, K., 2004. 20 best resources on globalization. *Health Policy and Planning*, 20(2), 137–139.

Missoni, E., Martino, A., 2011. L'insegnamento della salute globale. In Cattaneo, A. (Ed.), *Salute Globale. InFormAzione per cambiare*. 4° Rapporto dell'Osservatorio Italiano sulla Salute Globale. Pisa: Edizioni ETS, 21–34.

Missoni, E., 2013. Global health education in Italy. In Missoni, E., Tediosi, F. (Eds.), *Education in Global Health Policy and Management*. Milano: Egea, 21–29.

Missoni, E., Pacileo, G., 2005. *Elementi di salute globale. Globalizzazione, politiche sanitarie e salute umana*. (1st edition). Milano: Franco Angeli.

Missoni, E., Pacileo, G., 2016. *Elementi di salute globale. Globalizzazione, politiche sanitarie e salute umana*. (2nd updated edition). Milano: Franco Angeli.

Missoni, E., Pacileo, G., Giasanti, A., 2013. Teaching global health in a Faculty of Sociology: introducing a multidisciplinary, trans-cultural approach. In Missoni, E., Tediosi, F. (Eds.), *Education in Global Health Policy and Management*. Milano: Egea, 121–126.

Missoni, E., et al. 2013a. Teaching global health and development in a school of management and economics. In Missoni, E., Tediosi, F. (Eds.), *Education in Global Health Policy and Management*. Milano: Egea, 97–112.

Rieder, S., 2016. Interrogating the global health and development nexus: critical viewpoints of neoliberalization and health in transnational spaces. *World Development Perspectives*, 2(C), 55–61.

Rodin, J., 2015. Planetary health: A new discipline in global health. The Rockefeller Foundation. July 16. www.rockefellerfoundation.org/blog/planetary-health-a-new-discipline-in-global-health/.

Scholte, J.A., 2002. *What Is Globalization? The Definitional Issue – Again*. Coventry, Centre for the Study of Globalisation and Regionalisation (CSGR), Department of Politics and International Studies, University of Warwick; CSGR Working Paper 109/02.

Whitehead, M., 1990. *The Concepts and Principles of Equity in Health*. WHO, Reg. Off. Eur.: Copenhagen (EUR/ICP/RPD 414 7734r).

Unless otherwise indicated, all websites were accessed on 9 August 2018.

SECTION 1
Globalization, development and health

2 Development, globalization and health

2.1 The idea of development

Over the past decades, we have grown accustomed to the idea of a world divided into developed and developing countries, wherein "development" appears as the universally desired objective. Through a wide range of literature, the definition of "development" has been used to "encompass almost all facets of the good society, everyman's road to utopia" (Arndt 1987: 1). As a societal evolutionary process, development was hardly used as a concept before World War II. For example, the Covenant of the League of Nations, the predecessor of today's United Nations, and the first permanent International Institution (II), indicated the well-being and development of people living in countries "under the sovereignty of the States which formerly governed them" and that are "not yet able to stand by themselves under the strenuous conditions of the modern world", as a "sacred trust of civilization". The tutelage of those peoples was entrusted to "advanced" nations who would exercise it "as Mandatories on behalf of the League" (League of Nations 1919).

The first institution to explicitly include "development" in its mission was most likely the International Bank for Reconstruction and Development (IBRD), which is now part of the World Bank Group.

For the League of Nations, international cooperation meant the achievement of "international peace and security". By contrast, the Charter of the United Nations Organization, established in 1945, understood the notion of international cooperation as the resolution to global issues of economic, social, cultural or humanitarian nature, and included, among its aims, the promotion and respect of human rights and fundamental freedom for all. The UN Charter engaged all members in international economic and social cooperation in the pursuit of a "higher standard of living, full employment, and conditions of economic and social progress and development" as well as achieving "solutions of international economic, social, health, and related problems, and international cultural and educational cooperation; and universal respect for, and observance of human rights and fundamental freedoms for all" (UN 1945).

In line with that approach, Polanyi Levitt states that: "development in a meaningful sense implies a social and economic transformation to eradicate injustices of the past" (Polanyi Levitt 2012: 17).

In the aftermath of World War II, the reconstruction of Europe was among the most pressing issues. The launch of the Marshall Plan on the 5th of June 1947 responded to the dire need to restore the European economy that was battered by the war. The plan created a wide market for the American industry, and simultaneously created a political and economic bloc for nations allied with the USA that could prevent the spread of Soviet communism.

The Marshall Plan (officially known as the European Recovery Program – ERP) is commonly seen as the prototype of international aid. From the Marshall Plan and the Conference of Sixteen (Conference for European Economic Co-operation) emerged the Organization for European Economic Co-operation (OEEC) in 1948, with the intention to establish a permanent organization that would continue working towards a joint recovery program and, more importantly, supervise the distribution of aid. In September 1961, the OEEC was superseded by the Organization for Economic Co-operation and Development (OECD). The former Development Assistance Group (DAG), formed as a forum for consultations among aid donors on assistance to less-developed countries, was constituted as the Development Assistance Committee (DAC). Economic growth and the expansion of world trade were clearly spelled out as part of the OECD's aims and therefore linked with the idea of development.

Thus, the concept of development has been largely associated with the politics of development cooperation policies, and development studies have been limited to poor countries' economy and welfare, and to North-South relations. This approach entirely disregarded the global dimension.

Various authors refer to United States President Harry Truman's "Inaugural Address" on the 20th of January 1949 as the inauguration of the "era of development" and development aid (Rist 1997). In his speech Truman proclaimed

> a bold new program for making the benefits of our scientific advances and industrial progress available for the improvement and growth of underdeveloped areas ... a program of development based on the concept of democratic fair dealing.
> (Truman 1949)

The economic space replaced the concept of the world as a political space characteristic of the colonial era. According to a wide range of literature, the new discourse would serve for the emerging power of the USA to justify the dismantling of colonial empires and gain access to new markets (Rist 1997). As Truman stated, "The old imperialism– exploitation for foreign profit – has no place in our plans" (Truman 1949). Nevertheless, "donor" countries would still benefit from improved access to world resources.

> All countries, including our own, will greatly benefit from a constructive program for the better use of the world's human and natural resources. Experience shows that our commerce with other countries expands as they progress industrially and economically.
> (Truman 1949)

Development became the universal ideal that should guide the progress of the "underdeveloped" world, where, in this context, "underdeveloped" was being used as a term for "economically backward regions" and a state of deficiency, rather than a result of historical circumstances (i.e. colonial legacy effects).

The term "development" became a metaphor of economic growth measured through the increase of the gross domestic product (GDP), and economics towered over all other aspects of life and wellbeing.

It must be noted that GDP only measures economic transactions of goods and services. Goods or services that are exchanged free (presents, volunteering, etc.) do not contribute to growth measured through GDP. In addition, economic growth is not qualitatively neutral. Depending on the type of goods and services that contribute to GDP and its growth, their production cycle and their marketing, the impact on life conditions of the population (and life in general) may vary substantially. For example, a GDP based on the production of weapons or cigarettes has a very different social and health impact than one based on wealth created through food or cultural production. The production and marketing of processed food has a very different health, social and environmental impact than food produced according to "organic" or "bio" standards and consumed locally. In the technological era, an increase in production, leading to economic growth, is not necessarily associated with a rise in employment rates; rather, the opposite effect occurs. Not to mention the weakness of an economic growth based predominantly on financial dynamics, without increase in production.

A recent research paper showed a direct relation between economic growth and the incidence rate of cancer, which increases linearly with per capita income, even after controlling for population ageing, improvement in cancer detection, and omitted spatially correlated variables (Luzzati *et al.* 2018). While this observation does not allow for disentangling the role of lifestyle and environmental degradation on cancer, it is unequivocal that industrial production is linked to the introduction of carcinogenic pollutants. Thus, the effects of economic growth are necessarily different depending on the level of pollution of the production cycles and the renewability of energy resources utilized. In general, industry tends to "externalize" the impact of production, and therefore also its environmental and social costs, i.e. costs are transferred to the community and the State has to take on the burden of those costs. If those costs were accounted for as production costs, i.e. "internalized", goods resulting from non-sustainable productive processes and practice would lack profitability due to a substantial increase in their final price. As a consequence, companies would be pushed to increase their social and environmental sustainability. There are several ways in which government regulation can reduce detrimental externalities to consolidate the production and actual costs: legislation to force firms to internalize costs, imposition of taxes as high as the externalities produced by the firms, and pollution controls and emission standards which are environmentally sustainable (Hayes 2017).

The conceptualization of "development" as economic growth also serves as a good example of how the language of politics is closely linked to politics of language, specifically in the realm of North-South relations, where "use and abuse of the language of politics" is evident and "Concepts such as 'development,' 'justice' and 'cooperation' frequently have been associated with particular ideological agendas and not infrequently obscure the nature and content of political-economic relations and processes rather than illuminating them" (Petras and Veltmeyer 2001: 121).

Conceived in technocratic and quantitative terms, growth and aid were proposed as the only possible, paradigmatic answers, and "development" soon became "the password for imposing a new kind of dependency, for enriching the already rich world and for shaping other societies to meet its commercial and political needs" (George 1976: xvii).

During the 1950s, the international development agenda found support from the Modernization Theory, elaborated by Walt W. Rostow and other American economists. In his *The Stages of Economic Growth: A Non-Communist Manifesto* (1960), Rostow utilizes the "takeoff" concept as a metaphor to identify these five stages of growth leading to modernization: the traditional society, the pre-conditions for takeoff, the takeoff, the drive to maturity, and the age of high mass-consumption.

In those years, development attention focused on the establishment of urban-industrial nodes as the basis for self-sustained growth, assuming that in the long run the "trickle-down effect" would spread modernization from urban to rural areas. In the following decade, the importance of agriculture was reassessed, as there was a growing recognition that employment does not grow along with industrial production.

The UN declared the 1960s as the "development decade" as it called for industrialized countries to considerably increase their Official Development Aid (ODA) (see Chapters 4 and 13).

During the mid-1960s, the foundations of the classic development theory were also criticized. The dependency theory, developed mainly by Latin American scholars, such as Raúl Prebish, Fernando H. Cardoso, Theotonio dos Santos, Osvaldo Sunkel, André Gunder Frank and others, pointed out that the causes of under-development should be sought beyond domestic economic factors (Muñoz 1981). According to these scholars, the principal cause of underdevelopment depends on the structural position of countries that are considered backwards in the economic world, where resources tend to flow from the "periphery" of poor, underdeveloped states, into the "core" of wealthy states. This dynamic enriched the latter at the expense of the former through progressive deterioration in the terms of trade. In addition, the interests of bureaucratic and political elites of those "peripheral" countries would functionally converge with those of the elites of the developed countries, promoting distorted forms of development that encouraged investments in areas with no direct benefit for the population, e.g. military expenditures (Prebisch 1950) and mega-projects, which were often ill-conceived and enormously costly, exemplified in the Trans-Amazonic Highway in the 1970s. In 1964, the UN established the Conference on Trade and Development (UNCTAD) under the direction of Raúl Prebisch in order to address the problems of export-dependent peripheries.

In Africa, Julius Kambarage Nyerere, who served as the first president of Tanzania, decided to face "underdevelopment" in his country by making his fellow citizens rely mainly on their own forces. The Arusha Declaration (1967), passed by the Tanganyka African National Union (TANU) on the 5th of February 1967, promoted the concepts of self-reliance and self-centered development. The self-reliance approach proposes to undertake the "war against poverty and oppression" in Tanzania by attempting to move "the people of Tanzania (and the people of Africa as a whole) from a state of poverty to a state of prosperity". The Declaration indicated an alternative and autonomous, although not autarchic, way to development. This approach refused to rely on external aid and money provided through gifts and loans, as it "will endanger our independence". For Nyerere, the "foundation of development" was agriculture, the people and their hard work, where money is considered "one of the fruits of that hard work". Land, people, good policies and good leadership were the keywords of that strategy that oriented society "toward the development of man instead of material wealth" (Nyerere 1974: 32).

In the 1970s, the debate was fueled by the Movement for the New International Economic Order (NIEO) and the so-called "basic needs" approach. Both concepts were born from the observation that, despite the positive overall economic performance of the Third World, growth failed to alleviate poverty.

In 1972, the first Report of the Club of Rome[1] had already marked the existing "limits to growth" that demonstrated the quantitative restraints of the ecosystem. To avoid "the tragic consequences of an overshoot", the Report also called for "the initiation of new forms of thinking that will lead to a fundamental revision of human behavior and, by implication, of the entire fabric of present-day society" (Meadows *et al.* 1972: 185–196).

The so-called "North-South Dialogue" between industrial and developing countries led the United Nations General Assembly to adopt the Declaration for the Establishment of a NIEO (UN 1974), which focused on the restructuring of the world economy in order to allow greater participation by, and benefits to, developing countries.

A non-economic reinterpretation of "development" was attempted by the Dag Hammarskjöld Report in 1975. Through the initiative of the Hammarskjöld Foundation and the United Nations Environment Program (UNEP), coordinated by Marc Nerfin, a group of approximately a hundred people from all the parts of the world concluded that development should be endogenous, arising from within the culture of every society, and cannot be reduced to the imitation of developed societies as there is no universal formula for development. Instead, satisfying the basic needs of the poorest populations should come first. These communities would have to rely primarily on their own strengths to succeed. According to this concept, which is outlined in the report "What Now?", disadvantaged countries essentially depended on exploitation structures that originated in the North but were reproduced in the South by the leading classes who were both rivals and accomplices of the élites in industrialized countries (Rist 1997).

Even the president of the World Bank, Robert McNamara, underscored the need of "a serious reexamination of earlier growth strategies ... causing governments to focus more directly on ... the hundreds of millions of individuals whose basic human needs go unmet" (McNamara 1976).

The Basic Needs approach was adopted by the 1976 World Employment Conference. It placed priority on policies and programs that ensured access to clean water, nutrition, appropriate shelter, health care, education and security to the poorest populations (ILO 1976). During those years, modest reorientations clashed with the debt crisis of developing countries during the following decade and with the reaffirmation of the role of the market in the name of neoliberal principles.

The Reagan administration in the USA and the Thatcher government in Great Britain championed the neoliberal ideology, with the International Monetary Fund (IMF) and the World Bank (WB) implementing those principles globally. According to that approach, known as the Washington Consensus,[2] the state is the main obstacle to development and every barrier blocking any market penetration must be removed in developing countries. Instead of international aid, foreign investments should provide external resources to developing countries whose governments are considered inefficient, corrupt, and therefore incapable of a productive and efficient allocation of resources.

In response to the debt crisis, the WB and the IMF shared a similar perspective through the Structural Adjustment Programs (SAP), imposing neoliberal policies on developing countries with the effect of impeding their autonomous choices that, according to those financial institutions, "would end up damaging world trade" (Isernia 1995: 50).

Therefore, the global expansion of the neoliberal model entails large-scale privatizations, reduced taxation for the benefit of higher incomes, cuts in public spending and the dismantling of education, health and social systems, the financial deregulation and the free movement of capital, the uncontrolled exploitation of environmental resources and, lastly, export-oriented industrial production. Neoliberal policies led to the growth of inequalities and concentrated on the small sectors of the wealthy populations that emerged from the expansion of the economy.

The impact of structural adjustment policies on health and health systems is analyzed in further detail in Chapters 4 and 11.

Without questioning the assimilation of development with economic growth, some authors argued that the underlying production and consumption patterns should be reshaped in order to be compatible with respect for the concern for justice. In 1987, the Our Common Future Report, better known as the Brundtland Report, which is the name of the research group coordinator, introduced the concept of "sustainable development" defined as: "development that meets the needs of the present without compromising the ability of future generations to meet their own needs" (WCED 1987).

While recognizing the limits of the biosphere, the report introduced the possibility that future knowledge would still allow the continuity of economic expansion:

> The concept of sustainable development does imply limits – not absolute limits but limitations imposed by the present state of technology and social organization on environmental resources and by the ability of the biosphere to absorb the effects of human activities. But technology and social organization can be both managed and improved to make way for *a new era of economic growth*.
>
> (WCED 1987)

According to Rist, the idea of sustainable, "durable", development was just another masking operation to prevent the radical questioning of the effects of economic growth. It was an invitation to ensure lasting development, i.e. to make continuous and everlasting growth (Rist 1997).[3]

Around the 1990s, neoliberal policies were criticized. As a result, there was a growing need to redefine the meaning, goals and measurements for development.

The Nobel laureate Amartya Sen introduced the capability approach as a conceptual framework. In his view development is seen as the improvement of peoples' lives through the expansion of people's capabilities such as: to be healthy and well fed, educated, knowledgeable, and to participate in the life of the community. As Sen put it, human development is the process of enlarging a person's functionings and capabilities to function, the range of things that a person could do and be in his/her life (Sen 1989).

Sen's work inspired UNDP's first annual flagship report in1990, where the concept of "human development" was adopted. The report questioned whether economic growth and GDP were efficient indicators of a country's progress. "People are the real wealth of a nation. The basic objective of development is to create an enabling environment for people to enjoy long, healthy and creative lives" was the incipit of the first Human Development Report. "Excessive preoccupation with GNP growth and national income accounts has obscured that powerful perspective, sup-planting a focus on ends by an obsession with merely the means" (UNDP 1990). Human development was thus defined as "a process of enlarging people's choices", the most critical ones being identified in "leading a long and healthy life, to be educated and to enjoy a decent standard of living", with additional choices that included political freedom, guaranteed human rights and self-respect.

The Human Development Index (HDI) was proposed as a new indicator to measure progress, based on longevity, knowledge and decent living standards (UNDP 1990).

Without questioning the function of economic growth for development purposes, UNDP subsequently addressed the notion of inequality by saying that there can be no human development with unequal income distribution and low and poorly distributed social spending (UNDP 1999).

In its subsequent reports, UNDP introduced improved versions of HDI, as well as new composite indicators that measure aspects of human development, which the HDI does not reflect, such as inequality, poverty, human security or gender disparities.[4]

The process also fed into the international agenda for economic and social development.

Indeed, during the 1990s, widespread debate was sparked at various international summits,[5] which were aimed at redefining the world agenda for economic and social development, with the objective to centralize the world's attention on the fight against poverty. Debate centered on "Shaping the 21st Century: The Contribution of Development Co-operation", a report by the Organization for Economic Cooperation and Development that laid the foundation for what would lead to the Millennium Declaration in 2000 (OECD/DAC 1996).

At the end of the homonymous summit, The Millennium Declaration was signed by all heads of state and government in September 2000. The declaration attempted to reaffirm a human rights-based development approach with the commitment to "making the right to development a reality for everyone and to freeing the entire human race from want" (UN 2000: 1–2). It proclaimed the "fundamental values" of equality, freedom, solidarity, tolerance, respect for nature and shared responsibility, and recognized the unequal distribution of the benefits and costs of globalization (UN 2000: 2). This was the first time in development cooperation history that all countries and main actors in development agreed on what should be done and formally adopted common results that they intend to achieve on a global level (Vähämäki *et al.* 2011).

With the aim to transform the Declaration into a more operational tool, participants in the Summit decided to identify Millennium Development Goals (MDGs) to progress the development agenda. The MDGs should have shifted the emphasis on poverty defined as lack of income to the multidimensional feature of human poverty. The original aim of the MDGs was to overcome the narrow paradigm of growth and to focus on human, sustainable and fair welfare. However, the conventional and economistic vision of development prevailed, with economic growth as the primary force of poverty reduction (Vandemoortele 2010). The discussions focused on the identification of a limited number of goals and relatively limited indicators rather than on the analysis of deeper social transformations, neglecting issues surrounding inequalities and discrimination almost entirely (Teichman 2014). Thus, the MDGs and the targets set for 2015 lacked a systemic vision and did not take into account the social, economic and environmental determinants of the living and working conditions of the populations or consider issues such as equity in distribution and the access to resources (Fehling *et al.* 2013; Teichman 2014).

In addition, the MDGs once again interpreted "development" as an issue that was exclusively relevant for the poorest countries. These countries were not heavily involved in the creation of these goals and therefore did not have much of a say as to where aid would be allocated. Thus, most of those goals measured the progress of the global agenda in accordance with specific needs and rights (such as access to food, education, gender equality, maternal health, a limited number of diseases, access to water and sanitation, etc.), most of which have little importance to middle- or high-income countries which would mainly be involved as "donors" (Fehling *et al.* 2013).

The approaching 2015 deadline incited the process to redefine a future development agenda. Twenty years after the first summit on this issue, in June 2012 at the United Nations Conference on Sustainable Development ("Rio+20"), participating countries decided to pursue concrete action in favor of sustainable development, igniting an intergovernmental process for the formulation of new global targets, which led to the definition of the Sustainable Development Goals (SDG). The document "Transforming Our World: The 2030 Agenda for Sustainable Development" is the result of that process and was adopted in New York on the 25th of September 2015 by the United Nations Summit of the Heads of State and Government (UN 2015; UN 2015a).

The introduction of the ambitious document highlights the "historic" dimension of the agreement, which commits governments to adopt a comprehensive, far-reaching and people-centered set of 17 universal and transformative "indivisible" goals and 169 universal targets. The new statement takes the development discourse to a global dimension and affirms the universal value of the SDGs. These goals aim to put an end to poverty by 2030, combat inequalities, ensure lasting protection of the planet and its resources, and create the conditions for "shared prosperity" and "sustainable, inclusive and sustained" growth (UN 2015a). There remains some debate surrounding the SDGs, highlighted by the fact that this last aim is oft-considered an oxymoron, since sustaining (keeping constant) something dynamic (such as growth) is a contradiction in terms (Spaiser *et al.* 2017). For some authors the new agenda does not address the systemic and structural roots of increasing inequities, social exclusion and environmental disaster (Horton 2014).

2.1.1 *The attributes of development*

The idea of development remains strongly tied to economic growth. Growth has been proposed as the most desirable effect of "development" and has been converted into a "global faith" (Rist 1997).

In an attempt to improve the definition of development, different authors have felt the need to add new adjectives, but each of them has its own limitations. As Luciano Carrino suggests:

> The idea of a "human" development focuses on the individual's abilities and freedoms but leaves in the shadow the collective responsibility and the functioning of societies.
>
> The idea that development needs to be "sustainable" does not represent well its destructive impact on the environment and leaves in the shadow the governance issues of societies that should deeply change their lifestyles.
>
> The idea that it needs to be "social" denounces the exclusion dynamics that generate poverty and unemployment but leaves in the shadow the problem of how to successfully pursue good growth and a good redistribution of wealth.
>
> (Carrino 2014: 36–37)

Some authors even proposed combinations for more adjectives. According to Diesendorf (2001), a more precise definition would be "ecologically sustainable and socially fair development". The addition of adjectives, however, does not solve the real problem. None of the approaches described has ever questioned the underlying societal structure that fosters growing inequalities, while the dominant discourse has always managed to reduce development to pure rhetoric, replicating the myopic goal of economic growth.

2.1.2 Overturning the paradigm

In the attempt to tackle the paradigm of sustainable development, the idea of "de-growth" has emerged over the years, a new paradigm that emphasizes the fundamental contradiction between sustainability and economic growth. This paradigm argues that the path to a sustainable future lies in democratic and redistributive reduction of the biophysical dimension of the global economy (Asara *et al.* 2015). Correspondingly, a societal project is envisaged of voluntary equitable downscaling of production and consumption that increases human well-being and enhances ecological conditions at the local and global level in the short and long term: a process that should lead to a post-growth society counteracting the omnipresence of market-based relations in society in search of alternative world representations (Demaria et al. 2013).

According to Sèrge Latouche, ideas such as "sustainable development" are simply "patching things up so as to avoid having to change them". Thus, it is vital to break the "confusion between 'development' and 'growth' that is deliberately sustained by the dominant ideology". "Growth has become humanity's cancer" and trying to cure this "human-generated illness" requires us to "decolonize our imaginaries" dominated by growth, where growth means progress and no growth means going backwards. Nevertheless, de-growth should not be understood as a growth society with a decreasing GDP, but as a starting point for a paradigmatic change in the inspiring values of human society (Latouche 2010).

Equally challenging the quantitative measure of economic growth and referring to the biological concept of development (i.e. "a sense of multi-faceted unfolding; of living organisms, ecosystems, or human communities reaching their potential"), Capra and Henderson (2009) preferred to leave development aside and put an adjective to growth. They describe the idea of "qualitative growth" as a process that embraces social, ecological and spiritual dimensions.

One could agree with Carrino (2014), who, discussing the attempts at a "true" definition of development, writes that "there are no true and honest words: every time the purpose behind their use should be understood".

Furthermore, Amartya Sen, whose seminal research had inspired UNDP's introduction of the "Human development" concept, did not opt for a new wording for development or further adding adjectives. In the attempt to adhere to the positive vision that the word itself evokes, Sen later described development as "a process of expansion of human freedoms". Although Sen acknowledged the possible role of economic growth in determining a country's living conditions, he challenged the tendency to equate development with the growth of GDP, the increase in individual income, industrialization, technological progress, or the modernization of society. According to Sen, even though economic growth or individual income can be an important means of expanding the freedom of members in society, this freedom also depends on other factors such as social and economic arrangements (for example, the school system or health care), or political and civil rights (e.g. the ability to participate in public debates and deliberations) (Sen 1999).

It is not surprising that among the most important definitions of freedom, Sen addressed freedom in relation to preventable conditions of illness and avoidable deaths, identifying good health as an integral part of a good development. There is no need to demonstrate that good health fosters economic growth to support the cause of health (Sen 1999a).

Health, under the understanding of the WHO definition as a "complete physical, mental and social well-being", to which we will return to later, is one of the best indicators of development. In the process towards the adoption of the Agenda 2030, the Italian Global Health Watch (OISG) suggested adopting health as the central goal and proposed that relevant health indicators (such as Healthy Life Expectancy, HLE), even alone, could provide an adequate measure of progress (OISG 2014). Health and health care strictly coincide with the defense and promotion of human and populations' rights, and therefore adopting health as a main goal binds to the juridical obligation deriving from international commitments and governmental responsibilities (ICESCR 1966; WHO 2002).

From a health perspective, success in development is measured by "the ability to meet the needs of the last among men of goodwill, not in GDP's growth rate" (Becattini 2002: 195–196). From this, new global government responsibilities arise:

> If the world is a global village, then the village chief will demonstrate its government's ability to act in order to avoid that anybody, white, black or yellow, Christian, Buddhist or Muslim, is thrown without survival means, without a reason to live, without hope in the future, and therefore without rights and duties in the trash can of society, which refuses it, ... it is not about defining the excellent allocation of given material resources but about defining the optimal allocation of potential human development.
>
> (Becattini 2002: 196)

The progressive disappearance of physical, temporal and cultural distances, chiefly due to technological progress, is the basis for the metaphor of the "global village". Global interdependence also gives rise to the idea of the planet as humanity's common home with a "planetary destiny" shared among all living beings (Morin 2011). This notion calls for an "integral ecology" with shared responsibilities and responses to the damaging consequences of lifestyles, production and consumption (Pope Francis 2015).

Nevertheless, the new global scenario is becoming increasingly interwoven with local realities. Today, the development concept and its corresponding policies must reflect this multilevel dimension and the need for a "g-local" approach. The world can no longer be divided between industrialized and poor (or developing) countries. The world today is characterized by inequality among and within countries, where the majority of the poor are living in Middle-Income Countries (MIC). Therefore, even global studies that encompass global health must definitively leave behind the anachronistic North-South (Western) development perspective. Now, the focus needs to center on the interaction between global influences and local experiences, identifying the appropriate level (local, national and global) for policy-making and action in search of appropriate solutions.

2.2 What is globalization?

Conceptualizing "globalization" is not simple. The word gets both its proponents and opponents very excited, but what exactly is it? Is there a shared definition? What initiated it and when did it start?

In a broader sense, globalization is understood today as the growing integration and interconnection between human societies beyond geographical and political boundaries (Lee 2014).

Obviously this is not a new phenomenon. After all, things that are happening today have already happened in the past. However, the notion of interconnectedness received a strong push during the modern era through the increase of exploration and commercial relations between the 15th and the 18th centuries. Later, in the 19th century colonialism and new transport and communications technologies (e.g. railways, steam navigation, telegraph) further pushed economic integration, with commercial, migratory and capital flows peaking between 1870 and 1914. This trend was briefly interrupted by the First World War and the Bolshevik Revolution (McNeill 2001).

In other words, globalization is a multidimensional historical process or a set of intertwined processes with certain structural properties, which "at the micro level, deeply affects human beings directly, including their consciousness and everyday life" (Turner and Khondker 2010: 17).

Thus, the current globalization landscape incontrovertibly has similarities with the past, yet there are also substantial differences. These differences are mainly due to the dramatic increase in speed, volume and geographical extensions of cross-border interactions and flows during the 20th century. In other words, we must speak of the *acceleration of globalization* processes with more accuracy.

What are the driving forces behind this acceleration?

Technological progress has played a decisive role by making trade faster and lowering its costs. Because of this, information and communication technologies are also often referred to as the main contributors to globalization.

However, others argue that technological innovation is itself the result of the economic phenomena. For example, the expansion of capitalism is driven by thousands of producers constantly exploring new ways to reduce the costs of production factors (labor, raw materials, transport, etc.), and by the advantages that the new markets and economies of scale bring. Capitalism is also pushed forward by millions of new consumers wishing to access more goods and services at a lower price.

A third group of observers challenge the purely technological or economic nature of the acceleration of globalization: they consider it the result of prevailing neoliberal ideology since the 1980s and the related liberalization and deregulation policies of the market (Lee 2014).

All these factors most probably interacted in a complicated process of social, cultural, economic and political connectedness that requires a complex approach to better understand (Turner and Khondker 2010). Economic transformations are among the most obvious features of the current globalization process and can be useful to exemplify its scope.

Economic globalization is understood as "the removal of barriers to free trade and the closer integration of national economies" (Stiglitz 2002: IX). Through Stiglitz's definition, one can understand that it is the result of several events, among them being the birth of modern capitalism, colonialism, the abolition of the fixed exchange system, and the fall of the Berlin Wall. However, most authors would agree in recognizing that the normative and institutional bases of the liberalization of financial flows and the opening up of national markets to investment and foreign trade were promoted shortly after World War II with the creation of the Bretton Woods institutions (International Monetary Fund, IMF; the World Bank and the General Agreement on Trade and Tariffs, GATT) (Lee 2014).

The liberalization of capital flows introduced in the United States in the 1970s commenced the widespread deregulation of international financial markets. More and more accessible, fast and cost-effective information and communication technologies have facilitated the development of a globally integrated financial market, active 24/24, with transaction volumes measured in thousands of billions, growing four times faster than global GDP.

The phenomenal growth of global trade, at least until the 2009 global crisis, was fueled by processes such as the removal of artificial barriers to the movement of goods and services pursued through free trade agreements (Stiglitz 2002), the international promotion and the adoption of incentive policies for foreign direct investment by various states (Steiner and Alston 2002), the gradual withdrawal of the state (UNDP 1999) and the collapse of the Soviet Union and the Communist regimes (Galli 2001). It is the globalized economy that allowed the 2007–2008 financial crisis in the United States (resulting from Lehman Brothers' bankruptcy) to spread with heavy recessions and catastrophic GDP collapses in countless countries around the globe, particularly the Western world, hitting sovereign debt and public finance. The free movement of capital, which no longer has territorial limits, has undermined the capacity of states to anticipate a post-Westphalian situation, drawing attention to the need for new forms of global governance, including in the field of health (which will be discussed in Chapter 5) (Labonté 2014).

2.2.1 The three dimensions of the globalization process

As a result of globalization, social relations have undergone transformations in three essential dimensions: space, temporal and cognitive (Lee 2000).

2.2.1.1 The spatial dimension

The transformation of the space dimension refers to changes in the way people interact in physical and territorial space. Increasingly powerful and diffused communication tools have changed the way we meet one another and establish relationships. This has allowed for the creation of virtual communities and social networks no matter an individual's location. With transport and communication means that are available today, distance no longer acts as a barrier and the concept of geographical boundaries becomes increasingly blurred.

> It suddenly seems clear that the divisions of continents and of the globe as a whole were the function of distances made once imposingly real thanks to the primitiveness of transport and the hardship of travel.
>
> (Baumann 2002: 15)

Globalization is therefore a result of the crumbling boundaries in the various dimensions of the economy, information, ecology, technology, transcultural conflicts and civil society. Thus, globalization feels like something familiar, but difficult to grasp, that radically transforms daily life with a noticeable influence that forces everyone to adapt and find answers. Money, technology, goods, information and pollution cross these geographical boundaries as if they did not exist. Even people and ideas that governments would like to keep out of the country (illicit drugs, illegal immigrants, criticisms of human rights violations) find their way past such boundaries. Thus, globalization conjures away distance (Beck 1997).

With the "loss of boundaries" alongside the traditional world community of nation states, a powerful world society of non-state transnational actors, both private entities (businesses, foundations, non-governmental organizations, networks, social movements) and hybrids (multi-stakeholder alliances, initiatives and public-private partnership organizations), contribute to modifying the world's power and conflict structures. They all play a role in influencing policies and decision-making processes, a role which previously was an exclusive prerogative of international, i.e. intergovernmental, institutions.[6]

These new transnational actors have some common features. First of all, their logic and strategies go beyond the interests of individual countries or regions in which they operate and overcome the territorial principle of national states; they have offices and operate simultaneously in several countries. They often act in delimited areas, but are usually more effective than state administrations and, especially in the case of social movements, they may be more inclusive (Beck 1997).

2.1.1.2 The temporal dimension

Globalization also affects the temporal dimension: the use and value of time. Our lives are moving at speeds we have never experienced before. However, many are unaware victims. Migrants, refugees and displaced persons live in high-mobility situations, but with limited alternative choices.

Time also affects the community and concerns public health. Beside the spatial dimension, the spread of communicable diseases across national boundaries is achieved with unprecedented speed thanks to population mobility and the speed of transport. These cases are shown in outbreaks of infectious diseases such as the atypical pneumonia known as SARS that spread between 2002 and 2003, the avian influenza caused by H5N1 viruses that started in 2003, swine flu from the H1N1 virus in 2009, or the Ebola virus epidemic developed between 2014 and 2015. Climate change is also an example of the acceleration of global transformation processes. If current levels of fossil fuel consumption, as well as the development model and population growth, remain unchanged, the impact on the environment, and consequently on human health and life, will be drastic and irreversible.

2.2.1.3 The cognitive dimension

Globalization, understood as a transformative process that transcends state boundaries limiting the effectiveness of national and even international actions, also inevitably influences the image we have of ourselves and the world around us (cognitive dimension) (Lee 2001). The cognitive dimension of globalization concerns changes in the production and exchange of knowledge, ideas, laws, beliefs, values, cultural identities and other mental processes. Globalization changed our way of thinking and feeling about ourselves and the world around us. Mass media, educational institutions,

24 *Globalization, development and health*

expert committees, scientists, consulting companies and communication experts all contributed to this transformation (Lee 2000). A common example is that of global teenagers; they share ways of dressing, eating, musical tastes, and even language, even if they are geographically apart from one another (Lee 1999).

The ultimate target of the global market is not the huge mass of people who live with one dollar or less a day, but rather the middle-class adolescents of industrialized and semi-industrialized countries. This teenager demographic consists of one billion people who consume a disproportionate share of the family income. Large multinational corporations (Coca Cola, Marlboro, McDonalds, Nike, etc.), after having transformed their products into "global" brands since the 1980s, are now aiming to make them an integral part of daily life (Klein 2000).

The cognitive dimension is structurally tied to the cultural dimension that depends on our ability to interpret reality.

Together with the tendency towards a cultural and behavioral homogenization that the global markets promote, the declining importance of distances and the growing speed of communications also offer the opportunity for a dialogue among different cultures to connect, and for an evolution substantially different from the clash of civilizations that some people foresee (or even hope for) (Huntington 1996).

Identifying common denominators is vital to address a whole range of transnational and, thus, global health-related topics such as environmental protection, and the right to peace and development.

In various parts of the world and in countless cultural contexts, the topic of human rights, its implementation and its protection are discussed differently. Human rights can only benefit from the opportunity that globalization offers; millions of people are able to share news and information quickly.

The right to health, a second-generation right, was formally, and internationally, recognized for the first time with the 1948 Universal Declaration of Human Rights (art. 25). It is a fundamental point of reference for any discussion on the relationship between globalization and development. It is no coincidence that this right is the pillar of the World Health Organization's founding act.

Analyzing the impact of globalization on human health is a prerequisite for the development of global policies and strategies aimed at limiting and possibly avoiding its adverse effects.

2.3 The impact of globalization on human health

2.3.1 *Looking for a methodological framing*

After nearly seventy years, the World Health Organization's definition of health as a state of complete physical, mental and social well-being retains much of its validity. Although often debated and not free from criticism, the definition, adopted with the WHO Constitution at the International Health Conference held in New York in 1946, remains the reference. It focuses on a fundamental concept: the essence of health is well-being and not just absence of illness; not only physical well-being, but also mental and social. With such a broad concept, there are numerous and diverse factors that determine the state of health. It is not enough, therefore, to question the immediate causes of the disease, and the analysis must necessarily be extended to the identification of all factors influencing the state of health.

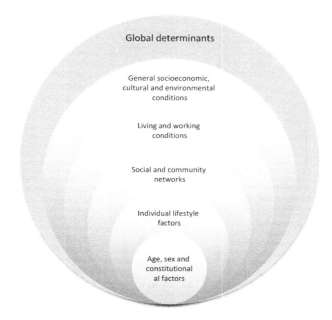

Figure 2.1 The determinants of health.
Source: based on Dahlgren and Whitehead (1991).

The determinants of human health are graphically represented in Figure 2.1.

At the center of the graphic are age, sex and constitutional (i.e. genetically determined) factors, which interact with other progressively more distal and modifiable factors such as individual lifestyles, social and community networks and socioeconomic, cultural and environmental conditions.

The analysis of the influence of globalization on human health, one of the defining components of global health studies, must therefore consider the specific interrelations between the phenomena linked to those determinants.

For a long time, public health experts have been trying to analyze the issue in more depth. For example, Yach (1998) linked a number of global transnational factors to some consequences and probable impacts on health status. Subsequently, Woodward and colleagues (2001) provided a more defined interpretative framework of the relationship between globalization and health, identifying the multiplicity of interactions and pathways through which global phenomena influence the distal and proximal determinants of health (Figure 2.2).

This framework is a reference point for all the others in this field. Its strength lies in its detail. This strength, however, is a weakness if the framework's intent is to communicate with policy-makers and the general public less acquainted with the nuances of the multiple pathways linking globalization and health (Labonté and Torgerson 2003). Labonté and Torgerson (2003) distinguished elements impacting the health outcomes on five levels: superordinate elements, global policy and economic contexts, domestic public policy contexts, community contexts, and household contexts. Huynen and colleagues (2005) show the impacts of globalization on distal determinants (health-related policies,

26 *Globalization, development and health*

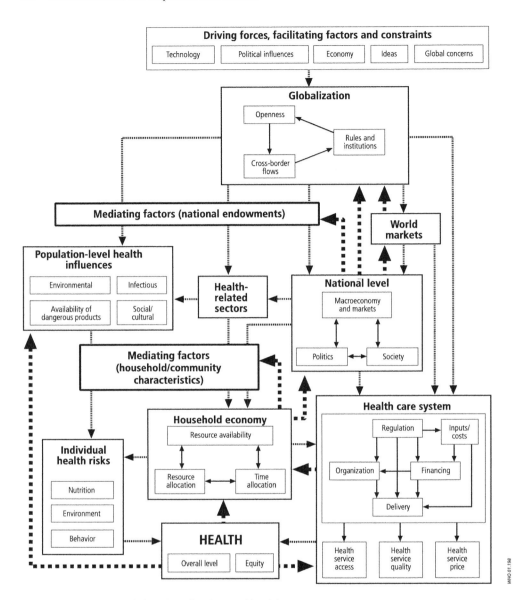

Figure 2.2 Framework for globalization and health.
Source: adapted from Woodward *et al.* (2001).

economic development, trade, migration, conflicts, social equity, social networks, ecosystem and services, and knowledge capital) and the mediated effects on proximal determinants (health services, social environment, lifestyle, physical environment). In recent years, great attention has been paid to the issue of social determinants of health. In 2005, the Commission on Social Determinants of Health (CSDH) was set up by the World Health Organization (WHO) to get to the heart of relationships between

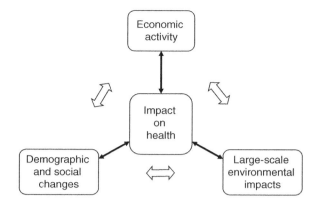

Figure 2.3 Influence on human health of changes related to globalization.
Source: adapted from McMichael (2012).

health and global complexity and as part of a comprehensive effort to promote greater equity in global health (Lee 2004). The CSDH was asked to summarize the evidence on how the structure of societies, through a myriad of social interactions, norms and institutions, affects population health, and what governments and public health can do about it (Solar and Irvin 2010). In the CSDH's perspective policies and interventions can be targeted at the micro level of individual interactions, at the meso level of community conditions, or at the broadest macro level of universal public policies and the global environment. According to McMichael, the processes of global change are wide and systemic (McMichael 2012). Remediating or adapting to these changes requires an understanding of dynamic systems, their complexity and associated uncertainties, and coordinated policy responses across relevant sectors. The relationships between these processes of change and human health are shown in Figure 2.3. The figure is a schematic representation of the three major domains within which globalizing processes and changes are occurring.

These exponential changes in demographic, economic, commercial and environmental indexes have been labeled the Great Acceleration: that is, the sharp increase in human population, economic activity, resource use, transport, communication and knowledge–science–technology that was triggered in many parts of the world following World War II and which has continued into this century (Costanza *et al.* 2007).

2.3.2 Is globalization good for your health?

Any framework is simply a modeling effort to render complexity into something more manageable and understandable. Frameworks are never comprehensive, and how frameworks organize complexity is determined by their purpose (Labonté and Torgerson 2003). Although all these models may vary at points, all stress that health outcomes and/or health inequities are shaped by multiple pathways that combine elements in many complex ways and that may function alone, simultaneously or in interaction with each other. What elements are included, what pathways they constitute, which pathways are involved, and how exactly they impact health inequalities may differ from one location to another and in time (Krumeich and Meershoek 2014).

After 17 years from Dollar's article (2001) entitled "Is globalization good for your health?" the question about "globalization and health" remains unanswered. There is no definite and unambiguous answer to this question. This depends on the fact that good health means different things to different people, and its meanings vary according to expectations and contexts. Moreover, the causality of human health is multi-factorial and many population health problems are invariably embedded in a global context (Huynen 2008), and there is also a variety of both negative and positive effects that are expected to influence our health in the future (Huynen *et al.* 2005).

Frameworks do not answer the question of whether globalization is good for health, they rather help to clarify the problems and pathways that link global phenomena and health, bearing in mind that health is both an individual and collective, local and global phenomenon that varies greatly depending on events and when and where they occur. The impact will be obviously different between well-off and disadvantaged countries and diverse population groups. A choice must also be made about the time frame of concern about the impacts of globalization: in the long run wealthier societies are healthier, albeit with wide variations in health status at a given level of income per capita. The issue of acceptable time raises the ethical question of how long is too long to wait (Labonté and Schrecker 2007).

A second issue is about the global distribution of risks. The distribution of risk largely follows a peculiar trajectory, with those living in developing countries being generally exposed to greater risk than residents of developed nations, primarily on account of less elaborate measures for the protection of the environment and human health and safety being available in less-developed countries (Beck 2016). The increasing complexity of our global society means that sustainable health cannot be addressed only from a single perspective, country, or scientific discipline. Changes in human health in the context of globalization are far more complex than health issues tackled in the past, and an extensive empirical work is needed to identify the relevant causal mechanisms underlying the influence of globalization on human health (Martens *et al.* 2010).

Notes

1 The Club of Rome is an organization convening notable scientists, economists, businessmen and businesswomen, high-level civil servants and former heads of state from around the world. Its mission is to promote understanding of the global challenges facing humanity and to propose solutions through scientific analysis, communication and advocacy. It was established in Rome in 1968 as an informal group at the invitation of Aurelio Peccei, a successful Italian industrialist, and Alexander King, an eminent Scottish scientist (Club of Rome 2018).
2 The Washington Consensus originally referred to a set of ten economic policy prescriptions considered to constitute the "standard" reform package promoted for developing countries by Washington DC-based institutions such as the International Monetary Fund (IMF), the World Bank and the US Treasury Department. The term was first used in 1989 by English economist John Williamson, but was later used in a broader sense, to refer to a more general orientation towards a strongly market-based, neoliberal macroeconomic approach.
3 The French translation of "sustainable" is "durable", which explains Rist's interpretation.
4 Among the new indicators the Inequality-adjusted Human Development Index (IHDI), the Gender Inequality Index (GII), the Gender Development Index (GDI) and the Multidimensional Poverty Index (MPI).

5 New York, 1990, on children; Rio de Janeiro 1992, on environment; Cairo 1994, on population issues; Beijing 1995, on women; Istanbul 1996, on habitat; Copenhagen 1995, on social development.
6 "Inter-national" relations refer to interactions among nation states, thus among their governments. Referring to non-state actors whose activities transcend the borders and the administrative authority of single national states, "trans-national" is a more appropriate attribute. According to Beck (2000), the emergence of global non-state actors envisages a "post-international" era.

References

Arndt, H.W., 1987. *Economic Development. The History of an Idea*. Chicago: The University of Chicago Press.
Asara, V., et al., 2015. Socially sustainable degrowth as a social–ecological transformation: repoliticizing sustainability. *Sustainability Science*, 7, 1–10.
Baumann, Z., 2002. *Globalization: The Human Consequences*. Columbia University Press.
Becattini, G., 2002. *Miti e paradossi del mondo contemporaneo*. Roma: Donzelli editore.
Beck, M., 2016. The risk implications of globalisation: an exploratory analysis of 105 major industrial incidents (1971–2010). *International Journal of Environmental Research and Public Health*, 13, 309.
Beck, U., 1997. *Was ist Globalisierung?* Berlin: Suhrkamp Verlag.
Capra, F., Henderson, H., 2009. *Qualitative Growth*. The Institute of Chartered Accountants in England and Wales, October.
Carrino, L., 2014. *Lo sviluppo delle società umane tra natura, passioni e politica*. Milano: Franco Angeli.
Club of Rome, 2018. The story of the Club of Rome. Available from: www.clubofrome.org/?p=375.
Costanza, R., et al., eds., 2007. *Sustainability or Collapse? An Integrated History and Future of People on Earth*. Dahlem Workshop Report 96. Cambridge, MA: MIT Press.
Dahlgren, G., Whitehead, M., 1991. *Policies and Strategies to Promote Social Equity in Health*. Stockholm: Institute for Futures Studies.
Demaria, F., et al., 2013. What is degrowth? From an activist slogan to a social movement. *Environ Values*, 22(2), 191–215.
Diesendorf, M., 2001. Models of sustainability and sustainable development. *IJARGE*, 1(2), 109–114.
Dollar, D., 2001. Is globalization good for your health? *Bulletin of the World Health Organization*, 79(9), 827–833.
Fehling, M., Nelson, B.D., Venkatapuram, S., 2013. Limitations of the Millennium Development Goals: a literature review. *Global Public Health*, 8(10), 1109–1122.
Galli, C., 2001. *Spazi politici – L'età moderna e l'età globale*. Bologna: Il Mulino.
George, S., 1976. *How the Other Half Dies. The Real Reasons for World Hunger*. Harmondsworth: Penguin Books.
Hayes, R., 2017. Internalizing externalities. Techniques to reduce ecological imprint of food products. In Steier, G., Patel, K.K. (Eds.), *International Food Law and Policy*. Cham: Springer.
Horton, R., 2014. Offline: why the sustainable development goals will fail. *The Lancet*, 383(9936), 2196.
Huntington, S.P., 1996. *The Clash of Civilizations and the Remaking of World Order*. New York: Simon and Schuster.
Huynen, M.M.T.E., et al., 2005. The health impacts of globalisation: a conceptual framework. *Globalization and Health*, 1, 1–12.
Huynen, M.M.T.E., 2008. *Future Health in a Globalising World*. Maastricht: Maastricht University Press.

ICESCR, 1966. *International Covenant on Economic, Social and Cultural Rights*. New York: United Nations. Available from: www.ohchr.org/Documents/ProfessionalInterest/cescr.pdf.

ILO, 1976. *Employment, Growth and Basic Needs: A One World Problem*. Geneva: International Labour Office.

Isernia, P., 1995. *La Cooperazione allo sviluppo*. Bologna: Il Mulino.

Klein, N., 2000. *No Logo: Taking Aim at the Brand Bullies*. Toronto: Random House.

Krumeich, A., Meershoek A., 2014. Health in global context; beyond the social determinants of health? *Global Health Action*, 7(1), 23506

Labonté, R., 2014. Health in all (foreign) policy: challenges in achieving coherence. *Health Promotion International*, 29(suppl 1), i48–i58.

Labonté, R., Schrecker, T., 2007. Globalization and social determinants of health: introduction and methodological background (part 1 of 3). *Globalization and Health*, 3, 5. doi:10.1186/1744-8603-3-5.

Labonté, R., Torgerson, R., 2003. *Frameworks for Analyzing the Links Between Globalization and Health*. STU/H&T/2003.2 Geneva: World Health Organization.

Latouche, S., 2010. *Farewell to Growth*. Cambridge: Polity Press.

Lee, J.W., 2004. *Address by the Director-General to the Fifty-seventh World Health Assembly*. Geneva: World Health Organization.

Lee, K., 1999. *The Global Context – A Review of Priority Global Health Issues for the UK*. London: The Nuffield Trust.

Lee, K., 2000. Global dimensions of health. In Parsons, L., Lister, G. (Eds.), *Global Health: A Local Issue*. London: The Nuffield Trust.

Lee, K., 2001. Globalization – a new agenda for health? In McKee, M., Garner, P., Stott, R. (Eds.), *International Cooperation and Global Health*. London: Oxford University Press.

Lee, K. 2014. Globalization. In Detels, R., Gulliford, M., Quarraisha Abdool, K., Tan, C.C. (Eds.), *Oxford Textbook of Global Public Health* (6th edn.). Oxford: Oxford University Press, 62–77.

League of Nations, 1919. The Covenant of the League of Nations.

Luzzati, T., Parenti, A., Rughi, T., 2018. Economic growth and cancer incidence. *Ecological Economics*, 146, 381–396.

McMichael, A.J., 2012. Globalization, climate change, and human health. *New England Journal of Medicine*, 368, 1335–1343.

McNamara, R.S., 1976. To the Board of Governors, 1976, Manila, Philippines, October 4, 1976. In McNamara, The McNamara Years at the World Bank, 337, quoted in Kapur, D., Lewis, J.P., Webb, R., *The World Bank. Its First Half Century*. Washington DC: Brooking Institution Press, 266.

McNeill, J.R., 2001. *Something New under the Sun*. New York: W.W. Norton & Company.

Martens, P., *et al.*, 2010. Is globalization healthy: a statistical indicator analysis of the impacts of globalization on health. *Globalization and Health*, 6, 16.

Meadows, D.H., *et al.*, 1972. *The Limits to Growth: A Report for the Club of Rome's Project on the Predicament of Mankind*. New York: Universe Books.

Morin, E., 2011. *La Voie. Pour l'avenir de l'humanité*. Paris: Librairie Arthème Fayard.

Muñoz, H., 1981. Introduction: the various roads to development. In Muñoz, H. (Ed.), *From Dependency to Development. Strategies to Overcome Underdevelopment and Inequality*. Boulder, CO: Westview Press, 1–11.

Nyerere, J.K., 1974. *Freedom and Socialism*. Oxford: Oxford University Press.

OECD/DAC, 1996. *Shaping the 21st Century: The Contribution of Development Co-operation*. Paris: OECD.

OISG, 2014. La salute al centro dell'agenda post 2015, Osservatorio Italiano sulla Salute Globale. Available from: www.saluteglobale.it/index.php/2014/09/02/la-salute-al-centro-dellagenda-post-2015/.

Petras, J., Veltmeyer, H., 2001. *Globalization unmasked: imperialism in the 21st century*. London: Zed books.
Polany Levitt, K., 2012. Rolling back the canvas of history: a contribution to the critical development studies project. In Cangiani, M. (Ed.), *Alternative Approaches to Development*. Padua: CLEUP.
Pope Francis, 2015. *Laudato Si'. Enciclica sulla cura della casa comune.* Città del Vaticano: Libreria Editrice Vaticana.
Prebisch, R., 1950. *The Economic Development of Latin America and its Principal Problems*. UN document: E/CN.12/89 Rev.1.
Rist, G., 1997. *Lo sviluppo. Storia di una credenza occidentale*. Turin: Bollati Boringhieri (original title in French: Rist, G., 1996. *Le Dévelopment. Histoire d'une croyance occidental*. Paris: Presses de la Fondation Nationale de Sciences Politiques).
Rostow, W.W., 1960. *The Stages of Economic Growth: A Non-Communist Manifesto*. Cambridge: Cambridge University Press.
Sen, A., 1989. Development as capabilities expansion. *Journal of Development Planning*, 19, 41–58.
Sen, A., 1999. *Development as Freedom*. Oxford: Oxford University Press.
Sen, A., 1999a. *Health in development. Keynote address by Professor Amartya Sen to the Fifty-second World Health Assembly*, A52/DIV/9 18 May 1999. Geneva: World Health Organization.
Solar, O., Irwin, A., 2010. A conceptual framework for action on the social determinants of health. *Social Determinants of Health Discussion Paper 2 (Policy and Practice)*. Geneva: World Health Organization.
Spaiser, V., et al., 2017. The sustainable development oxymoron: quantifying and modelling the incompatibility of sustainable development goals. *International Journal of Sustainable Development & World Ecology*, 24(6), 457–470.
Steiner H.J., Alston P., 2002. *International Human Rights in Context – Law, Politics, Morals*. Oxford: Oxford University Press.
Stiglitz, J.E., 2002. *Globalization and Its Discontents*. New York: W.W. Norton & Company.
Teichman, J., 2014. *The MDGs and the Issue of Inequality: The Enduring Power of Neoliberalism* (No. CCDS Working Paper #1), Toronto: Centre for Critical Development Studies (CCDS).
Truman, H., 1949. Truman's Inaugural Address, January 20, 1949 [Delivered in person at the Capitol], Harry S. Truman Library & Museum. Available from: www.trumanlibrary.org/whistlestop/50yr_archive/inagural20jan1949.htm.
Turner, B.S., Khondker, H.H., 2010. *Gobalization East and West*. London: SAGE.
UN, 1945. Charter of the United Nations. Available from: www.un.org/en/charter-united-nations/index.html .
UN, 1974. *Declaration for the Establishment of a New International Economic Order*. UN document: A/RES/S-6/3201.
UN, 2000.*United Nations Millennium Declaration*. UN document: Resolution A/RES/55/2, 18 September.
UN, 2015. *UN adopts new Global Goals, charting sustainable development for people and planet by 2030*, 25 September. Available from: www.un.org/apps/news/story.asp?NewsID=51968#.Vg6qFs4_Gm5.
UN, 2015a. *Transforming our world: the 2030 agenda for sustainable development*, New York: United Nations, 25 September. Available from: https://sustainabledevelopment.un.org/post2015/transformingourworld.
UNDP, 1990. *Human Development Report 1990. Concept and Measurement of Human Development*. New York: United Nations Development Program
UNDP, 1999. *Human Development Report 1999. Globalization with a Human Face*. New York: United Nations Development Program
Vähämäki, J., Schmidt, M., Molander, J., 2011. *Review: Results Based Management in Development Cooperation*. Working Paper, Riksbankes Jubileumsfond.

Vandemoortele, J., 2010. *Changing the Course of MDGs by Changing the Discourse*. Real Instituto Elcano; Area International Relations and Development, ARI 132/2010, 9 September.

WCED, 1987. *Our Common Future*. World Commission on Environment and Development. Oxford: Oxford University Press.

WHO, 2002. 25 questions and answers on health and human rights. Geneva: World Health Organization. Available from: http://whqlibdoc.who.int/hq/2002/9241545690.pdf.

Woodward D., Drager N., Beaglehole R., Lipson D., 2001. Globalisation and health: a framework for analysis and action. *Bulletin of the World Health Organization*, 79, 875–881.

Yach, D., 1998. The globalization of public health, I: threats and opportunities. *American Journal of Public Health*, 88, 735–738.

Unless otherwise indicated, all websites were accessed on 9 August 2018.

3 Global estimates of health indicators

3.1 Need and use of global health estimates

The increase in importance of global health has been accompanied by a heightened need for global estimates of health indicators. In the last decades, there has been a growing interest in timely data on health outcomes such as mortality rates, incidence and prevalence of diseases and risk factors, and for summary measures of population health that combine mortality and disability indicators. Global, regional, and country health indicators are required to assess development and health progress, to measure trends in population health, to evaluate the impact of global and national policies, and to inform global health policy decisions and resource allocation.

Global estimates of health indicators have been used for a long time. When the United Nations (UN) system was established, it required comparable data on member countries demographic and health trends. The United Nations Population Division (UNPD) was established in 1948 to produce routine estimates, for all countries, of population by age group and gender as well as fertility and mortality rates. Since then, all major global health commitments and declarations – from disease eradication initiatives, to the Alma Ata Declaration on Primary Health Care in 1978, to the more recent disease-specific global health initiatives – have required estimates of global health indicators (AbouZahr *et al.* 2017).

The approval of the MDGs in 2000 and then of the SDGs in 2015, with their several time-bound targets, further increased the need for comparable health statistics. The 17 SDGs comprise 169 targets and 230 indicators, including an overarching health goal that has 13 targets and around 34 health-related indicators that need to be monitored (United Nations 2015). Additionally, the SDGs put significant emphasis on equity, which can only be monitored with health indicators disaggregated by socioeconomic and demographic groups, geography and other dimensions.

UN agencies and academic organizations routinely publish estimates for child and adult mortality and priority causes, including HIV, TB, malaria, maternal mortality and major causes of child deaths. Global estimates of health indicators are used by development agencies to track progress towards international goals. Many donors, funding agencies and foundations use global estimates to track progress towards their own specific goals. They rely on global estimates to evaluate the impact of their actions, to advocate for their success, and to increase their visibility. These agencies use global estimates of health indicators not only to ensure comparability across countries, but also because they often perceive that country-reported data are of poor quality. Global estimates of health indicators are also used by global players to inform decisions on global health funding. Yet, these global decisions are not always consistent with priorities set by recipient countries that are typically taken using locally produced health indicators.

The recent increased focus on health policy and systems has generated a demand for global estimates of indicators for monitoring the progress towards global health goals related to the functioning of social health protection systems. For instance, the global focus on Universal Health Coverage requires comparable estimates on access to health services, inclusion in social health protection schemes such as health insurance programs, health financing indicators, impact on household financial condition and out-of-pocket payments for accessing needed health services (WHO and World Bank 2017).

Despite the increased demand for global estimates of health indicators, there remain challenges in the production of timely and high-quality estimates due to poor availability of country data, weak health information systems, high cost of data collection faced by low- and middle-income countries with tough budget constraints, weak logistic capacity of many countries, and governance and political issues (AbouZahr *et al.* 2017; Sankoh 2010; Brown 2015). In fact, the health information systems of many countries are not adequate to provide high-quality information on the health status of the population as a whole, on effective coverage of health interventions, and on health financing indicators. In several countries the investments in local capacity development for health information systems are minimal and global health donors have been traditionally reluctant to invest in this area. Furthermore, domestic policy-makers in low- and middle-income countries are not always interested in strengthening health information systems for producing global estimates of health indicators. The main reasons are competing priorities, lack of involvement in global-level initiatives and concerns that global health estimates could be then used to hold them accountable for meeting agreed global health targets.

As a consequence, global health players have been increasingly supporting the development of approaches for estimating demographic and health indicators with limited data. This led to international donors supporting the development and, in several countries, the implementation of household surveys such as, for instance, the Demographic and Health Survey (DHS) program and the Multiple Indicators Cluster Surveys (MICs) (see Box 3.1).

BOX 3.1 DHS and MICS programs

DHS program

The Demographic and Health Surveys (DHS) Program has collected, analyzed and disseminated representative data on population, health, HIV and nutrition through more than 300 surveys in over 90 countries. DHS supports several data collection options.

- Demographic and Health Surveys (DHS): Provide data for a wide range of monitoring and impact evaluation indicators in the areas of population, health and nutrition.

- AIDS Indicator Surveys (AIS): Provide countries with a standardized tool to obtain indicators for the effective monitoring of national HIV/AIDS programs.
- Service Provision Assessment (SPA) Surveys: Provide information about the characteristics of health facilities and services available in a country.
- Malaria Indicator Surveys (MIS): Provide data on bednet ownership and use, prevention of malaria during pregnancy, and prompt effective treatment of fever in young children. In most cases, biomarker tests for malaria and anemia are also included.
- Key Indicators Surveys (KIS): Provide monitoring and evaluation data for population and health activities in small areas – regions, districts, catchment areas – that may be targeted by an individual project. KIS can also be used in nationally representative surveys.

Source: https://dhsprogram.com/.

MICS program

The Multiple Indicator Cluster Surveys (MICS) have focused since 1995 on data on women and children worldwide. Close to 300 Multiple Indicator Cluster Surveys have been carried out in more than 100 countries, generating data on key indicators on the well-being of children and women, and helping shape policies for the improvement of their lives. Trained fieldwork teams conduct face-to-face interviews with household members on a variety of topics – focusing mainly on those issues that directly affect the lives of children and women. Countries use MICS results to report on their progress towards international goals. For example, MICS has generated data on the majority of Millennium Development Goal (MDG) indicators that can be measured through household surveys. Subsequent surveys in MICS6 will provide the baselines for the new Sustainable Development Goals.

MICS questionnaires are designed by implementing agencies, based on an assessment of a country's data gaps and needs. The starting point is the standard MICS questionnaires designed by UNICEF, in close coordination with partners and other international survey programs. All survey activities, from fieldwork to report writing, are carried out by the implementing agencies – with continuous technical support from UNICEF.

The number of topics covered has increased substantially over the years as demand for data has grown. In the fifth round, MICS is providing data on more than 130 internationally agreed-upon indicators. Over the years, MICS has pioneered the development of new measurement tools in areas including early childhood development, child discipline, hand washing, post-natal health care and low birthweight. Many of these tools have been adopted by other international survey programs.

Source: http://mics.unicef.org/.

These surveys aim to measure health status, health services utilization and behavioral and environmental risk factors, mainly in low- and middle-income countries. However, these surveys are not conducted in all countries on a regular basis and they have limitations for global and country monitoring. The estimates produced by these surveys can be representative of periods in the past, their sample size is often limited by funding available, and usually they represent the national level and not local administrative areas. The availability and consistency of survey and census data vary considerably between countries. So the comparability of most mortality indicators and those of disease incidence and prevalence is hard to assess. As a consequence, these household surveys can only partially compensate for the lack of reliable health information systems.

Global estimates of health indicators based on statistical modeling of the data available are therefore increasingly used. This trend has been fostered by impressive developments in methods developed to produce global estimates of health indicators, the new field referred to as the "science of global health estimates".

UN agencies such as the World Health Organization are increasingly active in the field of global estimates of health indicators. The WHO has published the World Health Statistics Annual Report since 1957 (until 1998) with data reported by countries that are considered official statistics on key indicators such as infant mortality and causes of death. Yet, the data reported by many countries were not always complete or reliable. As a consequence, the WHO started engaging in the production of global health estimates in collaboration with other UN agencies and academic institutions. The WHO flagship publication World Health Statistics offers online regular global health estimates that are rather complete. The WHO Global Reference List of 100 Core Health Indicators is a standard set of 100 indicators prioritized by the global community to provide concise information on the health situation and trends. Since 2016 the World Health Statistics have included indicator values for 34 health-related SDG targets for all countries. Some of these indicators are estimates generated with statistical models that use either past data or data from other countries (WHO 2016). The World Health Statistics Annual and the Global Health Observatory (GHO) data are in continuous development.[1] It is, however, hard to assess whether the figures reported in these statistics are reliable and comparable, even if it is possible to access detailed methodological information on the WHO website.

The shortcomings of available data led to the establishment of several technical reference groups aimed at supporting the independence and objectivity of global health indicators. The groups have been important contributors to global estimates of health indicators for children under 5 years old (e.g. the Child Health Epidemiology Reference Group, CHERG – see Box 3.2), for HIV/AIDS, tuberculosis, malaria, maternal health and other diseases and conditions. The WHO and the other global health programs regularly publish disease-specific epidemiological estimates and progress of interventions coverage such as the global tuberculosis report,[2] the world malaria report[3] or the UNAIDS Global AIDS monitoring report.[4]

BOX 3.2 Child Health Epidemiology Reference Group (CHERG)

The overall goal of CHERG is to develop and deploy new and improved evidence on the causes and determinants of maternal, neonatal and child morbidity and mortality, on intervention coverage, and on the effectiveness of interventions to inform and influence global priorities and programs.

The main purposes of the CHERG are

- advise WHO and other international organizations on the most appropriate methods and assumptions for their global, regional and country-level child health epidemiological estimates;
- advise researchers and public health officials on the different issues involved in the estimation of cause-specific morbidity and mortality; and
- publish papers, reports and reviews on child health epidemiology, especially on the distribution of causes of death.

Source: http://cherg.org/main.html.

More recently, the WHO, together with partner organizations, developed an international collaboration, the Health Data Collaborative, to improve measurement and accountability for global public health and to help countries to have strong health information systems following the Measurement and Accountability for Results in Health Summit (see Box 3.3).

BOX 3.3 The Health Data Collaborative (HDC)

"The Health Data Collaborative is a joint effort by multiple global health partners to work alongside countries to improve the availability, quality and use of data for local decision-making and tracking progress toward the health-related Sustainable Development Goals (SDGs)."

HDC aims to improve measurement and accountability for global public health and to help countries to have strong health information systems.

The Health Data Collaborative exists to empower countries to achieve the targets set out in the health-related SDGs, especially but not exclusively those in "Goal 3: ensuring healthy lives and promoting wellbeing for all at all ages". Its tasks include strengthening governance of health and statistics systems; innovations in birth and death registration; routine use of verbal autopsy to ascertain causes of death in out-of-hospital settings; methods for data quality assessment; and support for building country capacities for review, analysis, interpretation and communication of data.

Source: https://www.healthdatacollaborative.org/what-we-do/.

An increasingly leading player in the field of global health estimates is the Institute of Health Metrics and Evaluation (IHME). IHME is a private institute created in 2007 at the University of Washington in Seattle, USA, with funding from the Bill & Melinda Gates Foundation. It aims at "providing an impartial, evidence-based picture of global health trends to inform the work of policymakers, researchers, and funders".[5]

The IHME produces estimates and long-term projections for a vast number of global health indicators. It leads the revised Global Burden of Disease (GBD) study that quantifies the magnitude of health loss due to disease, injuries and risk factors globally.[6] The IHME has scaled up its innovative research infrastructure. It now employs over 300 people and it relies on a network of over 2000 collaborators.[7]

3.2 The Global Burden of Disease Study

The most used and influential global health estimates are currently produced by the Global Burden of Disease Study (GBD). The GBD is a systematic effort to quantify the comparative magnitude of health loss due to diseases, injuries and risk factors by age, sex and region for specific points in time. The first global burden of disease efforts were produced by academics at Harvard University and the WHO for the 1993 World Development Report, Investing in Health of the World Bank (IHME 2013). The WHO then produced annual updates during 1999–2002 and four-yearly updates from 2004. In 2012 IHME embarked on a revised version of the GBP producing estimates on premature death and disability for more than 300 diseases and injuries in 188 countries, by age and sex (GBD 2015 SDG Collaborators 2016). Since then the IHME has been producing yearly updates, and expanded the focus to global health financing indicators, global estimates of access to services, global estimates of quality of care, and forecasting estimations (GBD 2015 Mortality and Causes of Death Collaborators 2016).

The GBD produces regular estimates of all-cause mortality, deaths by cause, years of life lost due to premature mortality (YLLs), years lived with disability (YLDs) and disability-adjusted life years (DALYs) for a list of causes. The DALY is a metric designed to quantitatively measure the impact of various diseases and conditions on the productivity and well-being of people through a combination of mortality and morbidity estimates.

The GBD estimates are based on data of country health, mortality and covariate data, which are used as inputs to sophisticated mathematical and statistical models that generate global health estimates. The IHME is using the methods of the GBD to generate SDG indicators that can be used to monitor progress towards SDG targets.[8]

The GBD estimates are useful in giving an overall picture of mortality and morbidity in a country or region, of the major causes of burden of diseases and of how they changed over time. They are therefore potentially useful for country-level macro policy-making. However, these estimates are of limited value for policy and planning at subnational and local levels.

Given the SDGs focus on equity, requiring monitoring global health trends by stratifiers such as income, sex, age, race, ethnicity, geographical location and migration status, there is an emerging trend in producing local burden of disease estimates. In the last few years the IHME has been using advanced statistical methods such as Bayesian geospatial modeling to generate small area estimates that can be aggregated to administrative units such as districts. Small area health estimates can be used to identify potential overlooked priorities that may require additional evidence/data to be fully understood.[9]

3.3 Global health estimate challenges

The way global health estimates are produced, the institutions involved and their funding, reflects some of the contemporary challenges in global health governance. Currently global health estimates are largely produced by institutions based in high-income countries, funded by global health donors, and used mainly by the communities based at global levels or by academics in high-income countries. Although the countries, in particular low- and middle-income countries, are involved in the implementation of household surveys funded by global health donors, such as DHS or MICs, they are usually not involved in the production of global health estimates other than for providing data input. This lack of involvement in the production of global health estimates of the countries that own the data is a major challenge for the current science of global health estimate initiatives.

The recent investments in advanced statistical modeling, computation of uncertainty ranges and the production of compelling visualization of results mask the lack of high-quality data. As highlighted by Boerma *et al.* (2018)

> these advances could give the impression of abundant evidence that is actually based on very sparse empirical data. Unfortunately, global public health experts and academics are often oblivious to the limitations of these estimates and regularly over-interpret the numbers, especially if the estimates support their arguments.
> (Boerma *et al.* 2018)

One example is the evidence produced to monitor the MDGs health indicators. Mortality of children under 5 years and maternal mortality were the most important health indicators in the MDGs. Boerma *et al.* (2018) assessed the extent to which in the 2015 MDG assessments of achievements were based on predictions, by using the 2015 report by the UN and 2016 publications of IHME in *The Lancet*, and they found that

> Household surveys with birth histories were the most recent source of child mortality data for three-quarters of the 81 countries, generally a Demographic Health Survey (DHS) or Multiple Indicator Cluster Survey [....] The most recent empirical data collection efforts for child mortality on average ended around 3 years before the final MDGs reports in 2015 and, for maternal mortality, around 4 years before the 2015 MDGs reports. For vital events registration, the mortality data refer to the reporting year, but for surveys (and censuses) the period when deaths occurred was further back in time, as retrospective data are collected through birth histories for child mortality, and sibling survival histories for maternal mortality. [...] If we assume that survey data referred to deaths on average 2 years (child) and 3 years (maternal) before the data collection, only 38% of countries had child mortality data and 7% of countries had maternal mortality data for 2012 or beyond. The median year of the most recent datapoint for the 81 countries was 2010 for child mortality and 2008 for maternal mortality.
> (Boerma *et al.* 2018)

The reliance of global health estimates mainly produced in the North, with little involvement of other players, raises concerns about the validity and legitimacy of global health estimates. As described by Pisani and Kok (2017), the debate has been first on technical issues:

> Academics and health officials from several countries were confronted with estimates that they found hard to reconcile with the facts as they saw them [....] Experts working globally on specific disease areas questioned methods [..]
> (Pisani and Kok 2017)

and secondly on the role of global health estimates in shaping the global health agenda.

> Health data, including estimates, are produced by a variety of organisations whose mandates, aims, incentive structures, and institutional cultures differ. These differences shape both the processes through which data are collected and analysed and the interpretation of the results. Health data are often presented as 'objective' but, like all other knowledge, they are a construct that derives meaning from the very process of their construction.
>
> (Pisani and Kok 2017)

They then point out quite effectively that

> data and concepts in global health are institutionally and politically constructed: a health issue climbs up the international agenda because people deemed to be experts have used accepted methods to demonstrate its importance, and they have communicated this in forums that entrench that importance (and that influence funding decisions).
>
> (Pisani and Kok 2017)

Therefore, a challenge of the science of health estimates is in reconciling the need for global estimates, produced in an independent and objective manner, with the weak data available and the political interference that policy-makers may exert. Currently there seems to be a disconnection between the need and approaches of the institutions and players operating at global level and mainly based in high-income countries, and those of most low- and middle-income countries' governments.

Relying on global estimates poses questions of acceptability of the indicators at country level. In fact national governments may not accept global health estimates that are different from the data they use for national purposes. For instance, the WHO estimates are described as "official WHO figures" specifying that they "should not be regarded as nationally endorsed statistics of Member States". So the estimates are seen as external to countries themselves, primarily designed to meet the WHO mandate of providing information in relation to public health (AbouZahr *et al.* 2017).

At country level policy-makers often prefer using locally generated data to inform decisions and are reluctant to use global health estimates. This is sometimes due to the fact that country reported data often diverge from global health estimates. Most importantly, global health estimates are not that useful for informing national policy-making, which has to be informed by data not only at national level but also at the meso and local levels. Estimates based on complex modeling of limited data produced by international institutions are often mistrusted.

Additionally, the lack of interest in global health estimates by national policy-makers can be due to political considerations. In fact, political opponents, media and civil society could use global health estimates to challenge government statistics and policies. This problem is exacerbated when, as often happens, global health estimates are produced without or with little involvement of country officers. This tension is one of the reasons why often some of the most interesting data, in particular in the past, were not made publicly available.

The production of global health estimates should be increasingly based on high-quality national and subnational data and statistics. In the last few years, the global health community has called for high investment in strengthening health information systems and statistical systems at country levels (Laliberté 2002; Paris 21 2004; Health

Metrics Network 2008). Although some of these initiatives are promising, e.g. the National Evaluation Platform and the Data for Health Initiative (see Boxes 3.4 and 3.5), overall so far these initiatives have mobilized relatively little investment in institutional capacity to generate good-quality data and in data collection. In order to improve the availability of good-quality global health indicators it is urgently needed to increase investments in country health information systems and in international support for public health institutions in low- and middle-income countries to strengthen their knowledge and skills for data collection, analysis and interpretation (AbouZahr et al. 2017).

BOX 3.4 The National Evaluation Platform (NEP)

The NEP equips government decision-makers with the tools and skills to critically evaluate the state of maternal, newborn and child health and nutrition (MNCH&N) in their countries. Empowered with evidence, policy and program leaders can make strategic decisions that lead to maximum health and nutrition impact for women and children. The NEP provides a new way to assess the effectiveness and impact of MNCH&N programs, a systematic approach for identifying and a compiling health and nutrition data from diverse sources and ensuring that they are available for program evaluation, and a core set of analytical methods for developing evidence-based answers to countries' pressing program and policy questions and a commitment to building sustainable national capacity.

Source: https://www.nationalevaluationplatform.org/.

BOX 3.5 The Data for Health initiative

Fewer than half of all deaths around the world are registered with a cause of death, meaning that 29.4 million deaths go unrecorded each year. This lack of data means that many health policy decisions are made without adequate information. While there are reliable global numbers of leading causes of death, many individual countries lack the basic information they need to make informed decisions.

The lack of data disproportionately affects low- and middle-income countries, with 60% of these countries not reporting any data, covering 2 billion people. Additionally, nearly 40% of the 128 million babies born worldwide each year are not officially registered.

While our focus is on helping improve death data, we also help improve birth data in countries where we work.

The Data for Health initiative seeks to address this very issue and works to improve public health data so that governments are equipped with the tools and systems to collect and use data to prioritize health challenges, develop policies, deploy resources and measure success.

Data for Health partners with low- and middle-income governments (both national and city-level) to strengthen their public health data and improve the way they use this information to make policy decisions and public health investments.

> Data for Health initiative works with partner countries to:
>
> - **Collect data on deaths and births**, improving country-level ownership of health data.
> - **Conduct public health surveys** using gold-standard methods while testing new innovations to monitor major risk factors for early death.
> - **Use public health data to inform policy priorities**, especially by improving the ability to track trends and plan interventions at the national level.
>
> Source: https://www.bloomberg.org/program/public-health/data-health/#overview.

Notes

1 www.who.int/gho/en/.
2 www.who.int/tb/publications/global_report/en/.
3 www.who.int/malaria/publications/world-malaria-report-2017/en/.
4 www.unaids.org/en/resources/documents/2018/Global-AIDS-Monitoring.
5 www.healthdata.org/about/history.
6 www.healthdata.org/gbd.
7 www.healthdata.org/.
8 https://vizhub.healthdata.org/sdg/.
9 The most updated global burden of diseases estimates can be visualized here: www.healthdata.org/gbd.

References

AbouZahr, C., Boerma, T., Hogan, D., 2017. Global estimates of country health indicators: useful, unnecessary, inevitable? *Global Health Action*, 10(sup1). doi:10.1080/16549716.2017.1290370.

Boerma, T., Victora C., Abouzahr C., 2018. Monitoring country progress and achievements by making global predictions: is the tail wagging the dog? *The Lancet*. Available from: https://doi.org/10.1016/S0140-6736(18)30586-5.

Brown, G.W., 2015. Knowledge, politics and power in global health. Comment on 'Knowledge, moral claims and the exercise of power in global health'. *International Journal of Health Policy Management*, 4, 111–113.

GBD 2015 Mortality and Causes of Death Collaborators. 2016. Global, regional, and national life expectancy, all-cause mortality, and cause-specific mortality for 249 causes of death, 1980–2015: a systematic analysis for the Global Burden of Disease Study 2015. *The Lancet*, 388, 1459–1544.

GBD 2015 SDG Collaborators. 2016. Measuring the health related sustainable development goals in 188 countries: a baseline analysis from the Global Burden of Disease Study 2015. *The Lancet*, 388, 1813–1850.

Health Metrics Network & WHO, 2008. Framework and standards for country health information systems (2nd edn). Geneva: World Health Organization. Available from: http://apps.who.int/iris/bitstream/10665/43872/1/9789241595940_eng.pdf .

IHME, 2013. *The Global Burden of Disease: Generating Evidence, Guiding Policy*. Seattle, WA: Institute for Health Metrics and Evaluation. Available from: www.healthdata.org/sites/default/files/files/policy_report/2013/GBD_GeneratingEvidence/IHME_GBD_GeneratingEvidence_FullReport.pdf.

Laliberté, L., 2002. Statistical Capacity Building Indicators Final Report. PARIS21 Task Team on Statistical Capacity Building Indicators. Available from: www.paris21.org/sites/default/files/scbi-final-en.pdf.

Paris 21, 2004. A guide to designing a National Strategy for the Development of Statistics (NSDS). Paris 2004. Available from: http://siteresources.worldbank.org/SCBINTRANET/Resources/NSD_Guide-Nov04.pdf .

Pisani, E., Kok, M., 2017. In the eye of the beholder: to make global health estimates useful, make them more socially robust. *Global Health Action*, 10, 10.3402/gha.v9.32298.

Sankoh, O., 2010. Global health estimates: stronger collaboration needed with low- and middle-income countries. *Plos Medecine*, 7, e1001005.

United Nations, 2015. A/RES/70/1 – Transforming our world: the 2030 Agenda for Sustainable Development. Available from: https://sustainabledevelopment.un.org/index.php?page=view&type=111&nr=8496&menu=35.

World Health Organization and The International Bank for Reconstruction and Development, 2017. *Tracking Universal Health Coverage: 2017 Global Monitoring Report*. Geneva and Washington DC: World Health Organization and The World Bank. Available from: www.who.int/healthinfo/universal_health_coverage/report/2017/en/.

World Health Organization, 2016. World Health Statistics 2016: Monitoring Health for the SDGs, Sustainable Development Goals. 2016. Available from: www.who.int/gho/publications/world_health_statistics/2016/en/.

If not otherwise indicated, all websites were accessed on 9 August 2018.

4 The right to health and the evolution of public health strategies in the context of global development policies[1]

4.1 The global right to health

In 1946, the member states of the newly formed United Nations gathered in New York to draft and sign the constitution for the World Health Organization (WHO), which entered into force on 7 April 1948. With this document, the international community declared "the attainment by all peoples of the highest possible level of health" as the objective of the new organization and defined the mandate for the WHO to "act as the directing and coordinating authority on international health work" (WHO 1946).

By identifying health as a fundamental human right and defining it as "a state of complete physical, mental and social well-being and not merely the absence of disease or infirmity" it was implicitly recognized that promoting good health could not be achieved through medical care alone, nor solely through the control of diseases, but would, instead, require a much wider and intersectoral approach. Thus, the benefits derived from the knowledge of medical and health-related sciences must be extended to everyone, while the responsibility to appropriately select and implement health and social services for the health of citizens falls on the government (WHO 1946). Recognizing that the health of all people is an indispensable condition for the attainment of peace and security in the world, and citing that "unequal development in different countries in the promotion of health and control of disease" represents "a common danger", identifies both the global nature of health-related issues and their connections with international relations.

This idea is further reinforced in the Universal Declaration of Human Rights, Article 25, which states that

> every individual has the right to a standard of living adequate for the health and well-being of himself and of his family, including food, clothing, housing and medical care, and the necessary social services
>
> (United Nations 1948).

In addition, Article 22 of the Declaration recognizes the right of every individual to social security and to the realization of "economic, social and cultural rights indispensable for his dignity and free development of his personality" pursued "through a national effort and international cooperation in accordance with the organization and resources of each State" (United Nations 1948).

Thus, considering the WHO definition of health, in conjunction with the Universal Declaration of Human Rights, it is clear that health represents a right that cannot be fully guaranteed if it is not linked with the other fundamental rights that society as a whole is called upon to ensure.

The right to health and the conditions which are indispensable for its implementation are delineated in several international conventions. Due to the binding character of international agreements, the states whose legislative organs ratified the conventions have the obligation to guarantee the corresponding rights. All of the following international conventions make reference to the right to health: the International Covenant on Economic, Social and Cultural Rights (1966, which entered into force on 3 January 1976); the Convention on the Elimination of All Forms of Discrimination Against Women (1979, which entered into force on 3 September 1981), the Convention on the Elimination of All Forms of Racial Discrimination (1965, which entered into force on 4 January 1969) and the Convention on the Rights of the Child (1990, which entered into force on 2 September 1990). As we will discuss later, the commitment to the right to health has been reaffirmed in numerous world summits.

4.2 From disease eradication programs to health for all and primary health care

Until the mid-1980s the evolution of global health policies largely coincided with the WHO's role on the global scene; later the WHO had to progressively negotiate its role with a number of emerging global actors.

Despite its holistic definition of health, in its first period of existence the WHO oriented its action toward the development of disease control and eradication programs, such as the large-scale treatment of syphilis, and the malaria and smallpox eradication programs.

At that time the WHO and global health policies were also strongly influenced by the politics of the Cold War. The malaria eradication campaign and top-down interventions closely aligned with the political interests of the United States of America in promoting modernization and winning "hearts and minds" in the battle against Communism (Packard and Brown 1997). The Soviet Union seceded from the United Nations system in 1949 because they felt that the United Nations and the WHO were dominated by the United States (Lee 2009). The Soviet Union and other communist countries returned to the WHO in 1957, and two years later the global smallpox eradication program was launched, bringing together the interests of the two most powerful global players and making history as the only successful disease eradication program for a human disease[2] to this date (Brown *et al.* 2006). This period also brought the adoption in 1951 of The International Sanitary Regulations (renamed International Health Regulations [IHR] in 1969 and thoroughly reviewed in 2005 when the current International Health Regulations were adopted) (IHR 2008). The IHR were the only binding rules governing international health (apart from the Constitution of the WHO itself) until 2005, when the Framework Convention on Tobacco Control (FCTC) entered into force.

In the 1960s and 1970s, the political context was marked by the emergence of decolonized African nations, the spread of nationalist and socialist movements, and new theories of development (see Chapter 2). As a result, a "basic needs approach" was favored over top-down interventions, and the WHO shifted towards strategies more attentive to the development of basic health services, community participation and the immediate health needs of the population.

From 1973 to 1988, under the leadership of the Danish Director-General of the WHO Halfdan Mahler, the WHO was established as the "global health conscience", openly challenging the commercial practices of transnational pharmaceutical and food industries (Global Health Watch 2005).

In 1977, the World Health Assembly (WHA) adopted the goal of "Health for all by the year 2000" and the following year, with the Declaration of Alma-Ata, primary health care (PHC) was identified as the best strategy toward that objective.

PHC was viewed not only as an integral part of each country's health system, but also as important for the social and economic development of the country. The Alma-Ata Declaration was aimed a promoting equity and community participation through a focus on prevention and appropriate technologies and an integrated intersectoral approach to development (Alma-Ata 1978).

BOX 4.1 The Alma-Ata Declaration – excerpts

The Conference strongly reaffirms that health […] is a fundamental human right and that the attainment of the highest possible level of health is a most important world-wide social goal whose realization requires the action of many other social and economic sectors in addition to the health sector.

The existing gross inequality in the health status of the people […] is politically, socially, and economically unacceptable and is, therefore, of common concern to all countries […].

The people have a right and duty to participate individually and collectively in the planning and implementation of their health care.

Primary health care is essential health care based on practical, scientifically sound, and socially acceptable methods and technology made universally accessible to individuals and families in the community through their full participation and at a cost that the community and country can afford to maintain at every stage of their development in the spirit of self-reliance and self-determination. It forms an integral part both of the country's health system, of which it is the central function and main focus, and of the overall social and economic development of the community. It is the first level of contact of individuals, the family, and community with the national health system bringing health care as close as possible to where people live and work and constitutes the first elements of a continuing healthcare process.

An acceptable level of health for all the people of the world by the year 2000 can be attained through a fuller and better use of the world's resources […].

Source: Alma-Ata 1978. *Primary Health Care. Report of the International Conference on Primary Health Care*. Alma-Ata, USSR, 6–12 September 1978.

"For most, it was a true revolution in thinking" (WHO 2008), as stated by Mahler 30 years later,

> Health for All is a value system with primary health care as the strategic component. The two go together. You must know where you want your values to take you, and that's where we had to use the primary health care strategy
>
> (WHO 2008).

However, this broader developmental focus was soon challenged by several influential stakeholders. The WHO faced competing and powerful interest groups while Mahler's leadership toward policy change also led the WHO into much greater conflict than ever before (Walt 1994).

The implementation of PHC required rethinking health systems' organization and management, and redirecting policies, strategies and resource allocation (financial, physical and workforce), a task which faced a plethora of cultural and political barriers.

The focus on rural and on the most deprived urban population groups, on basic health services, and thus on the primary needs and pathologies of the poorest people, was met with resistance from the social hierarchy and power base in many countries. The economic, political and intellectual elite instead preferred to develop hospital health services that were highly specialized, costly and therefore unsustainable. Doctors' incomes, as well as their social and professional standing, were linked to their level of specialization and to technological sophistication, rather than to the value of the service they provided to patients. Indeed, in line with their training, health professionals have been historically more concerned about the clinical aspects of disease rather than about social determinants of health.[3] Ministries of Health had very little political weight for a host of reasons, not the least of which being that Ministries of Finance determined their budgets. Furthermore, even the countries that were more determined to introduce PHC had to face obstacles related to a lack of both financial and human resources, a plight affecting all developing countries (albeit to varying extents). The Alma-Ata Declaration was criticized for being too broad and idealistic and that the slogan "Health for All by 2000" was not feasible.

Only one year after Alma-Ata, a workshop entitled "Health and Population in Development" was hosted by the Rockefeller Foundation in Bellagio, Italy, and supported by the World Bank, with the Vice President of the Ford Foundation, the administrator of USAID and the Executive Secretary of UNICEF[4] in attendance. The meeting engendered the "Selective Primary Health Care" approach, which consisted of a series of interventions that were low-cost, pragmatic and limited in scope (Brown *et al.* 2006; Walsh and Warren 1979).

Selective Primary Health Care significantly narrowed the original, innovative approach and concentrated instead on the application of selective measures that

> should be aimed at preventing and managing those few diseases that cause the greatest mortality and morbidity and for which there are medical interventions of relatively high efficacy.
>
> (Walsh and Warren 1979)

The design and organization of programs would soon follow a top-down dynamic, a stark contrast to the bottom-up model of PHC, which instead prescribed decision-making by the local communities. These measures were selected according to questionable cost-effectiveness criteria. Under the strong influence of international organizations and bilateral agencies, this soon resulted in the reorganization of health systems into so-called "vertical programs". The fragmentation of public health activities created a complete detachment between these programs and development programs in other sectors (schools, production, environment, etc.).

"Vertical programs" dealt with individual diseases or conditions and were formulated at the central level, then implemented throughout the country (or throughout the world) in a uniform manner, and often with rigidly assigned resources. Sometimes, separate institutions were even set up for each program. For example, at that time, it was common to create special, independent bodies exclusively dedicated to malaria eradication, with exclusively assigned resources. Thus, a vehicle assigned to the malaria eradication program could not be used for immunization purposes. Similarly reporting procedures would be independent from the regular health services' information system. The resources designated for anti-malarial drugs could not be used for the purchase of any other medicine. With international agencies focused on specific and often autonomous, disease-oriented programs instead of cooperation and sharing between actors, there was often competition between them even when they were working toward similar objectives.

This disease- rather than health-oriented approach was often more concordant with the political and administrative needs of main donor countries and organizations, who had a strong influence on the choices of beneficiary countries. The relatively cheap yet highly visible and publicized campaigns typical of the selective PHC approach often served to mask the lack of political determination that was needed to overhaul the health system and improve overall health conditions.

This quite reductive, centralist approach was soon to become the dominant mind-set; attention was drawn away from health and health systems, and focused instead on the control of single diseases.

Under Mahler's leadership, the WHO also openly challenged the commercial practices of transnational baby food and pharmaceutical industries.

In 1979, an international meeting jointly hosted by the WHO and UNICEF, and involving representatives of governments, health organizations, companies and advocacy groups, called for the development of an international code of marketing. Two years later, the 34th World Health Assembly adopted the International Code of Marketing of Breast-milk Substitutes. The sole opposition vote came from the United States, which perceived the code as interference in global trade and marketing practices (Walt 1994).

The WHO also challenged the market logic through its "Essential Drug Program", a fundamental component of the PHC approach. The program was opposed by leading pharmaceutical companies, and, in 1985, as a demonstration of protest, the United States moved beyond a mere vote of opposition and, instead, decided to withhold its contribution to the WHO's regular budget (Godlee 1994).

This action followed a wider budgetary restriction imposed on the whole UN system. Claiming the "politicization" of UN agencies such as UNESCO and ILO, in 1982 major donors (the so called "Geneva group") imposed a "real zero growth"[5] policy on the regular budget of all UN organizations. In 1993 that policy was substituted by the even more austere "zero nominal growth" policy (Lee 2009).

In Chapter 7 we will specifically discuss the consequences of these decisions on the future strategy and management of the WHO.

4.3 The international financial institutions and health systems reform

As the selective PHC approach did not require significant investment in public health and system reorganization, it suited neoliberal macroeconomic policies that had started to take hold in the early 1980s. However, the 1980s brought not only new macroeconomic formulas to the global health scene, but also new actors and new challenges.

The debt crisis of the 1980s and the advent of neoliberal policies (see Chapter 2) played a critical role in launching the IMF and the World Bank (and their respective agendas) onto the global stage as major political players in the realms of crisis management, international development funding and general policy-making (including health), especially for low-income countries.

4.3.1 From the debt crisis to structural adjustment plans

Beginning in 1958, the major industrialized nations adopted the Bretton Woods financing system in which the value of currency was based on the gold standard.[6] However, in 1971, this system was abandoned when the then President of the United States, Richard Nixon, opted to unilaterally disengage the US dollar from the gold standard, preferring the accumulation of a deficit instead of increased monetary withdrawals. This decision was made, in large part, to alleviate some of the stress placed on the American economy by the inflation of the 1960s, but, above all, to alleviate the financial strain created by the ever-increasing cost of the Vietnam War. Thus, the dollar soon became a currency for speculation, primarily in the southern countries of the world; unfortunately, at the same time, the price of imports for these developing countries soared while the value of exports plummeted.

In 1973 through 1974, the situation was further compounded by the quadrupling of the price of oil as a consequence of the embargo that OPEC[7] countries targeted at nations perceived as supporting Israel during the Yom Kippur War. The embargo dealt a significant blow to industrialized nations but hit even harder those developing countries not producing oil. This oil price boom later prompted the subsequent recession in 1974–75. With their newfound wealth from petrodollars, OPEC nations began heavily investing in commercial banks. These banks, now experiencing an excess of liquidity from the increasing investments, began to invest in lending to developing countries, particularly those of Latin America and South East Asia, who, with the increase in oil price and the recession, were now "eager borrowers". These loans were made with extremely advantageous conditions for the borrowers, but were always linked to the market, thus were short-term and carried variable interest rates.

The types of loans, combined with rising inflation and the recession, trapped loan recipients in a vicious circle, in which new debts were generated by contracting additional loans specifically for the repayment of old debts,[8] thus, stimulating an ever-increasing export of capital.[9] In addition, in 1979, the Office of the Comptroller of the Currency (OCC), a division of the US Treasury Department, reinterpreted a key lending regulation; this decision most likely exacerbated the already shaky situation to a breaking point. The OCC claimed that no single borrower could occupy more than 10% of the lending capital of an institution, and, as many banks were already in violation of this rule, lending to developing countries was severely reduced (FDIC 1997). Thus, with debt consistently growing from 1973 to 1982, rising inflation[10] and cost of imports, combined with decreased exports and international donations, many developing countries faced insolvency. Despite the very public warning signs, it seems that very little was done to try to stem the inevitable. Thus, in 1982, Mexico was the first to openly declare that it was unable to repay the loans and fully opened the debt crisis. By the end of 1982, 40 countries were in arrears and by the end of 1983, 27 nations, including the four largest in Latin America that accounted for 74% of the debt (Mexico, Brazil, Venezuela and Argentina), were in debt-restructuring negotiations (FDIC 1997). The Bretton Woods institutions were called to contain the damage by binding the financial assistance for the indebted countries and access to credit with the application of a standard set of macroeconomic measures (known as the "Washington Consensus"), thus ensuring that obligations to private creditors were fulfilled after the eventual debt restructuring under the terms of the so-called Paris Club.[11] These restructurings were clearly designed to repair the capacity for indebted countries to honor the outstanding loans, rather than with the objective of improving the conditions of life for the populations. The Washington Consensus of deregulation, liberalization and privatization became the "universal prescription" (Polanyi Levitt 2012). The operational mechanisms to bring these objectives to fruition were termed Structural Adjustment Programs (SAP).

SAPs typically required the reduction and/or removal of direct state intervention in the economy's production and redistribution sectors. The conditions that SAPs envisaged included slashing public expenditure, with substantial cuts in the health, education and other welfare spending; liberalizing imports; removing restrictions on foreign investment; privatizing state companies and financial deregulation; devaluing currency; cutting wages; and weakening labor protection mechanisms. In essence, the elements within the SAPs served to destabilize many of each country's public organizations and institutions to make space for private, market-driven programs derived from Western models (Bello 2002).

4.3.2 Structural adjustment and health sector reform

The debt crisis, the advent of neoliberal macroeconomic policies, and structural adjustment programs all contributed to the rise in power of international financial organizations such as the International Monetary Fund and the World Bank, as they imposed these new programs on individual countries as a condition for Official Development Aid (ODA). The necessity for an outside force to stabilize the debt situation created the need for the IMF to act as the so-called "International Lender of Last Resort" (ILLR) (Devlin and Ffrench-Davis 1995) and the increased activity of the World Bank through SAPs enabled both organizations to take prominent roles in manipulating the direction of global health politics for the coming decades.

Adjustment policies had dramatic (and often debilitating) effects on large swaths of the population and forced social safety nets and welfare programs to be introduced alongside SAPs in order to dampen their impact.

Among the measures introduced to lessen the effects of SAPs, the World Bank promoted the construction in assisted countries of special national development or social funds. Ironically, these funds would provide resources to respond to the problems that SAPs were partially responsible for. While funds operated differently from country to country, they were all autonomous and independent from mainline government agencies, often with the creation of new ad hoc agencies, channeling funds to private non-profits for the implementation of social programs.

Although the World Bank financed them directly, governments eventually bore the costs of these programs that were being repaid through normal lending arrangements. Social funds thus represented a mechanism to subsidize with public funds the privatization of social services. The public sector and the social services it offered were dismantled while the "easy access" public resources from the non-profit sector facilitated the multiplication of both national and international NGOs. In an increasingly fragmented institutional environment, and competing among themselves for resources and visibility, NGOs were mostly unable to sufficiently meet the expectations and the social and health needs of the communities they intended to serve. Nevertheless, they soon became the preferred vehicle by which international aid would be disbursed (Hall and Midgley 2004).

The World Bank became increasingly involved in the health sector after 1979, when it created its own Population, Health and Nutrition Department (Ruger 2005).

In 1987, the World Bank published *Financing Health Care: an Agenda for Reform*, and since then has considered itself as a fundamental stakeholder in the field of global health policies (World Bank 1987). Developing countries were now pushed to adopt health sector reforms to address the collapse of their health systems, which occurred as a result of the SAPs. These health sector reforms prescribed a single recipe, which enforced user fees for health services, encouraged privatization of health services, promoted the introduction of private insurance schemes and fostered the decentralization of health-care management (Italian Global Health Watch 2008).

In 1993 the World Bank titled its annual flagship report *Investing in Health* (World Bank 1993). The report, which has been described as a "watershed in international health", gave legitimacy to the Bank as a new leader in global health (Ruger 2005). The Bank put renewed emphasis on a "selective" approach by means of a "minimum essential package" for the control of a limited number of diseases and continued advocating the privatization of health services. Both policies had severe consequences in terms of reduced access to health services, particularly for the poorest members of the population (Whitehead *et al.* 2001). During this time, attention focused on health system efficiency (with the utmost importance placed on costs), rather than on the impact of public health policies on the overall health condition. The issue now was not whether the economic resources destined for the health system were sufficient to respond to the public's needs, but rather how to limit public health spending independently of the effects on health.

Although the emphasis was placed on reform of the health sector, it did not correspond to a universal package of measures uniformly adopted by all major donors, nor an unambiguous, unified concept of reform. However, all of the reforms had a certain number of elements in common, in particular:

- linking the health sector reform to the reform of the public administration;
- promoting decentralization;
- reorganizing the Ministry of Health in the areas of regulatory bodies, guidance and control;
- expanding the financing options for the health systems to include user fees, community financing and health insurance;
- strengthening and reforming the systems of management, support and monitoring;
- liberalizing the policies toward the private sector and developing systems for a stricter collaboration with private service providers; and
- developing a system through which the user exercises major influence on the provision of health services (Cassels 1995).

These reforms remained the central topic of the international debate for the rest of the decade. Meanwhile, "the growing interdependence and globalization continued to test the control and strength of national health policies" (Walt 1998: 435).

Alongside its growing influence, the World Bank soon became the largest international donor in the health sector in middle- and low-income countries, significantly altering the scope of international health cooperation. In the sectors of "Health, Nutrition and Population", the World Bank provided USD 2.4 million in 1996, an amount equivalent to 11% of the money allocated to those respective areas for that year. This is even more significant when one considers that for the period between 1985 and 1993, the total amount of ODA allocated to the same sectors (excluding the contributions of the World Bank) reached only USD 2 million as well as the fact that, in the same time span, the budget of the WHO, including both obligatory and voluntary (extra budgetary) funds, did not exceed USD 800 million. With the size of its operations, the conditions imposed on countries in order to access credit, and the strategies adopted, the World Bank changed the sectorial priorities and the relationship between donors and beneficiaries at both global and national levels (World Bank 1997; Buse and Gwin 1998).

The increasing influence of the World Bank and the catapulting of the global health debate toward health system reforms also coincided with a "dark period" for both the WHO and global health in general following the end of Mahler's tenure (see Chapter 6). The leadership of the WHO as the "directing and coordinating authority on international health work" (WHO 1946) was increasingly challenged by the numerous players now claiming a role in the field of global health as well as the system of international and development banks and funds. Among these new actors were transnational companies (starting with those active in the biomedical, pharmaceutical and insurance sectors), traditional and emerging global philanthropies and a growing number of NGOs. Among the new private actors appearing on the global health scene at that time was billionaire Bill Gates. The William H. Gates Foundation, established in 1994, was further consolidated into the Bill & Melinda Gates Foundation and maintained global health among its top priorities, thus ensuring that the foundation would soon become the single most important non-institutional player in the global field, acting both directly and as a partner in the most important global initiatives.

In addition, free trade policies, negotiated and regulated in the context of the World Trade Organization (WTO), established in 1995, were increasingly interfering with access to biomedical products and health services.

Concomitant with the growth of the number of actors and international agencies, the Official Development Aid (ODA) at a global level was progressively reduced (17% between 1992 and 1997), and health seemed only a minor political interest (*The Lancet* 1998).

4.4 Local health systems and health promotion

Yet, despite the difficulties facing the WHO, and policies imposed by the Bretton Woods Institutions, a number of experiences kept alive the spirit of Alma-Ata and the need for systemic and integrated approaches.

In 1986, the Ottawa Charter on health promotion introduced the concept of "healthy public policies", highlighting the unavoidable influence of policies outside the health sector and the need to put health on the agenda of policy-makers in all sectors and at all levels (WHO 1986). The Ottawa Charter defined health promotion as "the process of enabling people to increase control over, and to improve, their health", and recognized that the health sector alone could not be held responsible for this, nor could governments face the task alone. In fact, beyond the actions of governments, health promotion demands a coordinated action by "other social and economic sectors, by non-governmental and voluntary organizations, by local authorities, by industry, and by the media". Going far beyond mere health care, health promotion requires policy-makers in all sectors and at all levels "to be aware of the health consequences of their decisions and to accept their responsibilities for health" and contribute to healthy public policies (WHO 1986). The Ottawa Charter was constructed through the debate on inter-sectorial action for health in the preceding World Health Assembly as well as on the progress made through the Declaration of Alma-Ata and the establishment of the WHO's targets for Health for All.

The following year at the Harare Conference in 1987, decentralization was again raised as a means of applying PHC, with districts promoted as the best way of iden-tifying the under-served populations and aligning appropriate health interventions (WHO 1987). Likewise, the concept of Local Health Systems (LHS), later proposed by the Pan American Health Organization (PAHO), signaled a renewed emphasis on equity and quality of service as well as democratization and social participation, with health, well-being and development viewed as integral concepts (Paganini and Chorny 1990).

4.5 Sectorial programs and poverty reduction strategies

In the mid-1990s, the World Bank began exploring new approaches to link sector lending to Sectorial Investment Programs (SIPs). The new approach was then shared with other bilateral and multilateral donors and in several countries a Sector-Wide Approach (SWAp) was adopted. Sector-wide programs were established with the involvement and co-financing of several donors, under the leadership of the national government and following common procedures. The often-abused rhetorical emphasis placed on put-ting the beneficiary country "in the driver seat" responded to the principles of "own-ership" of the country, coherence of the strategies and efficiency of the management systems, which were being proposed as part of a substantial change in the parameters of development aid (Hill 2002). That change was in line with the criteria included in the OECD/DAC's *Shaping the 21st Century* document recommending that donor coun-tries should shift the focus of their ODA from an individual and fragmented *project aid* approach, to new forms of *program aid* in support of national strategies and policies of the recipient countries. Coordinated interventions, integrated with national plans, possibly financed directly by supporting countries' national budgets, i.e. *general budget support*, would increase the efficiency of aid as a whole, emphasize the ownership of the partner country and reduce the burden of negotiating and managing separately with each donor (OECD / DAC 1996).

In those years, the development agenda started to put new emphasis on the fight against poverty. In 1999, the World Bank and the International Monetary Fund also started to hint at reducing poverty by including access to subsidized credit and debt relief in their Poverty Reduction Strategy Papers (PRSP), national plans that envisaged the involvement of a range of local public and private players (World Bank 2005). PRSPs became the general reference document for many other donors (bilateral and multilateral) also participating in cooperative interventions toward development goals. In particular, it seemed to naturally bring together the programs of development in the fundamental sectors for the fight against poverty, especially health and education. Program aid structured into SWAPs became an integral part of that policy.

4.6 Health returns to the center of the global debate

On the wave of the renewed attention toward the social component of development, after the decade of decay that followed Hafdan Mahler's charismatic leadership, the election of Dr. Brundtland, the experienced former Prime Minister of Norway, as the Director-General of the WHO in 1998 suggested that once again the organization could become the leading advocate for public health and the most competent organization to provide expertise, set standards and assist governments in strengthening health systems.

From the moment of her appointment, Brundtland defined four strategic directions for the WHO: reducing the burden of disease, reducing risks to health, creating sustainable health systems, and developing and enabling policies in the health sector. Taking a broader stance, she also declared the objectives of the organization should focus on combating poverty, underdevelopment and social inequalities (*The Lancet* 1998). In that sense, it seemed that the WHO would take a new lead in fostering "Healthy Public Policies" (i.e. orienting public policies in other sectors toward health objectives), a concept established in the Ottawa Charter (WHO 1986).

In the year 2000, the WHO courageously opened a new phase in the global debate by centering its annual report on health systems. The WHO defined a health system as "comprising all the organizations, institutions and resources that are devoted to producing health actions" and a health action as "any effort, whether in personal health care, public health services or through inter-sectorial initiatives, whose primary purpose is to improve health". The WHO measured the performance of different countries' health systems in achieving this objective by evaluating aspects such as equal opportunity in accessing health services, the pooling of risks, equity of financing and the responsiveness to expectations. It also highlighted the importance of inter-sectorial cooperation in achieving good health (WHO, 2000).

The WHO idea for a more integrated, inter-sectorial action toward health was also expanded in regional initiatives of the organization. A multidimensional and integrated approach for achieving health was at the center of the "Verona Initiative", which, under the patronage of the WHO's European Region, emphasized that "investing *for* health *is* investing in development". It is also interesting to note that, while there is no reference to economic growth in the final text of the declaration, "development" is interpreted as economic and social "prosperity" or "wellness". The same document claims that health must be the objective of policies in all sectors and, that health is the yardstick by which the effectiveness of interventions for development is to be measured (Verona Initiative 2000).

The integration of health interventions in a wider inter-sectorial development and fight against poverty approach was also reaffirmed in the *Reference Document on health initiatives in the context of fight against poverty* jointly produced by the WHO and OECD (OECD/DAC 2003).

In contrast with the broad outlook that the WHO advocated, in practice Brundtland openly supported "vertical" initiatives through Global Public-Private Partnerships (GPPPs) (see below and more in detail in Chapter 9) to face a variety of diseases and health issues, including the Stop TB initiative, Roll Back Malaria, Malaria Medicine Initiative, International Partnership against AIDS in Africa (IPAA), International AIDS Vaccine Initiative (IAVI) and the Global Alliance for Vaccines and Immunizations (GAVI). The WHO's promotion of partnerships and other interactions with the corporate sector represented an important shift in organizational policy (Deacon *et al.* 2003).

The WHO "Commission on Macroeconomics and Health", established in the year 2000 and led by Professor Jeffrey Sachs, added evidence to the direct relationship between economics and health and how investment in the latter may induce economic development (WHO 2001). Without negating the dogma of economic/GDP growth, the report, published one year later, challenged the idea that health was a consequence of economic growth, arguing instead that first improving health would consequently positively influence economic growth. For the first time in WHO history, a report sought to quantify the global resources necessary for a program of essential interventions to combat infectious diseases and nutritional deficits. In order to save 8 million lives per year (principally in low-income countries), the report calculated that an increase of at least USD 22 million per year in aid from wealthy developed countries would be necessary (the ODA for health in 2001 was USD 6 million). However, the Commission avoided explicitly questioning the dominant macroeconomic policies, structures and mechanisms that contributed to the increase of worldwide health inequities (Sanders and Chopra 2003). In addition, when it came to identify solutions, the Commission's report lacked originality and proposed interventions already on the global agenda. Without substantiating the recommendation, it gave its own blessing to the Global Fund to Fight AIDS, Tuberculosis and Malaria sponsored by UN Secretary-General Kofi Annan and G8 governments and proposed a new Global Health Research Fund to finance basic biomedical research (WHO 2001). In fact, the CMH Report stressed the role that public-private partnerships could play and cautioned the governing bodies of the WHO *not* to constrain the WHO's work by raising concerns about conflicts of interest (Deacon *et al.* 2003). Attentive analysis shows that strengthening of interactions with the private sector since the 1990s within the United Nations and its agencies, including the WHO, did not just happen by itself, come out of nowhere or go uncontested. It was strongly debated and largely was a result of constraints in UN funding, pressures from some member states and a strong commitment by Secretary-General Kofi Annan to take the UN in that direction (Deacon *et al.* 2003).

The role of the HIV/AIDS epidemic and a few other infectious diseases in bringing back health to the global policy agenda cannot be overestimated. The fact that, unlike other diseases of the South, HIV/AIDS also affected industrialized countries undoubtedly contributed to eliciting global attention. Besides HIV/AIDS, attention remained selectively focused on malaria, tuberculosis and a few other infectious diseases. Other conditions such as malnutrition, diarrhea and acute respiratory illnesses, which had attracted attention in the past and whose mortality rate was, and still is, very high, seemed to be forgotten; not to speak of the emerging burden of noncommunicable diseases (NCDs).

However, although security concerns had been influential in framing global health since the 1990s, as a result of the emergence of HIV/AIDS as a global threat and the subsequent newfound focus, in the year 2000, for the first time in its history, the UN Security Council showed an interest in health-related issues and included the theme of HIV/AIDS on its agenda.[12] This also contributed to the renewed link between health and the security agenda. A range of new health issues had joined infectious diseases traditionally perceived as the main security threats. Links between health and security were made at the UN Secretary-General's High Level Panel on Threats, Challenges and Change in 2002. Although other issues such as economic stability, international crises and humanitarian emergencies, chemical, radioactive and biological terror threats and environmental change were also identified as International Health Security Issues, the spread of emerging and re-emerging diseases (such as Avian influenza, in 1997; SARS, in 2002; H1N1 – swine flu – in 2009; Ebola, in 2014–2016; and most recently Zika, in

56 *Globalization, development and health*

2016, among others) continued to play a major role in the securitization of global health (McInnes and Lee 2012).

The control of infectious diseases also became an integral part of the poverty reduction debate. In June 2000, responding to a specific request from the G8 countries and with the intent of assessing progress toward poverty reduction goals and to outline a common vision for the way forward, the UN, OECD, IMF and WB jointly presented the report *A Better World for All*. Obstacles in the desired "development effort to pursue faster, sustainable growth strategies that favor the poor" were identified in the following succinct terms:

> Weak governance. Bad policies. Human rights abuses. Conflicts, natural disasters, and other external shocks. The spread of HIV/AIDS. The failure to address inequities in income, education and access to health care, and the inequalities between men and women [...], limits on developing countries' access to global markets, the burden of debt, the decline in development aid and, sometimes, inconsistencies in donor policies [...].
>
> (UN, World Bank, IMF and OECD 2000)

Regarding solutions, the report stated that the best way to overcome these obstacles was through "True partnership – and a continuing commitment to eliminate poverty" (UN, World Bank, IMF and OECD 2000).

That same year, health issues were also included in the G8 agenda. At their Okinawa summit, the group of leaders of the wealthiest countries included the fight against a few infectious diseases in their undertakings.

Taking a slightly broader approach, the European Union also declared its renewed and increased political and financial commitment to health as part of its development policy. Although reaffirming that health systems development and the fight against poverty are central to any strategy, the EU asserted that accelerated action was needed to control infectious diseases, highlighting the importance of partnerships with pharmaceutical companies and drug markets (Commission of European Communities 2000).

The year 2000 also brought the Millennium Summit to New York. Among the Millennium Development Goals (MDGs), health goals occupied an eminent position (Box 4.2).

BOX 4.2 Millennium Development Goals

Goal 1. To eradicate extreme poverty and hunger
Goal 2. To achieve universal primary education
Goal 3. To promote gender equality and empower women
Goal 4. To reduce child mortality
Goal 5. To improve maternal health
Goal 6. To combat HIV/AIDS, malaria and other diseases
Goal 7 To ensure environmental sustainability
Goal 8. To develop a global partnership for development

Source: www.undp.org/content/undp/en/home/sdgoverview/mdg_goals.html.

It should be mentioned that those goals and targets were mostly an update of the goals adopted in 1990 and largely missed by the year 2000. The new target was instead set for 2015 and the metrics were updated. For example, it was decided to reduce mortality by two-thirds in children under five (MDG 4), an update to the 1990 target, which was set at a one-third reduction by the year 2000. Additionally, a new goal was to reduce maternal mortality by three-quarters (MDG 5), a revision to the 1990 target of a 50% reduction by the year 2000. One entirely new goal was the control of HIV/AIDS, malaria and other infectious diseases (MDG 6).

Although the statement did not provide any concrete commitment regarding resources to be mobilized, the MDGs were at the origin of a significant increase in global resources for Development Assistance in Health (DAH) over the next 15 years, especially regarding three diseases under MDG 6 (see Chapter 13). Indeed, in the year 2000, the world was experiencing a climate of total disengagement of donor countries. The OECD/DAC countries' ODA was at the lowest historical levels (0.22% of their GDP in 2000, reaching 0.21% in 2001, the lowest level ever), thus, a new push was needed. According to the new agenda, the response should have come from the involvement of new actors through the development of a strong partnership with the private sector and civil society organizations committed to development and poverty eradication (MDG 8).

The idea of partnership understood as a social responsibility for development, shared among advanced and less advanced countries, later extended beyond traditional bilateral and multilateral actors to include the corporate sector and civil society, was soon translated into new organizational arrangements and the establishment of global public-private partnerships (GPPPs), i.e. more or less autonomous initiatives and organizations, devoted to specific issues, jointly funded and governed.[13]

The GPPP formula emerged between the end of the 1990s and the beginning of the new century. The model gained special momentum through the launch of the Global Alliance on Vaccines and Immunizations (GAVI) established in 2000 with an initial funding of USD 750 million of the Bill & Melinda Gates Foundation.

The creation of the Global Fund to fight HIV/AIDS, Tuberculosis and Malaria (GFATM) represented a paradigmatic case of political convenience prevailing over technical considerations. The initial proposal of the G8 Italian Presidency clearly envisaged an integrated approach to health; instead the following negotiations limited the scope of the future Global Fund to just three diseases (see Box 4.3).

BOX 4.3 Case study: politics-based evidence – the creation of the Global Fund to Fight HIV/AIDS, Tuberculosis and Malaria

At the beginning of 2001 the G8 Italian Presidency had circulated a relatively articulated agenda on health. Among others under the item *Health as a multifaceted issue in dealing with development*, the proposed Terms of Reference said:

> In Okinawa we reaffirmed the key role health plays in working towards economic prosperity and human progress. However we do not consider it sufficient to target only specific diseases. We have learned from past experience in the field that 'selective action' against diseases, in the absence of equitable, efficient and effective health systems, may not succeed in eradicating diseases

or improving general state of health. Access to proper heath services system appears to be the core issue. In particular, the need for effective health systems entails focusing on prevention, in the broader context of a comprehensive development approach, that gives priority to the improvement of people's life conditions.

(G8 Presidency 2001)

Furthermore that initial Italian Presidency's *Action Plan for Health Care* included: coordination efforts to intensify international action; support for national programs and priorities; measuring health progress; focusing action where needed the most; and global action for local access to key medicine and supplies. Regarding coordination, it said.

A higher degree of coordination amongst institutional partners is needed: we must pursue a common framework, which supports the mandate and stewardship of specialized international organizations, like the WHO and the specific assistance programs of the UN.

(G8 Presidency 2001)

Subsequently, following indications from the G7 financial ministers meeting that preceded the health experts meeting, the G8 Italian Presidency forced on the health experts group the introduction in the agenda of a World-Bank-administered Trust Fund for Health "in strict cooperation with the WHO to catalyze public and private contributions" and a management structure that "could be based on the model of the GEF (Global Environmental Facility)", i.e. with decisions taken through double majority: the majority of shareholders and the majority of countries. To ensure an adequate level of resources

The G7 should commit the initial start up of the Fund with a donation of USD 500 million, to match expected private contributions of an equal amount. The 1000 largest companies in the world would be invited to donate USD 500,000 each to this fund.

(G8 Presidency 2001a)

The proposal contained in the document, titled *Beyond debt relief*, was harshly criticized by representatives of civil society organizations, who considered it a

too simplistic, if not even insulting solution to complex problems. It lacks long term vision, and does not take into consideration the role corporate profits play on people's health needs. For this reason it should be dropped.

(Maciocco *et al.* 2001)

Others highlighting the doubtful scientific approach, governance issues and the economic inconsistency of the proposal, defined the document as a whole "only a recipe for building the empire" (Amalric 2001).

The new proposal of a new "Global Fund" became the hot issue of the following G8 health experts meeting held in Rome in March. While views differed on the approach to a new global fund, G8 health experts were in agreement in rejecting the establishment of new formal structures, suggesting instead that

Multiplicity of already existing initiatives should rather be brought under a common framework, and existing international institutions strengthened, while promoting mechanisms for higher efficiency.

(Missoni 2001)

Approximately one month later, the agenda was narrowed to the establishment of a new public-private partnership for the mobilization of resources and the management of the initiative now titled *Genoa Trust Fund for Healthcare*, where "a crucial role should be played by the contributions of the corporate sector and NGOs" (G8 Presidency 2001b). Mentioning NGOs was clearly a diplomatic opening to civil society; instead, in exchange for their financial contribution, transnational companies would have acquired the right to participate in the direction of the new facility, according to the arguable principle expressed in the document, that "Governance is the responsibility of those who provide and who use the funds" (G8 Presidency 2001b).

It must be pointed out that in parallel with the preparatory work for the G8 Genoa Summit, a number of other initiatives pointed in the direction of the establishment of some kind of global fund, mostly concerned with infectious diseases and specifically HIV/AIDS, especially in view of the UN General Assembly Extraordinary Session on AIDS to be held at the end of June in New York. Although among the options the strengthening of UNAIDS's role was considered, paradoxically, Kofi Annan, then Secretary-General of the United Nations, was among the strongest promoters of the constitution of a *Global AIDS and Health Fund* external to the United Nations, his argument being "Because I want others to join the fight", thus open to donor governments, but also to the private sector, foundations and individuals, with autonomous corporate governance representing them all (UN 2001).

The most contentious issue was the governance mechanism of the future fund. For example "Italy and others were aligned against the U.S. and those who didn't want it run by either the U.N. or World Bank" (Phillips 2002). Some authors have also argued that one aim of some proponents of this GPPP had been precisely "to undermine the role of the UN system in policy-making" (Deacon *et al.* 2003: 57).

Through negotiations among G8 leaders and the UN Secretary-General, any possible reference to a more systemic view of health and the complex issues at stake introduced in the G8 Agenda at the beginning of the year was dropped, and at the Genoa G8 Summit in July 2001 the Global Fund to fight HIV/AIDS, Tuberculosis and Malaria (GFATM) was launched.

After the initial spat among donors, GFATM was set up as a private foundation under Swiss law on 24 January 2002 (GFATM 2003).

Sources:
Amalric, F., 2001. *The unbearable lightness of G7 concerns for the South: A comment on Italy's "Beyond Debt Relief"*, Society for International Development, Rome, 13 March.

Deacon, B., et al., 2003. *Global Social Governance. Themes and Prospects*, Helsinki: Ministry of Foreign Affairs of Finland, Hakapaino Oy.

G8 Presidency, 2001. *Action Plan for health care. Terms of Reference*, 23 January.

G8 Presidency, 2001a. *Beyond Debt Relief*, February.
G8 Presidency, 2001b. *Genova Trust Fund for Health Care*, April.
GFATM, 2003. *Update on Legal Status for the Global Fund, The Global Fund to Fight AIDS, Tuberculosis and Malaria*. Report of the Governance and Partnership Committee, Fifth Board Meeting, ANNEX 6, Geneva, 5–6 June 2003.
Maciocco, G., et al., 2001. *Access to health and the G8 document 'Beyond Debt Relief'. The Perspective of Civil Society*.
Missoni, E., 2001. *A global fund for Health: the G8 present their human face?* Genoa Social Forum, Session on Right to Health and Trade Agreements, Genoa, 17 July.
Phillips, M.M., 2002. Infectious-disease fund stalls amid U.S. rules for disbursal. *The Wall Street Journal*, August 5.
UN, 2001. Secretary-General outlines plans for global aids fund, May 17. Available from: www.hri.org/news/world/undh/2001/01-05-17.undh.html.

With the launch of the Global Fund, the G8 established itself as an influential collective actor in global health, while the joint sponsorship of the UN Secretary-General and the G8 certainly contributed to the GPPP model becoming the dominant archetype in the international cooperation landscape.

The GPPP model was repeatedly proposed at every summit as the answer to the most varied and dramatic of world problems. Only in the health sector the number of GPPPs rapidly increased to surpass 90 different types of initiatives and organizations, fragmenting action and governance for health at all levels.

At the global level, the new model weakened the United Nations and their specialized agencies, further undermined their legitimacy and contributed to increased confusion in the overall direction and coordination of international development cooperation. New organizations involved recruitment of new staff and related costs (at international prices), new administrative costs and new procedures with additional burden on partner countries' institutions. In addition, in the governance of the new GPPPs, the commercial partners played a disproportionate role compared to the resources that it was assumed they would mobilize, which instead remained below expectations (Ruckert and Labonté 2014). Due to their selective approach and non-alignment with national procedures, they resulted in the weakening of health systems in addition to the limiting of sovereignty imposed on countries to access global funds. The GPPPs contributed to shaping the transformation of the organizational landscape of global health.

The 11 September 2001 tragedy suddenly changed the global scenario and the international agenda, as well as some donor countries' priorities.

At the Monterrey international conference on development financing, scheduled for 2001 but postponed to 2002, rich countries were urged once again to allocate 0.7% of their GDP to ODA – a goal set out in 1969 by the Pearson Commission on International Development (Pearson 1969) that later become a constant reference (Missoni and Alesani 2014) – however, US President George W. Bush emphatically expressed himself against the definition of "arbitrary levels" for ODA (Cevallos 2002).

The United Nations Special Session on Children scheduled from 19 to 21 September 2001 was postponed to May of the following year. Recognizing failure, that year UNICEF's flagship report stated that despite outstanding examples of progress for children in the last decade, most governments did not live up to the promises made at the 1990 World Summit for Children, and added: "the promises we make now are the promises we must keep. This time there is no excuse" (UNICEF 2002).

It is evident that the goals and commitments undertaken throughout international summits and conferences between the end of the second and the dawn of the third millennium were at risk of being purely rhetorical in the absence of a qualitative review of international cooperation between the North and South and its governance.

4.7 The right to health and commercial interests

The access to goods and health services, which as mentioned above could not be included in the 2001 G8 agenda, was increasingly linked to negotiations and multilateral agreements outside the health sector, and strongly influenced by the interests of the private commercial sector. For example, the access to many essential drugs in developing countries would depend on the outcome of negotiations on intellectual property rights, regulated by the TRIPs (Trade-Related Intellectual Property Rights) agreement, and the destiny of health services was in the hands of negotiators of the General Agreement on Trade in Services (GATS), both negotiated under the auspices of the World Trade Organization (WTO).

These agreements were discussed and signed by economic and financial representatives of governments and, although explicitly drawn to promote trade and business in relevant sectors, could inevitably influence the right to health and reduce the autonomy of government interventions in certain areas of public health such as access to essential goods and services.

The conflict between the interests of impoverished countries and those of the transnational pharmaceutical industry came to the forefront of public attention on 19 April 2001 when 39 transnational companies took the South African government to court questioning the implementation of the clauses foreseen in the TRIPs agreement, which allow for local production under compulsory licensing of patented drugs, and their parallel import. The case elicited a strong response of civil society activists who accused Big Pharma of pursuing profit at the expense of the lives of the millions of people unable to afford life-saving drugs in the developing world. Finally, the companies unconditionally dropped the case after carrying out intense negotiations aimed at securing a quiet exit from a case that left them mired in bad publicity (BBC News 2001).

A few months later, the "Doha Declaration on TRIPs and Public Health" signed at the end of the Fourth Ministerial Conference of the WTO, held in Doha in November 2001, clarified the interpretation of the above-mentioned TRIPs clauses giving member states the right to independently determine which situations represent a public health emergency, to issue compulsory licenses[14] for the production of patented medicines, and to determine upon which conditions such licenses could be granted. A subsequent "Decision on the interpretation of paragraph 6", adopted in August 2003, confirmed the right of countries without adequate production capacity to import compulsorily licensed pharmaceuticals from a third country in order to meet urgent health needs (Kerry and Lee 2007).

The Doha Declaration stopped short of putting an end to the negotiations around the modalities for the implementation of those principles, and the debate continued in the following years in the wider context of the WTO negotiations (the so-called Doha Round), which finally stalled mainly due to disagreement about agricultural issues. Nevertheless, in the period 2001–2014 there were at least 34 reported compulsory license instances. Of the instances, three concerned high-income countries, 26 concerned 18 developing countries, and three concerned Least Developed Countries (LDCs) (Hoen 2016).

Given the stalling of WTO negotiations, free trade negotiations soon shifted to bilateral and regional negotiations, such as those for the Trans-Pacific Partnership (TPP), the Transatlantic Trade and Investment Partnership (TTIP) and the Comprehensive Economic Trade Agreement (CETA) among many others. These trade agreements continue to be highly controversial for reasons including their potential negative impact on health, which can happen either directly through trade rules putting constrains on the provision of health services and access to drugs, or indirectly, through influence on social and environmental determinants of health (work, food, pollution, inequalities, etc.), as we shall see later (McNeill *et al.* 2017).

Commercial interests have challenged the right to health in other areas as well. The launch in 2003 of the WHO Framework Convention on Tobacco Control (FCTC), which entered into effect as international law in 2005, was a milestone in the history of corporate accountability and public health (Global Health Watch 2005). This initiative openly challenged the tobacco industry, which in turn harshly opposed it, finding support in the government of the United States, who actively worked to derail the treaty by trying to water down much of the document. The FCTC still remains one of the best examples of an attempt to defend the right to health through market regulation by using available WHO regulatory instruments as well as establishing appropriate alliances with civil society organizations defending public interests (Missoni 2015).

In 2005, the Sixth World Health Promotion Conference was held in Bangkok. It reaffirmed the principles already expressed in Ottawa (1986), but also established that "Effective mechanisms for global governance for health are required to address all the harmful effects of trade, products, services, and marketing strategies". It called upon governments to meet their responsibilities for health and recognized the role that can be exercised by communities and civil society through critical consumption. In addition, it called for the private sector to behave in an ethically and socially responsible manner and put forward the possibility of fostering this through appropriate national and international regulation, citing as an example the WHO Framework Convention on Tobacco Control (WHO 2005).

A new impetus for the idea of health as a fundamental human right also came from the renewed debate about social justice promoted by the WHO during the brief tenure of J. Wong Lee as Director-General of the Organization (2003–2006). Introducing the World Health Report 2003, Dr. Lee wrote "Today the global health situation raises questions about social justice" (WHO 2003: 3), and to find the right answers, in 2005 Lee established the Commission on Social Determinants of Health. The purpose of the commission, whose result would be presented in 2008, was to demonstrate the importance of health interventions and policies that improve the conditions in which people grow, live, work and age (CSDH 2008).

At that time, however, the prevailing idea was still that solutions to health problems were to be sought in market mechanisms and in the financial markets.

In 2003, the British government in its *UK Treasury Paper* presented the concept for an International Finance Facility (IFF) developed with the assistance of Goldman Sachs. IFF would serve the purpose of making immediately available large amounts of resources for initiatives managed by national and international institutions by placing

IFF bonds on international financial markets. The British presidency proposed the idea to the Gleneagle's G8 Summit in 2005, which launched a new public-private partnership, the International Financing Facility for Immunizations (IFFIm), which would apply that concept to support the purchase of vaccines managed by GAVI, relying on the World Bank for the treasury service to ensure safety and thus attractiveness of IFFIm bonds on the financial markets.

On the same occasion, Italy presented another market mechanism with the aim of encouraging the biomedical industry to invest in the search for a new vaccine. The so-called Advance Market Commitment (AMC) envisaged participating governments commiting the financial resources needed to ensure the purchase of vaccines that the private sector, driven by the guarantee of return on investment, would develop on the basis of agreed technical criteria (Calì and Missoni 2014).

The French President Chirac seized the opportunity of the World Economic Forum in January 2005 to announce an initiative (also supported by Brazil, Chile, Germany and Spain) to introduce a levy on airplane tickets and use the revenues for the purchase of biomedical products for the diagnosis and treatment of HIV/AIDS, malaria and tuberculosis in developing countries. The new public-private partnership named UNITAID was launched in September 2006 at the United Nations General Assembly (Silverman *et al.* 2013).

These initiatives, based on selective approaches, further contributed to the fragmentation of global health financing, and were evidently in contrast with the growing awareness about the need for strengthened health systems and wider health coverage for the most disadvantaged populations. They also disregarded the principles of ownership, alignment, harmonization, results and mutual accountability, adopted with the Paris Declaration on Aid Effectiveness in 2005 (OECD/DAC 2005). The Declaration, which called for donors to align their support, whenever possible, with recipient-country government priorities, was signed by more than 100 countries and international organizations and was followed three years later by the Accra Agenda for Action putting additional emphasis on ownership, 'inclusive partnerships' and results.

To face the challenge of fragmentation and increase coordination in Development Assistance in Health (DAH) a number of other initiatives were launched in the following years. Among them were the International Health Partnership,[15] launched by UK Prime Minister Gordon Brown in 2007 to apply the Paris Declaration principles to the health sector,[16] and the "H8", an informal group of eight health-related organizations (WHO, UNICEF, UNFPA, UNAIDS, GFATM, GAVI, the Bill & Melinda Gates Foundation and the World Bank) formed in 2007 to improve global coordination on the health-related MDGs (Moon and Omole 2013) (see also Chapter 13).

4.8 The renewed interest in a systemic vision

In 2008, on the thirtieth anniversary of the Alma-Ata Declaration, the need for a more holistic and systemic approach was raised by the World Health Report "Primary Health Care now more than ever" (WHO 2008a) and the Report of the Commission on Social Determinants of Health (CSDH 2008).

The World Health Report (2008) critically analyzed the way in which health care was organized, funded and managed in both rich and poor countries. It highlighted the factors interfering with health systems' functions, i.e. focus on hospital care, fragmentation resulting from programs' and projects' multiplication, and the pervasive commercialization of health care. In response, the report identified four interlocking sets of reforms that aimed to achieve universal access and social protection in order to improve health equity, reorganize service delivery around people's needs and expectations, secure healthier communities through better public policies, and remodel leadership for health around more effective government and the active participation of key stakeholders (WHO 2008a).

The Commission's report on social determinants, titled "Closing the gap in a generation: Health equity through action on the social determinants of health", examined the "toxic combination of bad policies, economics, and politics [that] is, in large measure, responsible for the fact that a majority of people in the world do not enjoy the good health that is biologically possible, and the political, social and economic forces that determine them" (CSDH 2008). The Commission identified 12 goals based on three principles of action: improve daily living conditions; tackle the inequitable distribution of power, money and resources; measure and understand the problem and assess the impact of action. The result was an agenda that aligned the broad principles of social justice and health equity with specific policy measures that could be supported by global action from governments, civil society, the WHO and other international organizations (Lee 2010).

That same year (2008), the G8 Toyako summit also focused on strengthening health systems (Reich and Takemi 2009). The following year at L'Aquila, eight years after the Genoa summit when the original systems approach had been deleted from the agenda and substituted with the launch of the Global Fund, the G8 (under Italian presidency) declared:

> 122. We promote a comprehensive and integrated approach to the achievement of the health-related MDGs, also maximizing synergies between global health initiatives and health systems ....
>
> 123. We also recognize the need to strengthen the link between health sector and other policies by promoting the strategic approach of "health as an outcome of all policies". We aim at addressing the key determinants of health through mutually reinforcing policies across sectors ....
>
> (G8 2009)

The World Health Assembly also put renewed emphasis on the social determinants of health, stressing that health improvement cannot be achieved by simply investing in specific health interventions, but requires an approach based on human rights and health as a fundamental right, as well as important economic and social changes (WHO 2009). In other words, this new vision must not treat global health and human rights as two separate entities, but rather as inextricably linked factors for humanitarian development.

Over 30 years after Alma-Ata, the systemic approach seemed to regain priority in the global agenda. Universal access to care was re-emerging as an important policy objective linked to the right to health and to the debate on strengthening health systems. In addition, the WHO World Health Report in 2010 was focused on "Universal Coverage" (WHO 2010).

The collapse of financial markets in the United States between 2008 and early 2009 rapidly expanded to the global financial market, resulting in a period of severe economic downturn. Those events affected the global political and humanitarian agenda. In 2010, both the G8 and G20 summits were held at Muskoka, in Canada. Much of the agenda was occupied by the need for the stabilization of the financial markets and resuming economic growth, which was also considered to be key for the achievement of the MDGs (G20 2010). In the Muskoka Declaration, the G8 countries acknowledged the slow advances in the improvement of maternal and reproductive health and launched the Muskoka Initiative with new financial commitments (USD 5 billion to be disbursed by 2015) for the reduction of maternal, neonatal and infant mortality in developing countries (G8 2010). Furthermore, as the crash of the financial markets impinged upon the progression of the MDGs, former UN Secretary-General Ban Ki-Moon assembled a special MDG Summit to form proposals for acceleration towards these goals (UN 2010).

The economic and financial crisis also negatively affected international aid flows. Nevertheless, overall development assistance for health slowed down but did not halt, as some donors' cuts in aid expenditure were offset by the counter-cyclical action of others. In addition, there remained a relatively steady flow from non-governmental actors – in particular the Gates Foundation – and from several GPPPs (IHME 2014).

Moreover, the overall landscape of development cooperation was rapidly changing as a result of several factors: (1) the progressive change in the economic and geopolitical equilibrium, with a growing role of emerging economies, particularly the BRICS (Brazil, Russia, India, China and South Africa) countries, (2) the constant push for more substantial private-sector involvement and the emphasis on the role of the market, (3) the distribution of poverty now no longer concentrated in the poorest countries and (4), regarding health, the steady increase in the burden of chronic noncommunicable diseases as a result of the epidemiological transition.

In 2011, at the Fourth High Level Forum on Aid Effectiveness of the Organization for Economic Cooperation and Development (OECD) held in Busan (Korea), participation was extended to political leaders, government representatives, parliamentarians, civil society organizations and representatives of the private sector, from both developing and donor countries. The over 3000 delegates met to review progress on implementing the principles of the Paris Declaration. They also discussed how to maintain the relevance of the aid effectiveness agenda in the context of the evolving development landscape.[17]

Busan represented a turning point with respect to the traditional North-South approach in international development cooperation. Now many developing countries engaged in the new aid-effectiveness agenda. Those that signed up included not only traditional partner countries (recipients), but also middle-income countries that acted as both recipients and donors. The BRICS group (Brazil, Russia, India, China, South Africa), which traditionally kept a distance from the OECD because they perceived it as Western-dominated, also endorsed the final document. They did not, however, commit in their capacity as donors to applying the principles of the Paris Declaration, considering them only as voluntary guidelines. From then on, a new global organization would be responsible for monitoring the results of development cooperation, the so-called Global Partnership for Effective Development Cooperation (GPEDC). The GPEDC is a multi-stakeholder platform, open to the participation of governmental actors, representatives of bilateral and multilateral organizations, civil society organizations and the private commercial sector, with the aim of strengthening the effectiveness of development cooperation. The mission of the GPEDC is to enforce aid effectiveness principles as defined in the Paris Declaration, exemplifying a further shift from the conventional donor–recipient mode to a development–partnership approach (Missoni and Alesani 2014).

66 *Globalization, development and health*

Although the GPEDC is more inclusive than the OECD Development Assistance Committee (DAC), some of the new and emerging actors in the development system still consider it to be an expression of the OECD and may look more favorably at the United Nations, specifically its Economic and Social Council (ECOSOC), as the appropriate center for the coordination of development policies. At the 2005 World Summit, Heads of State and Government recognized the need for a more effective ECOSOC

> as a principal body for coordination, policy review, policy dialogue and recommendations on issues of economic and social development, as well as for implementation of the international development goals agreed at the major United Nations conferences and summits, including the Millennium Development Goals

and called for the establishment of a high-level Development Cooperation Forum (DCF)

> to review trends in international development cooperation, including strategies, policies and financing, promote greater coherence among the development activities of different development partners and strengthen the links between the normative and operational work of the United Nations.
> (UN 2005)

The DCF was established in 2007 and would also provide a platform for member states to share experiences in formulating, supporting and implementing national development strategies. It was open to participation by all stakeholders, including the organizations of the United Nations, the international financial and trade institutions, regional organizations, civil society and private-sector representatives.[18]

As the 2015 deadline drew closer, the limitations surrounding the MDGs and the strategies used to attain their targets came under scrutiny, and the debate intensified about the future development agenda.

At the political level, an important hallmark in the process was the United Nations Conference on Sustainable Development (Rio+20) in 2012 (see Chapter 2). The Rio+20 conference established the United Nations High-level Political Forum on Sustainable Development (HLPF), which, after the launch of the "Agenda 2030 for Sustainable Development" (UN 2015), assumed the central responsibility of follow-up and review of the 2030 Agenda and its sustainable development goals (SDGs),[19] evidently taking into account the work of the DCF.

As part of the elaboration of the future global development agenda, the achievement of MDGs was assessed. According to the final UN report, despite "uneven achievements and shortfalls in many areas", there were "reasons to celebrate": lives of millions were saved and life conditions improved for many more (UN 2015a).

Many developing countries did not meet the target of the MDGs and were deemed to be "off-track"; nevertheless, some made remarkable improvement towards the targets.

Despite limitations, some success had been made around specific health-related targets.

Although the global under-five mortality rate declined remarkably by more than half, dropping from 90 to 43 deaths per 1000 live births between 1990 and 2015 (UN 2015), the result fell short of the goal envisaged by MDG 4 (reduce by two-thirds, between 1990 and 2015, the under-five mortality rate).

Since 1990, the maternal mortality rate has declined by 45% worldwide, and most of the reduction has occurred since 2000 (UN 2015). Initially, a 50% reduction was the target established in 1990 to be achieved by the year 2000; however, maternal mortality actually increased during this time. This result fell far from the MDG 5 target (reduce by three-quarters, between 1990 and 2015, the maternal mortality ratio).

With 30% of the global development assistance in health resources invested in controlling the HIV/AIDS epidemic, according to UNAIDS in 2015 new HIV infections had fallen by 35% since 2000 (and by 58% among children): "the world has exceeded the AIDS targets of Millennium Development Goal 6, halting and reversing the spread of HIV, and more and more countries are getting on the Fast-Track to end the AIDS epidemic by 2030 as part of the Sustainable Development Goals (SDGs)" (UNAIDS 2015).

The UN (2015) also acknowledged uneven achievements and shortfalls in many areas, stating there was unfinished work to be continued in the new development era.

As mentioned in Chapter 2, the MDGs lacked a system and global vision, and to address this gap there was a strong push towards a more inclusive and comprehensive agenda, contextualizing development processes with each country's national reality and priorities, an agenda now going beyond the traditional North-South approach. The "Agenda 2030 for Sustainable Development" (UN 2015), with its 17 "indivisible" Sustainable Development Goals (SDGs) (Box 4.4), may represent a new phase in development policies in an increasingly complex global context with unprecedented challenges.

BOX 4.4 Sustainable Development Goals

Goal 1. End poverty in all its forms everywhere

Goal 2. End hunger, achieve food security and improved nutrition and promote sustainable agriculture

Goal 3. Ensure healthy lives and promote well-being for all at all ages

Goal 4. Ensure inclusive and equitable quality education and promote lifelong learning opportunities for all

Goal 5. Achieve gender equality and empower all women and girls

Goal 6. Ensure availability and sustainable management of water and sanitation for all

Goal 7. Ensure access to affordable, reliable, sustainable and modern energy for all

Goal 8. Promote sustained, inclusive and sustainable economic growth, full and productive employment and decent work for all

Goal 9. Build resilient infrastructure, promote inclusive and sustainable industrialization and foster innovation

Goal 10. Reduce inequality within and among countries

Goal 11. Make cities and human settlements inclusive, safe, resilient and sustainable

Goal 12. Ensure sustainable consumption and production patterns

Goal 13. Take urgent action to combat climate change and its impacts

Goal 14. Conserve and sustainably use the oceans, seas and marine resources for sustainable development

Goal 15. Protect, restore and promote sustainable use of terrestrial ecosystems, sustainably manage forests, combat desertification, and halt and reverse land degradation and halt biodiversity loss

Goal 16. Promote peaceful and inclusive societies for sustainable development, provide access to justice for all and build effective, accountable and inclusive institutions at all levels

Goal 17. Strengthen the means of implementation and revitalize the Global Partnership for Sustainable Development

Source:
UN, 2015. *Transforming our world: the 2030 agenda for sustainable development.* New York: United Nations, 25 September.

The progress toward the achievement of the SDGs in general, and of "healthy lives and well-being for all at all ages" (SDG3) with its targets and actions in particular (Box 4.5), will be largely determined by the balance of forces involved and the vision that will prevail.

BOX 4.5 Health targets and actions for Sustainable Development Goal 3

3.1 By 2030, reduce the global maternal mortality ratio to less than 70 per 100,000 live births.

3.2 By 2030, end preventable deaths of newborns and children under 5 years of age, with all countries aiming to reduce neonatal mortality to at least as low as 12 per 1000 live births and under-5 mortality to at least as low as 25 per 1000 live births.

3.3 By 2030, end the epidemics of AIDS, tuberculosis, malaria and neglected tropical diseases and combat hepatitis, water-borne diseases and other communicable diseases.

3.4 By 2030, reduce by one-third premature mortality from noncommunicable diseases through prevention and treatment and promote mental health and well-being.

3.5 Strengthen the prevention and treatment of substance abuse, including narcotic drug abuse and harmful use of alcohol.

3.6 By 2020, halve the number of global deaths and injuries from road traffic accidents.

3.7 By 2030, ensure universal access to sexual and reproductive health-care services, including for family planning, information and education, and the integration of reproductive health into national strategies and programs.

3.8 Achieve universal health coverage, including financial risk protection, access to quality essential health-care services and access to safe, effective, quality and affordable essential medicines and vaccines for all.

3.9 By 2030, substantially reduce the number of deaths and illnesses from hazardous chemicals and air, water and soil pollution and contamination.

3.a Strengthen the implementation of the WHO Framework Convention on Tobacco Control in all countries, as appropriate.

3.b Support the research and development of vaccines and medicines for the communicable and noncommunicable diseases that primarily affect developing countries, provide access to affordable essential medicines and vaccines, in accordance with the Doha Declaration on the TRIPS Agreement and Public Health, which affirms the right of developing countries to use to the full the provisions in the Agreement on Trade-Related Aspects of Intellectual Property Rights regarding flexibilities to protect public health, and, in particular, provide access to medicines for all.

3.c   Substantially increase health financing and the recruitment, development, training and retention of the health workforce in developing countries, especially in least developed countries and small island developing States.

3.d   Strengthen the capacity of all countries, in particular developing countries, for early warning, risk reduction and management of national and global health risks.

Source:
UN, 2015. Transforming our world: the 2030 agenda for sustainable development. New York: United Nations, 25 September.

The acceleration of the globalization process and the hegemony of the neo-liberal ideology led to the progressive deregulation and liberalization of trade regimes, to extensive privatization and scaling back of the state. These processes have intensified the commodification and commercialization of vital social determinants such as health and social services, water and electricity. Unhealthy products are aggressively marketed by global industries (tobacco, alcohol, processed foods and beverages, etc.). Environmental deterioration is also a result of the dominant economic model, which also has a heavy impact on labor and working conditions (CSDH 2008).

Health no longer depends solely on the specific situation of the country where people live, but is largely determined by global forces acting outside the control of individual states, becoming an issue of foreign policy, global security, international trade, overall sustainability of development, democratic governance and human rights (McInnes and Lee 2013).

In the globalization process, two future visions oppose each other. In the first vision

> individuals, households, and national economies have to 'earn their keep' in the global market-place. This offers major opportunities for some, and major risks – exemplified by long-term unemployment, economic insecurity and marginalization, and catastrophic illness – for others. This vision does not preclude social policy interventions, but they must be justified in terms of the return on investment.
>
> (Labonté and Schrecker 2007)

The second vision seeks to limit the negative impact of the emerging global marketplace and incorporates such perspectives as: (1) institutionalized recognition of at least minimal access to the material prerequisites for health as a human right, (2) the recognition of governmental social obligations and the incorporation of new institutions for global governance, (3) a regulatory framework for global market forces that is people-centered rather than capital-driven, (4) public policies based on a vision of the world where people matter and social justice is paramount, and (5) the idea of a "global social contract" analogous to the social contract within industrialized countries that supports contemporary welfare states (Labonté and Schrecker 2007).

Which of the two visions will prevail will largely depend on the role played by the increasing number of very diverse actors and interactions in the global arena, which impact the vast array of social, economic, environmental and political determinants of health and the overall evolution of global health-related governance processes that will be presented in the following Section.

Notes

1 Christina Procacci contributed to a first draft of this chapter.
2 In 2011 a similar success was obtained in the domain of animal health with the eradication of rinderpest, not affecting humans. Available from: www.oie.int/ for-the-media/rinderpest/.
3 The training of health professional was (and still largely is!) highly influenced by a biomedical approach to health. In 1971 the eminent Italian biologist, medical doctor and editor Maccacaro wrote: "There is no medical graduate or specialization course that produces a primary care doctor, who is able to usefully insert himself in a urban or rural community, to take care of it, to understand its disease related problems and defend its right to health" (Maccacaro 1971).
4 Due to a non-written rule UNICEF's Executive Director has always been a US citizen.
5 A "zero real growth" approach allows adjustments for inflation.
6 Under the Bretton Woods system the dollar was made the "reserve currency" with an official fixed exchange rate with gold (USD 35 per ounce). Member states were required to establish a parity of their national currencies in terms of the reserve currency and to maintain exchange rates within plus or minus 1% of parity. Thus all currencies linked to the dollar had a fixed value in terms of gold and central banks could exchange dollar reserves into gold at that official fixed exchange rate.
7 Organization of Petroleum Exporting Countries
8 The service of debt is essentially composed of returning a portion of the borrowed capital plus the interest.
9 1981 represented the first year in which there was a negative balance between new loans to developing countries and the repayment of debt – the net exportation of capital was about 7.2 million US dollars; in 1985, that figure was 10 times greater (IMF, 1986).
10 The loans were primarily made in US dollars, and the value of the dollar rose 11% in 1981 and 17% in 1982, making it extremely difficult for recipient countries to repay loans as the power of their domestic currency was severely reduced.
11 The Paris Club is an informal group of public creditors, existing as an analogous body to the London Club of private creditors, created to find coordinated solutions to the difficulties of payment in indebted countries, through renegotiation of the loan agreements (e.g. duration of payment scheme).
12 In 2014 the UN Security Council dealt for the second time with a health issue: the Ebola epidemic in Western Africa.
13 For a classification of GPPPs and the description of their governance see Chapter 9.
14 A compulsory license is issued by a government to allow the national manufacturing of a product without the consent of the patent holder.
15 The IHP soon expanded to include other initiatives with a similar vision and became known as the IHP and Related Initiatives (IHP+), which in 2016 was transformed in the UHC2030 partnership, to take into account the SDGs. See Chapter 13.
16 Eight donor countries (Canada, France, Germany, Italy, the Netherlands, Norway, Portugal, UK) and 11 other global actors (African Development Bank, Bill & Melinda Gates Foundation, European Commission, GAVI, GFATM, UNAIDS, UNFPA, UNICEF, WHO, World Bank, UN Development Group) originally signed the IHP launching document. See: http://webarchive.nationalarchives.gov.uk/+/; www.dfid.gov.uk/news/files/ihp/default.asp.
17 See: Fourth High-Level Forum on Aid Effectiveness; www.oecd.org/dac/effectiveness/fourthhighlevelforumonaideffectiveness.htm.
18 See: www.un.org/ecosoc/en/development-cooperation-forum.
19 See: https://sustainabledevelopment.un.org/hlpf.

References

Alma-Ata, 1978. *Primary Health Care. Report of the International Conference on Primary Health Care*. Alma-Ata, USSR, 6–12 September 1978.

BBC News, 2001. SA victory in Aids drugs case. April 19. Available from: http://news.bbc.co.uk/2/hi/africa/1285097.stm.
Bello, W. 2002. *Il futuro incerto. Globalizzazione e nuova resistenza.* Milan: Baldini & Castoldi.
Brown, T. M., Cueto, M., Fee, E., 2006. The World Health Organization and the transition from 'international' to 'global' public health. *American Journal of Public Health*, 96(1), 62–72.
Buse, K., Gwin, C., 1998. The World Bank and global cooperation in health: the case of Bangladesh. *The Lancet*, 351, 665–669.
Cali, M.L., Missoni, E., 2014. La finanza innovativa. La partecipazione italiana a IFFIm e AMC. *Sistema Salute*, 58(4), 440–452.
Cassels, A. 1995. *Aid Instruments and Health systems development: an analysis of current practice.* WHO/SHS/NHP/95, 6.
Cevallos, D., 2002. Cumbre de Monterrey concluye sin decisiones. *IPS*, México. 22 March 2002.
Commission of the European Communities, 2000. *Communication of the Commission to the Council and the European Parliament. Accelerated action targeted at major communicable diseases within the context of poverty reduction.* Brussels, 20/9/2000 COM(2000), 585.
CSDH, 2008. *Closing the gap in a generation. Health equity through action on the social determinants of health.* Final Report of the Commission on Social Determinants of Health. Geneva: World Health Organization.
Deacon, B., et al., 2003. *Global Social Governance. Themes and Prospects.* Helsinki: Ministry of Foreign Affairs of Finland, Hakapaino Oy.
Devlin, R., Ffrench-Davis, R., 1995. The great Latin America debt crisis: a decade of asymmetric adjustment. *Revista de Economia Politica*, 15(3), 117–142.
FDIC, 1997. *History of the 80's – Lessons for the Future Vol. 1: An Examination of the Banking Crises of the 1980's and Early 1990's.* Chapter 5: pp. 191–210. Federal Deposit Insurance Corporation, Div. of Research and Statistics.
G20, 2010. G20 Toronto Summit Declaration.G20 Annual Summit. Toronto, Canada, June. Available from: www.g20.utoronto.ca/2010/to-communique.html.
G8, 2009. G8 Leaders Declaration. Responsible leadership for a sustainable future. L'Aquila. Available from: www.g8.utoronto.ca/summit/2009laquila/2009-declaration.html.
G8, 2010. G8 Muskoka Initiative. Recovery and new Beginnings. Muskoka, Canada, June. Available from: www.g8.utoronto.ca/summit/2010muskoka/communique.html.
Global Health Watch, 2005. *Global Health Watch 2005–2006. An alternative world health report.* London: Zed Books.
Godlee, F., 1994. WHO in Retreat; is it losing its influence? *BMJ*, 309, 1491–1495.
Hall, A., Midgley, J., 2004. *Social Policy for Development.* London: Sage.
Hill, P.S., 2002. The rhetoric of sector-wide approaches for health development. *Social Science & Medicine,* 54(11), 1725–1737.
Hoen, E., 2016. *Private Patents and Public Health: Changing Intellectual Property Rules for Access to Medicines.* Amsterdam: HAI. Available from: http://apps.who.int/medicinedocs/documents/s22475en/s22475en.pdf.
IHME, 2014. *Financing Global Health 2013. Transition in an Age of Austerity.* Seattle, WA: Institute for Health Metrics and Evaluation.
IHR, 2008. *International Health Regulations (2005).* Geneva: World Health Organization.
IMF, 1986. *World Economic Outlook.* April, Washington DC.
Italian Global Health Watch, 2008. From Alma-Ata to the Global Fund: The History of International Health Policy. *Social Medicine*, 3, 36–48.
Kerry, V.B., Lee, K., 2007. TRIPS, the Doha declaration and paragraph 6 decision: what are the remaining steps for protecting access to medicines? *Globalization and Health*, 3, 3. Available from: http://doi.org/10.1186/1744-8603-3-3.
Labonté, R., Schrecker, T., 2007. Globalization and social determinants of health: Promoting health equity in global governance (part 3 of 3). *Globalization and Health*, 3, 7.
Lee, K., 2009. *The World Health Organization.* Abingdon: Routledge

Lee, K., 2010. How do we move forward on the social determinants of health: The global governance challenges. *Critical Public Health*, 20(1), 5–14.

Maccacaro, G. 1971. Una facoltà di medicina capovolta, intervista. *Tempo Medico*, November, 97.

McInnes, C., Lee, K., 2012. *Global Health and International Relations*. Cambridge: Polity Press.

McNeill, D., et al., 2017. Viewpoint. Political origins of health inequities: trade and investment agreements. *The Lancet*, 389, 760–762.

Missoni, E., 2015. Degrowth and health: local action should be linked to global policies and governance for health. *Sustainability Science*. doi:10.1007/s11625-015-0300-1.

Missoni, E., Alesani, D., 2014. *Management of International Institutions and NGOs. Framework, practices and challenges*. Abingdon: Routledge

Moon, S., Omole, O. 2013. *Development Assistance for Health: Critiques and Proposals for Change*. Working Group on Financing. Paper 1. London: Chatham House.

OECD/DAC, 1996. *Shaping the 21st Century: The Contribution of Development Co-operation*. Paris: OECD.

OECD/DAC, 2003. *Poverty and Health*. DAC guidelines and reference series. Paris: OECD-WHO 2003.

OECD/DAC, 2005. *Paris Declaration on Aid Effectiveness*. High Level Forum. Paris, February 28 – March 3.

Packard, R.M., Brown, P.J., 1997. Rethinking health, development and malaria: historicizing a cultural model in international health. *Medical Anthropology*, 17, 181–194.

Paganini, J.M., Chorny, A.H., 1990. Los sistemas locales de salud: desafíos para la década de los noventa. *Boletín de la Oficina Sanitaria Panamericana*, 109(5–6), 424–448.

Pearson, L.B., 1969. *Partners in development: Report of the Commission on International Development*. London: Praeger.

Polanyi Levitt, K., 2012. Rolling back the canvas of history: a contribution to the critical development studies project. In Cangiani, M. (Ed.), *Alternative Approaches to Development*. Padua: CLEUP.

Reich, M., Takemi, K., 2009. G8 and strengthening health systems: follow-up to the Toyako summit. *The Lancet*, 373, 508–515.

Ruckert, A., Labonté, R., 2014. Public–Private Partnerships (PPPs) in global health: the good, the bad and the ugly. *Third World Q*, 35(9), 1598–1614.

Ruger, J.P., 2005. The changing role of the World Bank in Global Health. *American Journal of Public Health*, 95, 60–70.

Sanders, D., Chopra, M. 2003. Globalization and the challenge of health for all: a view from sub-Saharan Africa. In Lee, K. (Ed.), *Health Impacts of Globalization: Towards Global Governance*. Basingstoke: Palgrave Macmillan.

Silverman, R., Fan, V., Glassman A., 2013. *UNITAID. Background paper prepared for the Working Group on Value for Money: An Agenda for Global Health Funding Agencies*. Center for Global Development.

The Lancet, 1998. The Brundtland era begins. *The Lancet*, 351, 381.

UN, 1948. Universal Declaration of Human Rights. Available from: www.un.org/en/universal-declaration-human-rights/.

UN, 2005. Resolution adopted by the General Assembly on 16 September 2005.60/1. 2005 World Summit Outcome. General Assembly, Sixtieth Session, United Nations A/RES/60/1. Available from: www.un.org/en/ga/search/view_doc.asp?symbol=A/RES/60/1.

UN, 2010. UN Summit on the Millennium Development Goals. New York: United Nations, 20–22 September. Available from: www.un.org/en/mdg/summit2010/news.shtml.

UN, 2015. Transforming our world: the 2030 agenda for sustainable development. New York: United Nations, 25 September. Available from: https://sustainabledevelopment.un.org/post2015/transformingourworld.

UN, 2015a. *The Millennium Development Goals Report 2015*. New York: United Nations.

UN, World Bank, IMF, OECD, 2000. A better world for all. 26 June 2000. Available from: www.paris21.org/sites/default/files/bwa_e.pdf.

UNAIDS, 2015. Aids the numbers by 2015. Geneva: UNAIDS.

UNICEF, 2002. *The State of the World's Children.* New York: UNICEF.

Verona Initiative, 2000. The Verona Challenge: investing for health is investing for development. Arena Meeting III, 5–9 July 2000, Verona, Italy.

Walsh, J.A., Warren, K.S., 1979. Selective primary health care: an interim strategy for disease control in developing countries. *New England Journal of Medicine*, 301, 967–974.

Walt, G., 1998. Globalization of international health. *The Lancet,* 351, 434–437.

Walt, G., 1994. *Health Policy. An Introduction to Process And Power.* London: Zed Books.

Whitehead, M., Dahlgren, G., Evans, T., 2001. Equity and health sector reforms: can low-income countries escape the medical poverty trap? *The Lancet*, 358, 833–836.

WHO, 1946. Constitution of the World Health Organization. In WHO, 2014. *Basic Documents* (48th edn). Geneva: World Health Organization.

WHO, 1986. The Ottawa Charter for Health Promotion, First International Conference on Health Promotion. Ottawa, 21 November 1986. Available from: www.who.int/healthpromotion/conferences/previous/ottawa/en/.

WHO, 1987. Interregional Meeting on Strengthening District Health Systems, Harare, 3–7 August 1987.

WHO, 2000. *The World Health Report 2000.* Geneva: World Health Organization.

WHO, 2001. *Macroeconomics and Health: investing in heath for economic development. Report of the Commission on Macroeconomics and Health*, chaired by Jeffrey D. Sachs. Geneva: World Health Organization.

WHO, 2003. *The World Health Report 2003.* Geneva: World Health Organization.

WHO, 2005. The Bangkok Charter for Health Promotion in a Globalised World. 6th Global Conference on Health promotion, Bangkok, Thailand, August 2005.

WHO, 2008. Primary health care comes full circle, *Bulletin of the World Health Organization*, 86 10), 747–748.

WHO, 2008a. *World Health Report 2008. Primary Health Care (Now More Than Ever).* Geneva: World Health Organization.

WHO, 2009. Sixty-second World Health Assembly. Resolution 62.14. Geneva: World Health Organization.

WHO, 2010. *World Health Report 2010. Health Systems Financing: The Path to Universal Coverage.* Geneva: World Health Organization.

World Bank, 1987. Financing Health Services in Developing Countrie: An Agenda for Reforms. Washington DC: The World Bank Group.

World Bank, 1993. *World Development Report 1993: Investing in Health.* Oxford: Oxford University Press.

World Bank, 1997. *Sector Strategy. Health, Nutrition, & Population.* The Human Development Network. Washington DC: The World Bank Group.

World Bank, 2005. *Issues and Options for Improving Engagement Between the World Bank and Civil Society Organizations.* The World Bank, March.

If not otherwise indicated, all websites were accessed on 9 August 2018.

SECTION 2
Global governance and health

5 Global governance in health

5.1 Introduction

With the acceleration of the globalization process and the emerging role of transnational non-state actors, traditional policy-making processes and the international coordination and steering mechanisms faced new challenges. Governance processes became progressively more inclusive, involving a much broader range of public and private actors pushing for a *multi-stakeholder* approach.

The term governance has been used to refer to multiple concepts. Here we will focus on two of them: (a) organizational/institutional governance, which identifies legislative and policy requirements, conventions and other expectations designed to ensure accountability, decision-making, proper management and efficient use of resources, and (b) international regimes and global governance, including the management of complex transnational inter-organizational networks and international regimes, traditionally defined as sets of explicit or implicit principles, norms, rules and decision-making procedures around which actors' expectations converge in one or more given areas of international and transnational relations (Missoni and Alesani 2014).

In Chapter 4, we identified a number of stakeholders globally influencing health-related policies. In the following chapters we will try to examine in greater detail the objectives, functions and organizational governance of the major health and health-related global actors, and how they interact in determining "principles, norms, rules and decision-making procedures" (i.e. governance) which impact health determinants and health systems at the global level.

5.2 From international to global health governance, and global governance *for* health

Historically, health governance has been limited to the national and subnational level and national authorities have assumed primary responsibility for the health of the population in the country. Especially with the expansion of trade beyond national borders, nation states felt the need to establish common international rules to prevent the spread of disease, including for example the adoption of quarantine practices. We can refer to these as the early forms of cooperation on health matters between two or more countries, or as the origins of International Health Governance. During the nineteenth century the process of building institutional structures, rules and mechanisms to systematically protect and promote human health across national borders led to a consolidated mechanism of international health governance, including the creation of the International Sanitary Conference in 1851, the International Sanitary Bureau (later the Pan American Sanitary Bureau) in 1902, the Office International d'Hygiene Publique (OIHP) created in Paris in 1907, and the Health Organization of the League of Nations, established in 1920. After World War II, the establishment of the World Health Organization (WHO) in 1948 as the UN specialized agency for health, with its pledge to universality, although strongly defined by the sovereignty of its member states, opened a new period in international health governance, and represented the first step toward a more complex system of interactions beyond international relations (Dodgson et al. 2002). The WHO Constitution allowed for official relations with non-governmental organizations (NGOs) and professional groups beyond national governments and, according to Brown et al. (2006), naming the new organization the *World* Health Organization also raised sights to a worldwide "global" health perspective.

Over the last decades, the number of intergovernmental organizations active in the field of health has grown dramatically. The elaboration of international public health norms and policies is the result of the contribution of a growing number of multilateral organizations. In particular, in addition to the WHO, in the United Nations system there has been increasing involvement by several funds and programs (e.g. UNICEF, UNFPA, WFP), other entities such as UNAIDS, and specialized agencies (e.g. ILO, FAO, World Bank).

In addition, the role of old and new private actors (non-profit, non-governmental agencies; foundations; and for-profit organizations, including pharmaceutical, food and other industries) has grown considerably, including with the creation of hybrid entities such as coalitions, alliances and all sorts of more or less structured public-private partnerships, having a powerful impact on international health policy.

The defining feature of international health governance has been the primacy given to the state, although non-state actors and interests have always been present. By the late twentieth century, with the growing impacts of globalization on health determinants and outcomes, that primacy was challenged and the concept of global health governance (GHG) emerged (Dogson et al. 2002). Since then the term has been widely used by both scholars and practitioners, but with considerable variation in its definition and how it is applied, also largely due to the ongoing vagueness of the term global health that we discussed in Chapter 1. Lee and Kamradt-Scott (2014) identified three distinct uses of the term GHG: (a) globalization and health governance (i.e. "the institutional actors, arrangements and policy-making processes that govern health issues in an increasingly globalized world"); (b) global governance and health (i.e. "how global governance institutions outside the health sector have influenced the broad social determinants of health"); and (c) governance for global health (i.e. "what governance arrangements are needed to further agreed global health goals").

The first concept of GHG, possibly the most commonly used, is primarily concerned with the health-related actors that govern collective responses to such issues, and can be summarized as: the actors, regimes, interactions and policy-making processes that govern issues of transnational and global relevance in health systems and public health services.

In this context, there are multiple mechanisms (political and economic) which allow national states to address global health policies, though their detailed analysis is outside the scope of this textbook. In brief, it is evident that some countries, particularly the United States and others participating in the G7/G8, still play a predominant role in guiding global policies (obviously not only in health), while the role of emerging economies, including the so-called BRICS (Brazil, Russia, India, China and South Africa) as well as the G20 group in general, is rapidly growing. Indeed, the geopolitical weight of state actors still determines the dynamics and the limits of international, rather than global, governance, in a scenario where the formal and informal veto powers of dominant states still represent the effective limit for a concerted global action (Held and McGrew 2003). But it is equally true that the opinion or vote expressed by individual governments is always influenced, to a greater or lesser extent, by states which are "strong powers" as well as by national and transnational private interests. Indeed, there has been long-standing shift of power from intergovernmental organizations to the private sector, though a world with greater interdependence would rather require the former to play a more important role (Taylor 2002).

Over the last decade or so, there has been an increased focus on recognizing the importance of the social, economic, political and environmental determinants of health that are influenced by decisions made in other global policy-making arenas (such as those governing international trade, environment, migration) (Lee and Kamradt-Scott 2014). The need to protect and promote health in global governance processes outside the global health system led to the concept of "global governance *for* health" (Frenk and Moon 2013).

Both global health governance and global governance *for* health are basically based on two approaches: the legislation-based approach typical of trade and investment agreements (the so-called "hard law") involving economic sanctions for those who do not respect the rules; and the moral norms derived from internationally recognized human rights (so-called "soft law") characterized by the absence of rules binding partners to their commitments, as in the case of international declarations and resolutions, whose implementation relies more on domestic civil society pressure than international censure and rules (Labonté 2014).

Although the idea of global governance is understood as a collaborative process among involved actors, power relations continue to play the main role in the definition of the political agenda because certain states hold final decision-making authority. Thus, states' foreign policy priorities and practices are central to health protection and promotion in multilateral negotiations and policy-making. This has given risen over the last decade to the concept of "Global Health Diplomacy" (GHD).

Without entering into the wider debate about the definition of the term GHD, used rather vaguely to encompass almost any relationship between foreign policy and global health (McInnes and Lee 2012), two main uses can be identified. The first and more common use of GHD maintains a strong "normative" dimension focusing on how other foreign policy goals can be linked to advance health globally (e.g. adapting trade policy to positively discriminate in favor of healthy foods, or imposing financial transaction taxes to reduce the destabilizing effect of short-term capital flows and to finance health development in poorer countries). A second use is linked to the *Realpolitik* line of advancing states' interests using health as a means to enhance other foreign policy goals (e.g. using economic costs of excess disease burdens to strengthen commitments to climate change targets, or increasing health aid to reduce the risk of conflict in strategically important countries or regions) (McInnes and Lee 2012; Labonté 2014). Labonté (2014) is right in saying that the first use "is aligned more closely with global health" as it goes beyond the interests of a single country; however, diplomacy – and consequently GHD – still refers to governments' foreign policy and the "method of influencing the decisions and behavior of foreign governments and people through dialogue, negotiation, and other measures short of war or violence" (Encyclopaedia Britannica 2018). Thus, we prefer to use the term "global governance" when referring to the complex interactions that involve both states and non-state actors. As countries remain the final decision-makers, the relationship between health and countries' foreign policy is critical to global health, which represents a "pressing foreign policy issue of our time" (Oslo Ministerial Declaration 2007), as expressed in the Oslo Declaration signed by the Ministers of foreign affairs of Brazil, France, Indonesia, Norway, Senegal, South Africa and Thailand. For the same reason, international institutions represent the main global governance forum, as we will see in the following chapters.

5.3 Global health governance map

In 2002, Dodgson, Lee and Drager drew up a first map of global health governance, trying to position actors according to their influence in terms of authority and leadership. In their map the "WHO and the World Bank are shown as central because they represent the main sources of health expertise and development financing respectively" (Dodgson *et al.* 2002).

Along with these two institutions, in the center of the map they placed the United States, arguably the single most influential governmental actor. Curiously, although recognizing that some of the other numerous actors such as the Bill & Melinda Gates Foundation "have become highly prominent in recent years" (Dodgson *et al.* 2002), Dodgson and colleagues did not include those emerging organizations on their map.

After one and a half decades the scenario is quite different. The emergence of new actors with significant political and economic power has occurred as a result of an unresolved structural weakness of the WHO still struggling to define its role in the new context. The WHO's reduced credibility and sustainability have arguably contributed to member states themselves, in particular the largest donors, showing inconsistency between their global health and development cooperation policies. For the latter, they declare their commitment to aid effectiveness principles requiring the reduction of existing aid fragmentation; meanwhile they undermine those principles by promoting and supporting a plethora of new players which tend to undermine the credibility and sustainability of the WHO, of whom the same donors request greater efficiency. Member states may have one set of priorities expressed in the WHO's own governing forums, while their funding to the WHO and other institutions may reflect a different set of priorities (Liden 2014).

Today Dodgson and his coauthors' map (2002) needs to be redrawn with a center extremely crowded with old and new actors, and with an attempt to render graphically the increased and often interlinked external influences on traditional actors (Missoni 2017) (Figure 5.1).

The subjects that will be described in some detail in the following chapters do not all participate directly in formal governance processes; however, with different weight and responsibility they all contribute to determining the direction of these processes. Although a number of them claim significant institutional/organizational innovation, a rethinking of the traditional bureaucratic model of post-war intergovernmental organizations is still lacking, and institutions still seem to be rather disconnected from the reality of a globalized world and the need for wider and more equitable representation and involvement:

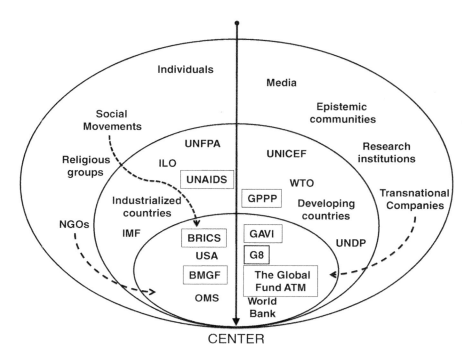

Figure 5.1 Global health governance. Arrows show increased centrality of actors. Actors in boxes were not present in the original map.
Source: Missoni 2017; adapted from Dodgson *et al.* 2002.

Globalization has created new collective health needs which cross old spatial, temporal and cognitive boundaries. In response, we need GHG institutions which represent the many, not the few; are sufficiently nimble to act effectively in a fast-paced world; and capable of bringing together the best ideas and boundary spanning knowledge available.

(Lee 2017)

References

Brown, T.M., Cueto, M., Fee, E., 2006. The World Health Organization and the transition from 'international' to 'global' public health. *American Journal of Public Health*, 96(1), 62–72.
Dodgson, R., Lee, K., Drager N., 2002. *Global Health Governance. A conceptual review*, Discussion Paper n. 1, Centre on Global Change & Health, London School of Hygiene & Tropical Medicine – Dept of Health & Development, World Health Organization.
Encyclopaedia Britannica, 2018. Available from: www.britannica.com/topic/diplomacy.
Frenk, J., Moon, S., 2013. Governance challenges in global health. *New England Journal of Medicine*, 368(10), 936–42
Held, D., McGrew, A., 2003. *Globalismo e antiglobalismo*. Bologna: il Mulino.
Labonté, R., 2014. Health in all (foreign) policy: challenges in achieving coherence. *Health Promotion International*, 29(Suppl. 1), i48–i58.

Lee, K., 2017. Business as usual: a lack of institutional innovation in global health governance. Comment on "Global health governance challenges 2016 – are we ready?" *International Journal of Health Policy Management*, 6(3), 165–168.

Lee, K., Kamradt-Scott, A., 2014. The multiple meanings of global health governance: a call for conceptual clarity. *Globalization and Health*, 10, 28. doi.org/10.1186/1744-8603-10-28.

Lidén, J., 2014. The World Health Organization and global health governance: post-1990. *Public Health*, 128(2),141–47. doi:10.1016/j.puhe.2013.08.008.

McInnes, C., Lee, K., 2012. *Global Health and International Relations*. Cambridge: Polity Press.

Missoni, E., 2017. Chapter 21 – Global health. In Klassen, T.R., Cepiku, D., Lah, T.J. (Eds.), *Handbook of Global Public Policy and Administration*. Abingdon: Routledge, 229–240

Missoni, E., Alesani, D., 2014. *Management of International Institutions and NGOs. Framework, practices and challenges*. Abingdon: Routledge

Oslo Ministerial Declaration, 2007. Global health: a pressing foreign policy issue of our time. Ministers of Foreign Affairs of Brazil, France, Indonesia, Norway, Senegal, South Africa, and Thailand. *The Lancet*, 369(9570), 1373–1378.

Taylor, A.L., 2002. Global governance, international health law and WHO: looking towards the future. *Bulletin of the World Health Organization*, 80(12), 975–980.

Unless otherwise indicated, all websites were accessed on 9 August 2018.

6 International institutions
The United Nations system

6.1 Introduction

In the wider context of international organizations, we define international institutions (IIs) as organizations based on a formal instrument of agreement between three or more governments of national states (i.e. "multilateral" organizations) and that possess a permanent secretariat. Being established with an international formal agreement among nation states, IIs have autonomous international legal personality, which confers on them legitimacy and provides them with an international mandate to operate. Membership may include non-state actors, but these cannot exercise a veto power on collective decisions. IIs have their own budget, with no single member state or other organization in control of more than 50% of the funding (Missoni and Alesani 2014).

Treaties and agreements among nation states have existed for centuries; however, the kind of formal institutions to which we are referring here were established in the aftermath of the Napoleonic Wars in the nineteenth century. In the second part of the twentieth century the complexity and the number of IIs grew considerably to over 250 organizations, including the UN system, several regional organizations, and "supranational" institutions to whom member states delegate vast areas of sovereignty, as is the case of the European Union (Missoni and Alesani 2014).

Many IIs play a role in global health governance and/or in other domains of international public policy with an impact on health. In this chapter we will limit our attention to the organizations in the United Nations system (including the UN organization itself, with its organs, subsidiary organs, Funds and Programs, the Specialized Agencies and the related organizations) with special focus on those with a significant role in global health.

6.2 The United Nations Organization

6.2.1 *The origins*

Toward the end of World War II, the Allied forces promoted the establishment of an international organization with a universal vocation tasked with a collective security system to prevent new armed conflicts. The League of Nations, whose founding agreement was signed in 1919 and which lacked the support of the most powerful countries to deal with the crises between the two wars, had remained largely inactive since the beginning of World War II. The League was formally dissolved on 18 April 1946, and part of its assets and functions were transferred to the newly established United Nations Organization (UNO).

Since 1941, F.D. Roosevelt and W. Churchill, in agreeing on the Atlantic Charter, had included some of the principles that would lead to the reorganization of world assets at the end of the conflict; among them the rejection of war as a mean of international dispute settlement, and the hypothesis of a permanent system of collective security. Still during the conflict, 26 countries at war adopted the United Nations denomination (Washington Declaration of 1942), and after several diplomatic steps, a permanent organization was established on 25 April 1945 in San Francisco at the United Nations International Conference, with the participation of the countries which by 1 January 1945 had declared war on Germany and Japan. The Conference ended on 26 June 1945, with the approval of the United Nations Charter (UN 1945), which entered into force on 24 October 1945, after the end of the conflict. The United Nations Organization, which today has 193 Member States, was born.

Since the establishment of the organization in 1946 there have been many proposals, studies and discussions around the question of reform. Today the UN faces a broad reform agenda with the objective of strengthening the UN's contribution to the 2030 agenda for sustainable development. On the basis of a mandate received from the General Assembly (UN 2018) the current UN Secretary-General Guterrez proposed a wide range of measures for enhancing the capacity of the system to tackle conflict and sustain peace and for improving the UN's accountability and internal management and ability to deliver. The emphasis is on increasing collaboration within and among the three UN pillars (development, human rights, peace and security), also through strengthening integrated planning and risk management and simplifying procedures. The agenda also includes a realignment of UN bodies with the 2030 agenda for reducing overlap and enhancing synergy and coherence.

6.2.2 Structure and functions

The mission and the activity of the United Nations are guided by the purposes and principles contained in its founding charter. The UN Charter – with the binding value of an international treaty – includes among the Organization's purposes the maintenance of international peace and security; the development of friendly relations among nations based on respect for the principle of equal rights and self-determination of peoples; the achievement of international cooperation in solving international problems of an economic, social, cultural or humanitarian character, and in promoting and encouraging respect for human rights and for fundamental freedoms for all without distinction as to race, sex, language or religion; and to be a center for harmonizing the actions of nations in the attainment of these common ends.

The main organs of the UN are the General Assembly, the Security Council, the Economic and Social Council, the Trusteeship Council, the International Court of Justice and the UN Secretariat.

The United Nations General Assembly (UNGA) is the main deliberative, policy-making and representative organ of the UN. All 193 Member States of the UN are represented in the UNGA, each with a right to one vote, making it the only UN body with universal representation. The UNGA is not of a permanent nature; rather it is convened in ordinary or special sessions, the latter being convened by the Secretary-General, who proceeds at the request of the Security Council or of the majority of the Member States.

Each year, in September, the full UN membership meets in New York for the annual UNGA session. Decisions on important questions, such as those on peace and security, admission of new members and budgetary matters, require a two-thirds majority of the UNGA. Decisions on other questions are by simple majority. Decisions are expressed in the form of recommendations to the Member States or to the Security Council. The UNGA can only intervene at the request of the Council itself. Each year the UNGA elects a President to serve for a one-year term of office. Health is featured prominently in UNGA's discussions, and resolutions adopted have wide-reaching implications for health. In the past, world leaders have gathered at high-level meetings and special sessions to take action on communicable diseases, AIDS and Ebola. Other health issues have also been discussed (such as malaria, maternal health, universal health coverage, noncommunicable diseases, road traffic accidents and autism). Starting in 2008, Global Health and Foreign Policy have been regular items on the UNGA agenda. In September 2011, the United Nations General Assembly held a high-level meeting on the prevention and control of noncommunicable diseases (NCDs). A follow-up high-level meeting was held in 2014, and the next comprehensive review on progress made towards the prevention and control of NCDs was held in September 2018 (WHO 2017; UN 2018a). Malaria is also a regular item on the agenda of the UNGA and every year a resolution is adopted on the progress on its control in developing countries.

The Security Council (SC) has primary responsibility for the maintenance of international peace and security. It has 15 members, 10 non-permanent members elected every two years by the UNGA on a geographical basis, and five permanent members (China, France, United Kingdom, Russia and the United States of America). Each member has one vote. However, decisions on substantive matters require nine votes, including the concurrent votes of all five permanent members.[1] All Member States are obligated to comply with the Council's decisions. The SC takes the lead in determining the existence of a threat to peace. It calls upon the parties to a dispute to settle it by peaceful means and recommends methods of adjustment or terms of settlement. In some cases, the SC can resort to imposing sanctions or even authorize the use of force to maintain or restore international peace and security. The SC has a presidency, which rotates monthly. On three occasion the SC passed a resolution concerning health issues: twice on the HIV/AIDS epidemic in 2000 (UN 2000) and in 2011 (UN 2011), and more recently on occasion of the Ebola epidemic in 2014 (UN 2014). On these and other health-related issues the SC also issued other documents such as presidential statements, council letters and press releases.[2]

The Economic and Social Council (ECOSOC) is the principal body for coordination, policy review, policy dialogue and recommendations on economic, social and environmental issues, as well as implementation of internationally agreed development goals. It serves as the central mechanism for activities of the UN system and its specialized agencies in the economic, social and environmental fields, supervising subsidiary and expert bodies. It has 54 members, elected by the UNGA for three-year overlapping terms. Among other health issues, following the Political Declaration adopted by the above-mentioned High-Level Meeting on NCDs in 2011, the ECOSOC called for the establishment of the Task Force on the Prevention and Control of Noncommunicable Diseases by expanding the mandate of the existing Ad hoc Inter-Agency Task Force on Tobacco Control. The Task Force was established by the UN Secretary-General in June 2013 and placed under the WHO's leadership. Its terms of reference were adopted by ECOSOC in July 2014.

86 *Global governance and health*

The International Court of Justice (ICJ) is the principal judicial organ of the United Nations. Its headquarters are in the Hague (Netherlands). The Court's role is to settle, in accordance with international law, legal disputes submitted to it by states and to give advisory opinions on legal questions referred to it by authorized United Nations organs and specialized agencies. The World Health Organization (WHO) has agreed to furnish any information which may be requested by the International Court of Justice (Article 34 of the Statute of the Court) and may request advisory opinions of the International Court of Justice on legal questions arising within the scope of its competence (WHO 2014). Among the few health-related issues brought to the attention of the ICJ there was the WHO's request for an opinion of the ICJ about the use of nuclear weapons and international law.[3]

The Trusteeship Council, which has not operated since 1994,[4] was established to provide international supervision to the processes toward the independence of Trust Territories that had been placed under the administration of seven Member States.

The Secretariat constitutes the administrative apparatus of the United Nations; it carries out the day-to-day work of the UN as mandated by the UNGA and the organization's other principal organs. The Secretary-General is the chief administrative officer of the organization and is appointed by the UNGA on the recommendation of the SC for a five-year, renewable term. The Secretary and staff of the Secretariat do not represent any state, including their country of origin, and act exclusively on an individual basis. The Secretariat is organized along departmental lines, with each department or office having a distinct area of action and responsibility. Among those more relevant to global health there are the Department of Economic and Social Affairs (UNDESA) and a number of coordination mechanisms such as the Chief Executive Board for Coordination (CEB) and the Office for the Coordination of Humanitarian Affairs (OCHA).

UNDESA is in charge of the development pillar of the UN Secretariat and is the prime instrument for strengthening the coordination role of UN inter-governmental bodies on social, economic and related matters. UNDESA's work program can be categorized into three areas: norm-setting, data and analysis, and capacity-building. UNDESA also hosts the secretariat for the High-level Political Forum on Sustainable Development (HLPF) for the follow-up and review of the 2030 Agenda for Sustainable Development. It provides support to ECOSOC, and cares for the relations with relevant stakeholders in and outside the UN system, including with the corporate sector and civil society.

Due to its complexity the UN system also needs solid organizational governance and management coordination. The CEB brings together the executive heads of 31 specialized organizations to "deliver as one" at the global, regional and country levels. Three "pillars" support it: The High-Level Committee on Programs (HLCP), the High-Level Committee on Management (HLCM) and the United Nations Development Group (UNDG). While HLCP and HLCM work mostly at headquarters and policy level, promoting system-wide coordination of core programs and administrative regulations and procedures, UNDG is mainly responsible for coordinating operational activities at the country level.

Coordination of humanitarian assistance is ensured through OCHA, which brings together multiple actors also from outside the UN system, to ensure a coherent response to emergencies. OCHA also serves as the secretariat for critical inter-agency coordination mechanisms. The cluster approach was introduced in 2005 to ensure that there is predictable leadership and accountability in all main sectors or areas of humanitarian response, and to strengthen system-wide preparedness and technical capacity to respond to humanitarian emergencies. WHO and the World Food Program (WFP), for relevant logistics, provide leadership in the health cluster. UNICEF leads the nutrition cluster (as well as education) (Missoni and Alesani 2014).

Regarding funding, modalities differ among the various agencies of the United Nations system. These can be divided in two large groups: "assessed" and "non-assessed" organizations. The former includes the United Nations Secretariat and the specialized agencies (see below), which can count on a regular budget made up by mandatory contributions by all their Member States. These are budgetary contributions "assessed" on the basis of a UN scale of ability to pay (based on GNP and population). Budgetary resources are normally complemented by voluntary "extra-budgetary funding" (EBF), which donors often earmark for specific initiatives or areas of activity of the organization.

Non-assessed organizations, which include funds and programs of the UN, are entirely funded through voluntary contributions, which organizations generally subdivide into "core" and "non-core" resources. The former are funds made available for the essential, structural functions of the beneficiary UN entity, which can administer them according to the organization's needs and priorities. In other words, core resources are non-earmarked. Instead, "non-core" resources are earmarked funds, which are often justified in terms of "value for money" from the donors' perspective but may greatly influence the organization's priorities and limit its autonomy.

> This is surely intended to stimulate management by results and competition for resources among organizations but could also result in fragmentation and pose a threat to the multilateral nature of organizations.
> (Missoni and Alesani 2014: 25)

6.2.3 Subsidiary organs and other entities

Alongside the main organs, a number of other entities have been established over the years, such as subsidiary organs, functional and regional commissions, committees, funds (e.g. UNFPA, UNICEF) and programs (e.g. UNDP, WFP), and other bodies (e.g. UNAIDS) and entities (e.g UNHCR), as well as research and training institutions. All these entities are not autonomous organizations; thus, they lack a representative organ (i.e. an Assembly); indeed, the representative function lies in the United Nations General Assembly,[5] not in their executive boards.

Although subordinated to the UN organization, funds and programs are immediately controlled by distinct intergovernmental bodies – usually called Executive Boards – and derive most of their financial resources from sources other than the UN regular budget. Thus "they are somewhat more akin to specialized agencies than to 'subsidiary organs' such as UN commissions and committees" (Missoni and Alesani 2014: 21). They are generally led by an executive director appointed by the Secretary-General of the United Nations, and report to the Executive Board on financial, administrative and program matters.

Several of these UN entities directly or indirectly include in their mandate public health issues, and often have joint programs with the WHO, and participate in the United Nations Development Group (UNDG) and other United Nations joint programs (such as UNAIDS) and in several global initiatives and public-private partnerships that we will describe later. Entities specifically devoted to humanitarian intervention, such as the WFP and the United Nations High Commissioner for Refugees (UNHCR), necessarily include health care while others such as the United Nations Population Fund (UNFPA) and the United Nations Fund for Children (UNICEF) also play a role in advocating, defining and promoting health policies.

The United Nations Population Fund (UNFPA)[6] describes itself as "the lead UN agency for delivering a world where every pregnancy is wanted, every childbirth is safe and every young person's potential is fulfilled" (UNFPA 2017). As part of its wider mandate UNFPA addresses population and development issues, with an emphasis on reproductive health and gender equality, within the specific context of the Program of Action of the International Conference on Population and Development (ICPD), dating back to Cairo 1994, and the findings of the 20-year review endorsed by a Special Session of the General Assembly in September 2014. UNFPA receives overall policy guidance from the UN General Assembly and ECOSOC. It reports to its governing body, the UNDP/UNFPA Executive Board, on administrative, financial and program matters. UNFPA works in close collaboration with many other development and humanitarian agencies (particularly WHO, UNICEF, UNDP and UNAIDS) in the field.

The United Nations Children's Fund (UNICEF) was established by the UN General Assembly on 11 December 1946 as an Emergency Fund to assist children in European countries in the post-war period. In 1953 UNICEF became permanent, with a mandate aimed at childhood in Africa, Asia and Latin America, and is now orienting its action on the basis of the principles enshrined in the 1989 UN Convention on the Rights of the Child, the first legally binding international convention to affirm human rights for all children. UNICEF's tasks concern the protection of children and their rights; the assistance to contribute to meet their basic needs and broaden their opportunities to reach their full potential; the mobilization of political will and resources to help states to ensure due priority to children and to strengthen their capacity to do so; the response to emergencies to alleviate the suffering of affected children and their care-taker; the promotion of equal rights for women and girls and the support for their full participation in the development of their communities; the commitment to the achievement of development goals, peace and social progress recognized by the United Nations Charter. Improving the health of the world's children is a core UNICEF objective. Historically it significantly contributed to progress in immunization, nutrition, control of diarrhea, pneumonia and malaria, improving access to quality care for newborns and pregnant women, child health in emergency settings, and strengthening health systems to better serve the needs of women and children.

6.2.4 The specialized institutions

As we have mentioned in the introduction to this chapter, the UN system includes a number of specialized agencies (or institutions), such as the World Health Organization (WHO), the International Labor Organization (ILO) and the World Bank Group. These are autonomous organizations established through a separate international agreement and founding charter or constitution, signed and ratified by all their Member States, thus subject solely to their own rules and procedures, without the United Nations organization being able to decide in any way about their existence and operations.

Thus, specialized agencies have their own legal personality, membership, organs, rules and financial resources. Specialized agencies are brought into relationship with the UN through bilateral agreements, which normally include aspects concerning the coordination of their respective programs and activities. The General Assembly of the United Nations can make observations on the specialized agency's budget but cannot intervene on it.

In the following sections specialized agencies which are more relevant or influential in global health (mainly the World Health Organization and the World Bank) will be analyzed more closely. However, one must not underestimate the role of other UN specialized agencies whose mandate and activity maintain important links to populations' health and its determinants, such as food policy and nutrition in the case of the Food and Agriculture Organization (FAO), or social protection policies, including health coverage, and the protection of human rights at work, in the case of the International Labor Organization (ILO).

6.3 The World Health Organization

6.3.1 The origins

The World Health Organization (WHO) is an international institution, based on the principle of universality, established as a specialized agency of the United Nations, with 194 Member States. WHO's Headquarters are in Geneva.

WHO origins date back to April 1945 when during the Conference to set up the United Nations representatives of Brazil and China proposed establishing an international health organization, and to convene a conference to frame its constitution. One year later, on 22 July 1946, the International Health Conference, held in New York City, adopted the Constitution of the World Health Organization, signed by representatives of 61 countries. The Constitution came into force on 7 April 1948,[7] with the ratification by the 26th signing government. The first Director-General of the WHO was George Brock Chisholm, who held the post from the Organization's origin in 1948 until 1953, when he was replaced by the Brazilian Marcolino Candau.

While WHO was established in the aftermath of World War II, the predecessors of the organization have long-seeded roots. The first organization mandated to monitor health status internationally was established in 1907: the Bureau International d'Hygiène Publique in Paris collected epidemiological data from its member states. A similar agency was founded in 1902, the Pan American Sanitary Bureau, which carried out many of the same functions for the Americas. Finally, the most direct predecessor of the modern day WHO is the League of Nations Health Organization, which was established by the League of Nations.

6.3.2 Functions and structure

WHO's overall goal as defined in Article 1 of its Constitution is "the attainment by all peoples of the highest possible level of health" with a broad definition of health as "a state of complete physical, mental and social well-being and not merely the absence of disease of infirmity". Health is recognized as "one of the fundamental rights of every human being" and governments are responsible for the health of their peoples (WHO 2014).

While the Constitution lists 22 functions of the WHO, these can be divided into six fundamental areas:

1. Coordination and Advocacy, including: to establish and maintain effective collaboration with the United Nations, specialized agencies, governmental health administrations, professional groups and such other organizations as may be deemed appropriate; to promote cooperation among scientific and professional groups; to propose conventions, agreements and regulations, and make recommendations with respect to international health matters.
2. Support to Countries, including: to assist Governments, upon request, in strengthening health services; to furnish appropriate technical assistance and, in emergencies, necessary aid upon the request or acceptance of Governments; to provide or assist in providing, upon the request of the United Nations, health services and facilities to special groups.
3. Promotion of Global Health, including: to advance work to eradicate diseases; to promote the improvement of nutrition, housing, sanitation, recreation, economic or working conditions and environmental hygiene; to promote the prevention of accidental injuries; to promote maternal and child health and welfare, and to foster activities in the field of mental health.
4. Global Information, including: to establish and maintain administrative and technical services, including epidemiological and statistical services; to provide information, counsel and assistance, and to assist in informing public opinion.
5. Research and Training, including: to promote and conduct research, and to promote improved standards of teaching and training; to study and report on administrative and social techniques affecting public health and medical care from preventive and curative points of view, including hospital services and social security.
6. Setting Standards, including: to establish and revise international nomenclature of diseases; to standardize diagnostic procedures; to develop and promote international standards with respect to food, biological, pharmaceutical and other similar products.

When deemed necessary, WHO can implement these functions in cooperation with other specialized agencies.

The World Health Assembly (WHA) is the supreme normative and decision-making body for the WHO. The WHA meets annually in May in Geneva, Switzerland, and is attended by delegations from all 194 Member States. Delegations from Member States consist of not more than three delegates, who are often the most qualified in their technical competence in the field of health and, preferably, represent their national health administration. Territories or groups of territories that are not responsible for the conduct of their international relations may be admitted as Associate Members by the Health Assembly.[8]

In addition to these official delegates, representatives from other relevant international organizations and NGOs are invited to the WHA as observers, can contribute with their own statements, but have no voting power. The WHA is assisted by a General Committee and two Main Committees (Committee A – to deal predominantly with program and budget matters; Committee B – to deal predominantly with administrative, financial and legal matters). In addition to these two main committees, the Health Assembly may establish such other committees as it may consider necessary. The WHA determines the overall policies and direction of the organization, including the supervision of the financial policies and review/approval of the proposed program budgets. The WHA is also responsible for determining each Member States' mandatory contribution. The WHA works in close conjunction with the Executive Board, which it advises on actions requiring further study, investigation or report. The WHA appoints the Director-General, "on the nomination of the Board on such terms as the Health Assembly may determine". Current rules of procedure allow the Board to nominate up to three candidates (WHO 2014).

The WHA exercises its authority through the adoption of three instruments: recommendations, conventions or agreements, and regulations.

Recommendations are addressed to the Member States and are adopted by simple majority voting. Although not binding, the recommendation is a legal act with moral force and political value. In practice, with the exceptions mentioned below, to date the WHO normative activity has been exclusively based on this type of resolution. Even in the case of the adoption of "Codes", such as the International Code of Marketing of Breast-milk Substitutes, the instrument used was a non-binding recommendation.

Art. 19 of the WHO Constitution provides the WHA with the authority to adopt conventions or agreements with respect to any matter within the competence of the organization. In order to be adopted, conventions or agreements require a majority of two-thirds and come into binding force for each Member after ratification in accordance with their constitutional processes. The only example of such a Convention in WHO's history is the Framework Convention on Tobacco Control (FCTC) (FCTC 2003).

Finally, the WHA has the authority to adopt regulations concerning issues listed in article 21 of the WHO Constitution, such as sanitary and quarantine requirements, nomenclatures with respect to diseases, causes of death and public health practices, and standards for international use, including with respect to the safety, purity and potency of biomedical products commercialized internationally, and their advertising and labeling. Such regulations may be adopted by a simple majority and shall enter into force for all Member States following the announcement by the Assembly, unless a Member State notifies its rejection or its willingness to make reservations. The only example of the use of this type of instrument is the International Health Regulations (IHR 2008).

BOX 6.1 The International Health Regulations

The International Health Regulations (IHR 2005) are an international binding agreement which aim to prevent, protect against, control and respond to the international spread of disease while avoiding unnecessary interference with international traffic and trade. The IHR (2005) are also designed to reduce the risk of disease spread at international airports, ports and ground crossings. They entered into force on 15 June 2007 and are binding on the 194 WHO Member States.

A first set of International Sanitary Regulations adopted by the WHA in 1951 was replaced by and renamed the International Health Regulations in 1969. The 1969 Regulations were subject to minor modifications in 1973 and 1981. The 1969 IHR were primarily intended to monitor and control six serious infectious diseases: cholera, plague, yellow fever, smallpox, relapsing fever and typhus. Under the IHR (1969), only cholera, plague and yellow fever remain notifiable, requiring states to notify WHO if and when these diseases occur on their territory.

With their narrow scope (just three diseases), their dependence on official country notification, and their lack of a formal internationally coordinated mechanism to

92   Global governance and health

> contain international disease spread, the IHR 1969 were not equipped to address the growing and varied public health risks that resulted from increased travel and trade in the last quarter of the twentieth century. This led to their revision.
>
> In May 2001, the World Health Assembly adopted resolution WHA 54.14, Global health security: epidemic alert and response, in which WHO was called upon to support its Member States in strengthening their capacity to detect and respond rapidly to communicable disease threats and emergencies.
>
> In May 2003, the WHA established an intergovernmental working group (IGWG) open to all Member States to review and recommend a draft revision of the International Health Regulations. The final text was adopted by the WHA at its 58th meeting in 2005.
>
> Under article 21 of the WHO Constitution, all WHO Member States were automatically bound by the new IHR because they did not affirmatively opt out within a limited time period and only a very small number made reservations. According to the procedures established in the IHR (2005), reservations are evaluated by other WHO Member States within a defined time period. Because one-third of the other states did not object to the reservation(s), the Regulations entered into force on 15 June 2007 for the states that filed them subject to the reservation(s).
>
> The IHR (2005) cover existing, new and re-emerging diseases, including emergencies caused by non-infectious disease agents. Through a new legal framework, the IHR (2005) ensure a rapid gathering of information, a common understanding of what may constitute a Public Health Emergency of International Concern (PHEIC) and the availability of international assistance to countries. According to the IHR (2005) a PHEIC refers to an extraordinary public health event which is determined, under specific procedures:
>
> (a) to constitute a public health risk to other States through the international spread of disease; and (b) to potentially require a coordinated international response.
>
> Timely and transparent notification of events combined with a collaborative assessment of the risks by the concerned State and WHO, along with effective risk communication, will reduce the potential for international disease spread and the likelihood of unilateral imposition of trade or travel restrictions by other countries. Under these rules, WHO, as a neutral authority, with critical technical expertise and resources and an extensive communications network, can assess information, recommend actions and facilitate or help coordinate technical assistance, when needed, that is tailored to events as they unfold.
>
> Source: WHO, Frequently asked questions about the International Health Regulations (2005). Available from: www.who.int/ihr/about/faq/en/.

Except for the aforementioned cases, as well as in the case of the modification of the Constitution, which requires a two-thirds majority, the Assembly shall take its decisions by a simple majority and each Member shall be entitled to one vote. However, as in most cases in the United Nations Organization, most WHA decisions are not subject to voting but are agreed by consensus.

Though the WHA has formal decision-making power, priority-setting and other decisions may be strongly influenced through informal processes. Among others, richer

Member States may exert their influence through earmarked voluntary contributions. The financial and technical capacity of Member States also determines their ability to participate equally and fully in the decision-making process.

The Executive Board (EB) is composed of 34 members, technically qualified individuals in the field of health, of which at least three are elected by the regional committees of the WHO. Members are elected for three-year terms and each year one-third of EB members change and are replaced by a newly elected group. The Executive Board meets twice a year, in January and May, and oversees the implementation of decisions and resolutions made by the WHA. Member States retain the power to respond to the proposals and actions of the EB (within one year) in the form of a report to the WHA. More specifically, the Executive Board prepares the agenda for the WHA, drafts the general Plan of Work (PoW), advises the WHA on proper responses and facilitates these actions, and nominates the Director-General. Though the WHA is the formal decision-making body, in necessary cases and emergency situations the EB may proceed autonomously, adopting the necessary measures, while still respecting both the functions and financial resources of the WHO.

The Secretariat is the administrative and technical organ of the WHO responsible for implementation of the policies. The Director-General, who is the chief technical and administrative officer of the Organization and is subject to the authority of the Executive Board, leads the secretariat. The current Director-General is Dr. Tedros Adhanom Ghebreyesus. He was appointed in May 2017, and succeeded Dr. Margareth Chan.

The secretariat of the WHO is composed of more than 7000 people working at the Headquarters in Geneva and in 150 WHO offices in countries, territories and areas, six regional offices, and the Global Service Center in Malaysia.

In addition to the secretariat, the WHO works directly with many collaborating centers; these are accredited national centers of excellence that may provide technical and scientific guidance.

Furthermore, the WHO is divided into six regions: Africa (AFRO), Americas (AMRO/PAHO), The Eastern Mediterranean (EMRO), Europe (EURO), Western Pacific (WPRO) and Southeast Asia (SEARO). In each region Member States and associated members participate in the Regional Committee, which is in charge of electing the Regional Director, who leads the regional office, with a high degree of independence, autonomy and decision-making power. It is interesting to note that regional membership may not always coincide with geographical location. Israel, for example, is a member of the EURO group due to the inability to cooperate effectively with the Arab States of the EMRO.

The American Region actually represents an anomaly in the system in that the Pan American Health Organization (PAHO) pre-dates the WHO. The International Sanitary Bureau (predecessor of the current PAHO) was established in Washington DC on 2–4 December 1902. The Pan American Sanitary Bureau (PASB) is the secretariat of the PAHO and simultaneously serves as the Regional Office for the Americas of the World Health Organization.[9]

As any specialized agency of the UN, the WHO has its own budget. The regular budget of the Organization is financed through Member States' assessed contributions. In addition, the Organization may receive extra-budgetary funds through additional voluntary contributions from Member States as well as from other international organizations, national public bodies, non-governmental organizations, foundations and other private entities.

provided that the conditions attached to such gifts or bequests are acceptable to the Health Assembly or the Board and are consistent with the objective and policies of the Organization.

(WHO 2014)

A small number of high-income countries provide most of the WHO's regular budget, or core funding. In addition, within its regulations, the WHO attempts to maintain autonomy by enforcing the rule that no single country can contribute more than one-third of the total Regular Budget Funding (RBF): even with this provision, the US remains the largest single source, providing 22%[10] of the RBFs (Lee 2009). Since the freezing of RBFs in the 1980s (see Chapter 5), WHO has seen an increase in the proportion of EBFs largely earmarked by donors for special purposes. Financial aspects have been under review as part of an extensive reform of WHO over the last years and will be discussed later in this chapter.

6.3.3 The evolution of WHO's role as the directing and coordinating authority in global health

In 1948, the Member States of the newly formed United Nations gathered together to create the World Health Organization, with the mandate to "act as the directing and coordinating authority on international health work" toward the objective of "the attainment by all peoples of the highest possible level of health" (WHO 2014).

Naming the new organization as the World Health Organization also raised sights to a worldwide "global" health perspective (Brown *et al.* 2006). The evolution of global health policies (see Chapter 5) is largely coincident with that of WHO's role in the global scenery, which in turn was strongly influenced by the personality and leadership of its Directors General.

The first period was one of establishment and consolidation of the new organization under the directorship of Brock Crisholm (1948–1953) and Marcolino Gomez Candau (1953–1973). As mentioned, until 1957 when the Soviet Union returned to the UN and WHO, WHO and the world's health policies were strongly influenced by the politics of the Cold War (Lee 2009) and action largely focused on the control of major infectious diseases. The first adoption of the International Sanitary Regulations (1951) according to article 21 of the Constitution belong to that period.[11]

Under the charismatic leadership of Director-General Hafdan Mahler (1973–1988) the WHA adopted the goal of "Health for all by the year 2000" and with the Alma-Ata Declaration (1978) Primary Health Care (PHC) became the focus of global health strategies toward that objective. In the same period the WHA adopted the International Code of Marketing of Breast-milk Substitutes, launched the "Essential Drug Program" and convened the first International Health Promotion Conference, which concluded with the Ottawa Declaration (WHO 1986). With this broader developmental focus came new dangers. WHO had to face competing and powerful interest groups and Mahler's leadership for change in policy direction also led WHO into much greater conflict than before (Walt 1994). UNICEF's sudden shift toward a selective PHC approach with the sponsorship of the World Bank, USAID and the Rockefeller Foundation, described as "a bowing to pressure from the US government which dismissed Health for All and PHC as too political" (Lee 2009:81), led to growing tensions between WHO and UNICEF. The main reaction to WHO initiatives was the freezing of WHO's regular budget and the decision of the United States to withhold their contribution to WHO's regular budget. The financial challenge that WHO had to face gave a start to a significant change in the way global health priorities were defined.

Since the middle of the 1950s EBF had increased in support of disease control and eradication programs. However, the most significant growth of EBF occurred from the 1970s onward, with a crucial shift from predominant reliance on the regular budget – drawn from Member States' assessed contributions – to greatly increased dependence on EBF. The WHA had no say over the use of EBF, which were pledged by "Donors" according to their own priorities, soon giving rise to a number of vertical programs, with a variable degree of independence from WHO's institutional decision-making structure. In 1970, EBF accounted for 20% of total WHO expenditure, by the beginning of the 1990s extra-budgetary funds already represented 54% of WHO's total budget (Brown et al. 2006), and that percentage would progressively grow over the years to reach 79% in 2007 (WHO 2008), becoming the most visible obstacle to WHO autonomy.

Mahler's tenure was followed by a "dark period" (Missoni 2006) under the mandate of the Japanese Hiroshi Nakajima (1988–1998). A "poor communicator, autocratic in style, and prone to inappropriate patronage appointments" (Lee 2009: 100), Nakajima failed to come up with convincing responses to the challenges posed to world health and to WHO during this period, and he alienated WHO staff and partners through his management style and high-profile disagreements (Global Health Watch 2005). His re-election in 1993 was highly controversial, with accusations of corruption and reports of economic threats to countries that would not support the Japanese candidate (Lee 2009). The loss of leadership of WHO coincided with the advent of "hard-nosed neoliberalism that had come to permeate many international organizations, including the World Bank and the IMF, along with many bilateral aid agencies" (Lee 2009: 82). The increasing influence of other actors in global health, especially the World Bank, and the emerging – during the late 1990s – of global public-private partnerships as a new approach to improve the delivery of worldwide vertical initiatives for a number of health problems, progressively undermined WHO authority. WHO became over-centralized at headquarters and regions, top-heavy, poorly managed and bureaucratic, and its image also reached a very low level because of suspicions of corruption among its staff (Smith 1995).

> The key voice that might have spoken out against this rising tide of neoliberal economism, the WHO, was hampered by its own internal problems, notably weakened leadership with the departure of Mahler.
>
> (Lee 2009: 84)

If donors were unduly influencing the WHO's policy agenda through earmarking of EBF, that influence was probably made possible because of the WHO's own lack of strategic vision. By the end of the 1990s, the reform of the organization was high on the agenda. Thus, the election as Director-General of Gro Harlem Brundtland, a former Norwegian prime minister with a prominent international career, was welcomed with hopes for WHO's renewal (Lee 2009) and marks the beginning of a third period, one of reform.

Brundtland needed to reaffirm WHO's role as a directing authority in global health, but also to reorganize the organization internally.

From the moment of her appointment, Brundtland defined four strategic directions for WHO: reducing the burden of disease, reducing risks to health, creating sustainable health systems, and developing an enabling policy in the health sector (Brundtland 1998).

During her mandate WHO brought back focus on health systems, starting with focusing its annual report on the issue (WHO 2000), which had the merit of also measuring systems' performance through equity and health impact lenses, but was also criticized especially from a methodological point of view (Richardson *et al.* 2001; Braveman *et al.* 2000; Williams 2001). The intersectoral focus was reinforced through the "Commission on Macroeconomics and Health", which added evidence to the direct relation between economy and health and how investment in the latter may induce economic development (WHO 2001). Notwithstanding that wider outlook, in practice Brundtland openly supported "vertical" initiatives to face a variety of specific diseases and health issues and their implementation through global public-private partnerships (GPPPs). The promotion within WHO of partnerships and other interactions with the corporate sector also represented an important shift in organizational policy (Deacon *et al.* 2003). Considering the difference between the objectives of WHO and those of corporate partners, and the increased dependence of WHO on private funds, Ford and Piedagnél (2003) anticipated that those interactions could potentially further undermine WHO independence.

One could imagine that WHO was looking for alternative, pragmatic ways to regain its position and get needed resources. Brundtland's head of cabinet, David Nabarro, reportedly declared:

> We certainly need private financing. For the past decade governments' financial contributions have dwindled. The main sources of funding are the private sector and the financial markets. And since the American economy is the world's richest, we must make the WHO attractive to the United States and the financial markets.
> (Motchane 2002)

But that policy of submitting the WHO to the dictates of global liberalization turned out to be ideological, not practical: WHO did not establish interactions it would coordinate; rather, it offered unconditional support to partnerships that would reduce WHO's role to one of a purely technical advisory capacity for those new international entities.

However, one of the undoubted achievements of Brundtland's tenure went in the opposite direction with the launch of the WHO Framework Convention on Tobacco Control (FCTC) in 2003, which entered into effect as international law in 2005 (see Box 6.2).

On the internal front, Brundtland's program of reform started at Geneva Headquarters aiming at a flatter structure, better communication and more transparency. A multitude of Programs were reorganized in nine "clusters", each led by an executive director, together forming the Director-General's "cabinet". Brundlandt's move to bring in prominent professionals perceived to be somehow linked to the World Bank was considered highly controversial. Her attempt to introduce corporate culture in the organization (fixed-term appointments, performance-monitoring and results-based management) had to face the internal progressive loss of enthusiasm and diffuse fear of job insecurity "in large part a reflection of the increase of EBFs received for short-term projects" (Lee 2009:106).

At the end of her mandate, "overstaffing in some divisions co-existed with understaffing in others; individuals with debatable competence maintained high-ranking positions; and hundreds of skilled employees were trapped in short-term contracts" (Benkimoun 2006).

Funding constraints remained a fundamental problem, and although negotiating with donors could limit earmarking to the cluster level, this led to competition among clusters to attract available resources. When Brundtland announced that she would not run for a second term, reforms were far away from being completed, and among other issues the complex relationship between headquarters and WHO Regions had not even been considered. Regions were reportedly inefficient and bureaucratic, duplicating expertise available at the headquarters in Geneva, and excessively bound up in regional politics (Godlee 1994).

Putting health high on the global agenda, including the achievement that health was represented in three out of eight Millennium Development Goals (MDGs), was another accomplishment that should be credited to Gro Harlem Brundtland's leadership, and there is wide consensus that her most significant legacy was the increased attention of major actors to health issues (Lee 2009).

BOX 6.2 The Framework Convention on Tobacco Control (FCTC)

The Framework Convention on Tobacco Control (FCTC) openly challenged the tobacco industry, establishing a milestone in the history of corporate accountability and public health (Global Health Watch 2005). Before the adoption of the initiative for FCTC by the World Health assembly in 1999, international tobacco corporations Philip Morris/Altria, British American Tobacco and Japan Tobacco International had already sought to weaken and bury the treaty. This was pursued by staging events to divert attention from the public health issues raised by tobacco use, attempting to reduce budgets for the scientific and policy activities carried out by WHO, putting other UN agencies against WHO, seeking to convince developing countries that WHO's tobacco control program was a "First World" agenda carried out at the expense of the developing world, distorting the results of important scientific studies on tobacco, and discrediting WHO as an institution.

Evidence was gathered by an Expert Committee established by WHO. The Committee found that the tobacco industry regarded the World Health Organization as one of their leading enemies, and that the industry had a planned strategy to "contain, neutralise, reorient" WHO's tobacco control initiatives (Zeltner *et al.* 2000). The tobacco industry considered the treaty to be an unprecedented challenge to the industry's freedom to continue doing business. Although the transnationals had developed a common industry-wide approach to resisting government legislation and regulation, they were opposed to WHO formulating an international response to an international problem. Among other things they accused WHO of "creating an additional layer of bureaucracy and regulation in a policy area where national governments are competent to act" (Saloojee and Dagli 2000).

On the other side, the global tobacco treaty process showed the potential of an alliance with civil society and public health advocates. NGOs provided technical

> assistance to government delegates, monitored and exposed tobacco industry abuses such as interference in public health policy, and generated direct pressure on tobacco transnationals including through boycott tactics targeting tobacco-related industries.
>
> Among the member states, the US Government worked throughout the FCTC negotiating process to dilute the treaty. Yet the developing world, led by a block of 46 African nations and supported by CSOs, notably allied in the Framework Convention Alliance (FCA), united to push for positions that would prevent the spread of tobacco addiction, disease and death.
>
>> The WHO's close collaboration with CSOs both during negotiation of the FCTC and its subsequent implementation, has been a notable departure from the organization's traditional focus on ministries of health.
>
> After its adoption by the 56th World Health Assembly in May 2003, the WHO Framework Convention on Tobacco Control (WHO FCTC) was open for signature until 29 June 2004. One hundred and sixty-eight states signed the WHO FCTC during this period, expressing their willingness to become a Party to the Convention. Countries wishing to become a Party, but that did not sign the Convention by 29 June 2004, could do so by means of accession, which is a one-step process equivalent to ratification. In accordance with Article 36 of the WHO FCTC, the Convention entered into force on 27 February 2005, 90 days after the fortieth state had acceded to, ratified, accepted or approved it. To date, the last Party was Mozambique (entry into force: 14 July 2017). While the Bush Administration finally signed the FCTC in May 2004, the US is notably absent from the list of countries that have ratified the treaty (FCTC 2017).
>
> (Lee 2009)

Dr. Lee Jong-Wook of South Korea succeeded Brundtland in 2003. With "extensive experience of the WHO at all three levels of the organization", Lee was reportedly a "compromise candidate" who had been "sidelined by the Brundtland administration to a relatively obscure position", and his election "reflected divided opinions on Brundtland's tenure" (Lee 2009).

He opened his mandate with a renewed focus on "Health for All", and with a wide outlook. The World Health Report 2003 "Shaping the future", the first published under his term as Director-General, reaffirmed the need for strengthening health systems, and advocated to do so by building on the values and practices of primary health care; it drew upon notions of responsiveness to population needs and stewardship toward pro-equity health systems. The report was considered "refreshing in its attempt to offer an integrated approach to improving health" (Walt 2004). The report also discussed Lee's flagship initiative to treat three million people with AIDS with antiviral therapy by the year 2005 (known as "3 by 5"), a goal that many would consider unreachable; in fact this target was not achieved.

Although his dramatic passing away in 2006 prematurely interrupted Lee's term of office, he left behind some important results. Probably the most remarkable initiative of Dr. Lee was the launch, in March 2005, of the Commission on Social Determinants of Health. Chaired by Michael Marmot, the Commission brought together leading scientists and practitioners to provide evidence on policies that improve health by addressing the social conditions in which people live and work and to collaborate with countries to support policy change and monitor results (WHO 2017a). He also managed to restart the process of revising the International Health Regulations, completed in 2005. And under his tenure, the WHA adopted the Global Strategy on diet, physical activity and health, nevertheless suffering harsh criticisms for having a complacent attitude towards the food industry. Although Lee was personally resolved to resist the US influence, he suffered the pressure put on WHO by the USA[12] (Benkimoun 2006).

Internally he continued the reform program of his predecessor, with particular attention to transparency of administrative and budgetary procedures and increase of expenditure in regions and countries rather than at headquarters. In moving forward with the reform of recruitment procedures, with a scheduled termination of 200–300 short-term contract positions, he faced the first ever work stoppage at WHO headquarters due to a strike by several hundred personnel and was severely criticized for his approach[13] (Benkimoun 2006).

After the sudden passing away of the late Director-General Lee Jong-Wook, the international health community looked with hope to the commitment of the new Director-General, Dr. Margaret Chan, to work tirelessly "to make this world a healthier place" and to foster a "noble system of ethical values" (Chan 2006). When she first addressed the EB she prudently stated that she would continue ongoing reforms at the WHO and that changes would be gradual and carefully managed (Lee 2009).

In her vision, in the context of unprecedented global interest and investment in health, where "WHO is not alone in the drive to improve health", unprecedented challenges could only be addressed through well-directed and coordinated global collaboration, which "gives WHO a clear role" (Chan 2008). Two years later, she clearly downgraded WHO's role. Despite WHO's mandate as the "directing and coordinating authority on international health work",

> In today's crowded landscape of public health, leadership is not mandated. It must be earned. And it must be earned through strategic and selective engagement. WHO can no longer aim to direct and coordinate all of the activities and policies in multiple sectors that influence public health today.
>
> (Chan 2010)

According to a former senior officer of the WHO, one major weakness of Dr. Chan was her tendency of "leading from behind", "shown by her unwillingness to stand up to Member States and instead looking to them for consensus and guidance" (Huang and Meltzer 2016).

She would indeed lack strategic vision and innovation and take a "safety approach". She attracted major criticism regarding the WHO's management of a number of crises, such as the H1N1 "swine flu" epidemic in 2010, when the organization was accused of lack of transparency (Flynn 2010), and later when she demonstrated "an overall lack of accountability throughout and after the 2014 Ebola crisis" (Huang and Meltzer 2016) and insisted on WHO being just a "technical agency" (Gostin and Friedman 2014).

Her mandate lasted ten years, being confirmed for a second five-year term in 2012. During her tenure, health remained high on the global agenda, although WHO continued to struggle with its internal reform process.

On the 30th anniversary of the declaration of Alma-Ata (and the 60th of the establishment of WHO), the need for a holistic approach to health and health systems was marked by the publication of WHO's World Health Report 2008, which re-focused the agenda on primary health care (WHO 2008a), as well as the Report of the Commission on Social Determinants of Health (CDSH 2008). Addressing the 60th World Health Assembly after one and a half years in her position, Margaret Chan seemed to challenge the strong vision of some influential actors in global health (such as The Bill & Melinda Gates Foundation), emphatically stating that "investment in technology and interventions alone will not automatically 'buy' better health outcomes" (Chan 2008). According to the Director-General, more investment should have been made in institutional capacity and systems for delivery; to that effect she insisted on a "return to primary health care" and its values, principles and approaches (Chan 2008).

The adoption of the WHO Global Code of Practice on the International Recruitment of Health Personnel was a milestone of Chan's mandate. In 2004 the WHA passed a resolution mandating that the WHO Director-General develop a code of practice on the international recruitment of health personnel, which was increasingly challenging the sustainability of health systems in developing countries (WHO 2004). In the following years the international community and major donors repeatedly urged the WHO to accelerate the development and adoption of the code of practice to tackle at the root the constant drain of health professionals from poor countries and its devastating impact on the health systems of source countries. In addition, widespread concerns were increasingly raised about unethical and unfair recruitment practices. The 63rd World Health Assembly finally adopted the non-binding code in 2010. The code established "voluntary principles and practices for the ethical international recruitment of health personnel" that Member States should refer to in "establishing or improving the legal and institutional framework" for the international recruitment of health personnel (WHO 2010).

Prevention and Control of Noncommunicable Diseases was included in the UN agenda and was supported by the Political Declaration of the High-Level Meeting of the United Nations General Assembly in 2011, later translated into WHO's "Global Action Plan for the Prevention and Control of Noncommunicable Diseases 2013–2020". The WHA also welcomed the report of the Commission on Ending Childhood Obesity (2016) and its six recommendations to address the obesogenic environment and critical periods in the life course to tackle childhood obesity. The implementation plan to guide countries in taking action to implement the recommendations of the Commission was welcomed by the World Health Assembly in 2017 (WHO 2017a). WHO's new emphasis on NCDs and the control of their social determinants was challenged by powerful economic forces, as Dr. Chan bravely stated on more than one occasion.

> Efforts to safeguard public health face opposition from a different set of extremely powerful forces. Many of the risk factors for noncommunicable diseases are amplified by the products and practices of large and economically powerful forces. Market power readily translates into political power.
> ...
> When public health policies cross purposes with vested economic interests, we will face opposition, well-orchestrated opposition, and very well-funded opposition.
> (Chan 2013)

Crisis management was definitively among the weakest points of Dr. Chan's tenure. The H1N1 influenza pandemic in 2009 was declared the first ever "public health emergency of international concern" (PHEIC) in application of the revised 2005 International Health Regulations (IHR). WHO was heavily criticized for keeping secret the identities of the members of the emergency committee who advised the Director-General on the actions to be taken to address the epidemic. The decision to keep the members' identities secret fostered suspicions about WHO decision-making and its possible collusion with vaccine manufacturers in light of the fact that the decision to grade the outbreak as "pandemic" triggered vaccine orders and activated silent contracts (Flynn 2010).

In 2014, WHO announced the Ebola epidemic in West Africa, three months after the outbreak began in December 2013, but did not declare the outbreak to be a "public health emergency of international concern" (PHEIC) until 8 August the following year. This delay between the WHO being made aware of the epidemic and declaring it a PHEIC has been the subject of considerable criticism, exposing the weaknesses in the WHO's approach to accountability (Eccleston-Turner and McArdle 2017).

But the reform process particularly marked Dr. Chan's tenure and especially her second term. In 2009, WHO faced financial crisis when Member States were confronted with the problem of the increasing "carry-over".

> WHO was borrowing against future revenues to maintain its operations. There was self-righteous finger-wagging from many of the rich Member States, whose insistence on maintaining the freeze on assessed contributions (ACs) was the fundamental cause of the crisis.
>
> (Global Health Watch 2014)

In December 2010, a former Assistant Director-General of the WHO named Jack Chow, considering the organization as "outmoded, underfunded and overly politicized", put forward a provocative question: "Is the WHO becoming irrelevant?" (Chow 2010). Indeed, as described in previous chapters (see Chapter 5), while an unprecedented level of global funding had been directed to health issues over the last two decades, the increase was mostly driven by vertical initiatives for the control of HIV/AIDS and a few other diseases. This was associated with the mushrooming of new organizations and global public-private ventures, bilateral programs and the rise of non-state actors (particularly the Bill & Melinda Gates Foundation) that often overshadowed WHO. Finally, WHO had to face priority-setting and planning constraints imposed, among other reasons, by the way it is financed.

Since the freezing of RBFs in the 1980s, WHO has seen an increase in the proportion of EBFs largely earmarked by donors for special purposes. Since 2007 EBFs have represented around 80% of the total budget of the organization. In 2010, more than 50% of EBFs came from Member States and 21% from the United Nations and other intergovernmental organizations, though a significant 26% came from private donors, including foundations (18%), NGOs and other institutions (7%) and the corporate sector (1%). The Bill & Melinda Gates Foundation (with a contribution of $220 m) was the second largest donor after the USA ($280 m) (WHO 2011). Over 86% of the voluntary contributions had no degree of flexibility and lacked predictability, challenging WHO's priority-setting, planning and implementing capacity. In fact, while the WHO could exert discretionary control over the RBF, donors increased their control over planning and management through EBFs. In addition, the already scarce RBFs suffered from arrears to the WHO from a number of countries, including the United States, whose arrears in 2010 were equivalent to about 5% of WHO's Regular Budget (WHO 2011a). Correcting this situation and avoiding the possibility of member states and non-state donors using the financial leverage to influence WHO's strategies was of paramount importance and represented an obvious priority.

Given the above-mentioned imbalance between assessed and voluntary contributions, it is not surprising that the idea of reform, for many years on the WHO agenda, gained extra speed and scope in 2011. Under the agenda item titled "The Future of Financing for WHO", the 64th WHA actually stealthily included a broader reform plan without analytical considerations and rationale for the far-reaching agenda that was now proposed, and that could reshape the way in which the organization operated, was governed, made decisions and was financed, and possibly its overall role in the global public health arena. The report touched upon seven issues: focusing core business;[14] increasing organizational effectiveness; improving results-based management and accountability; human resource policy, planning and management; strengthening financing, resource mobilization and strategic communication; WHO's effectiveness at country level; and WHO's role in global health governance (WHO 2011b).

With respect to the questioned relevance of WHO in today's world, the latter was possibly the most compelling issue, encompassing all the others. It was no surprise that the attention of many observers, especially those expressing the views of civil society, committed to a stronger WHO "playing a leading role in global health governance" (PHM 2011).

The reform process was marked from the beginning by strong tensions and distrust. Among other criticisms, the WHO was accused of not providing timely details of reform plans, of "cozy[ing] up to private industry" and of being too deferential to the Bill & Melinda Gates Foundation, whose financial contribution to the reform process was then unveiled (Hawkes 2011).

This debate encouraged a Member State-driven process, resulting in the adoption of a more transparent and inclusive consultative process for the finalization of a reform plan along three lines: (a) programmatic reform, to improve health outcomes; (b) governance reform, to increase coherence in global health; and (c) managerial reform, in pursuit of organizational excellence (Missoni 2011).

Regarding the program, in May 2013 the 66th WHA approved the Twelfth General Program of Work for the six-year period 2014–2019, describing six priorities (Box 6.3), "focused on the actions and areas where the Organization has a unique function or comparative advantage, and financed in a way that facilitates this focus" (WHO 2017b).

BOX 6.3 WHO priorities for the period 2014–2019

- Advancing universal health coverage
- Health-related Millennium Development Goals
- Addressing the challenge of noncommunicable diseases
- Implementing the provisions of the IHR (2005)
- Increasing access to essential, high-quality, safe, effective and affordable medical products
- Addressing the social, economic and environmental determinants of health.

Starting with the biennium 2014–2015, the Program Budget included a new organization-wide results framework structured around six categories and 30 program areas. The program would now identify the activities required to deliver the agreed outputs and achieve the related targets, improving accountability and facilitating a systematic way to monitor performance, reflecting the adoption of a result-based management (RBM) approach. In addition, priorities identified in country cooperation strategies would be more closely linked with the outcomes of WHO strategic and biennial planning. It was also the first time in history that the WHA approved the entire Program Budget; prior to this, the Assembly only approved Assessed Contributions.

Aiming to match the results and deliverables as agreed in WHO's biennial Program Budgets with resources available to finance them and to achieve full funding of the Program Budget, the "financing dialogue" was introduced, reaffirming principles of alignment, transparency, predictability, flexibility and broadening the donor base.

> The financial dialogue aims to change what was a somewhat opaque process of bilateral negotiations into a more open, transparent and collective discussion of how the budget agreed by Member States can be financed in a way that is both stable and predictable.
>
> (Cassels *et al.* 2014)

Despite improvement, financing the program budget remained a challenge.

> The increase in predictability of funding from 62% at the beginning of the biennium 2012–2013 to 83% at the beginning of the biennium 2016–2017 has not been sustained and funding levels for the Program budget 2016–2017 have not improved further.
>
> (WHO 2017b)

Most important gaps in funding were in the area of health emergencies, which was funded only to 56%, and noncommunicable diseases, funded only to 55% (WHO 2017b).

The governance component of the reform covers two aspects. The first concerns organizational governance, i.e. the way WHO is governed by its Member States and the functioning of its governing bodies and the linkage among them (including between the regional and the global level). The second element is concerned with WHO's role in global health governance. "Progress has been slow on both counts" (Cassels *et al.* 2014).

Regarding organizational governance, some steps forward were made in optimizing, harmonizing and aligning regional and global Governing Bodies, and the procedures and criteria for the election of the Director-General and Regional Directors were also harmonized and made more transparent. Regarding transparency and accountability, after two years of intergovernmental negotiations the highly debated issue of collaboration with non-state actors (NSA) led to the adoption of the Framework of Engagement with Non-State Actors in 2016 (FENSA) (WHO 2016).

Although presented as "one of the most transparent frameworks introduced in a UN agency" (WHO 2017c), the adoption of FENSA left unsatisfied a vast majority of civil society organizations (CSOs) that rejected the outcome of the WHO Member States negotiations. CSO advocacy included calls to strengthen WHO safeguards against undue influence from the private sector and develop an effective conflict-of-interest policy to protect WHO from the undue influence of global philanthropy and corporations (CSOs 2016).

Finally, regarding the managerial reform, major progress was made towards "strengthening oversight and accountability through the setup of the Compliance Risk and Ethics department and the Evaluation Office, the implementation of a risk management framework, the definition of a whistle blowing policy, a disclosure and management of conflicts framework, accountability compacts and letters of representation between the Director General and senior staff" (WHO 2017c). A human resources strategy was also defined, and staff rules and regulations were updated with the implementation of a new performance management system.

In May 2017, the new Director-General, Tedros Adhanom Ghebreyesus from Ethiopia, was appointed for the first time in the history of the organization through a very open and inclusive electoral process. Dr Ghebreyesus envisions a WHO "that belongs to all, equally. [...] efficiently managed, adequately resourced and results driven, with a strong focus on transparency, accountability and value for money". In his vision, the global commitment to sustainable development is perceived as "a unique opportunity to address the social, economic and political determinants of health and to improve the health and well-being of people everywhere". In Dr Ghebreyesus's vision, "an enhanced and independent WHO [...] maximizes inclusive partnerships, and ensures collective priority setting with all stakeholders". He has committed to "champion country ownership, so that countries are at the table, as full and equal partners, to guide and make the decisions that will affect the health of their populations" (Ghebreyesus 2018).

Indeed, the independence of WHO remains an open issue. According to important sectors of civil society, the current reform program

> does not address the real requirements as regards changes in WHO's capabilities and approach. It is not based on any coherent conception of WHO's role in confronting the global health crisis, nor a realistic account of the structures and dynamics of global (health) governance. Rather the reform identifies and seeks to address specific management weaknesses, many of which can be traced in part to the policy of zero nominal growth and the absurd funding situation WHO is in.
>
> (Global Health Watch 2014)

The reform process has not addressed the role of WHO in challenging the social and economic roots of the global health crisis. In summary, it is difficult to say if today WHO is better equipped than before to reaffirm itself as "the coordinating and directing authority" and

> to reposition itself in a leading role in the wider global health governance scenario, supported by the necessary resources and trust to fully exert it. Trust that can only be built on its capacity to act independently from external undue influences, in the sole interest of public health and peoples' right to "the attainment of the highest possible level of health".
>
> (Missoni 2011)

While there are many health institutions which are global in scope, WHO remains the only multilateral institution with the political legitimacy and dedicated mandate to promote and protect health.

6.4 The Bretton Woods institutions: the International Monetary Fund and the World Bank

6.4.1 The origins

In July 1944, a United Nations Monetary and Financial Conference took place at Bretton Woods (New Hampshire, USA) aiming to reorganize the world economy and to prevent new crises like the one leading to the Great Depression in the 1930s. The Conference resulted in a few agreements, named after the site of the event, and established a regulation system for international exchange rates, which characterized the second post-war period until 1971.

The Bretton Woods agreements marked the beginning of the International Monetary Fund (IMF) and of the International Bank for Reconstruction and Development (IBRD), the first of the five institutions that today constitute the World Bank Group. The idea of a system of organizations that could control the global economic situation belongs to John Maynard Keynes and Harry Dexter White, one of the closest advisers to President Roosevelt. The original project also included the establishment of an International Trade Organization (ITO) in order to develop cooperation among countries on a multilateral – and basically global – basis in relation to the three main forms of economic integration: monetary (maintaining the stability of international exchange rates, a main responsibility of IMF), financial (supporting capital investments in production, under the control of the World Bank) and commercial (a responsibility to be given to the ITO, which was never established due to an insufficient number of ratifications of the agreement). The Bretton Woods agreements limited the mandate of the IMF and the World Bank to the management of issues linked to capital deficiencies. The gold standard was reintroduced in a new formula of equivalence with the dollar. It was established that the value of each national currency would be set according to gold or to the equivalent in US dollars;[15] fluctuations would only be allowed up to 1% and any devaluation higher than 10% would require the approval of the IMF. The dollar became the reference currency of a system based on free movement of goods and capital.[16]

The Bretton Woods system's founding criteria were abandoned in 1971, when the United States of America released the dollar from gold convertibility. The devaluation of the US currency produced, especially in developing countries, a sudden increase in import prices and the fall in value of exports. The new situation pushed OPEC[17] member countries to double the price of oil. The huge gains from controlling the price of oil resulted in vast amounts of dollars (*petrodollars*) deposited in commercial banks. To ensure the mobility of that excess in liquidity, these banks began to offer extremely advantageous loans to developing countries, initiating the mechanism leading to a debt crisis in the early 1980s, when unsustainable interest rates made the debt unsustainable. With the collapse of the Bretton Woods system and the introduction of flexible exchange rates, the attention of the IMF moved from the monitoring and management of international liquidity, to the control of countries' internal macroeconomic policies and the structural elements of their markets. The IMF would now offer loans tied to specific conditions and strict macroeconomic stabilization plans, i.e. Structural Adjustment Plans (SAP) imposed on indebted developing countries.[18]

The above-mentioned events implied three major amendments to the original text of the agreement establishing the IMF. In 1969 "Special Drawing Rights"[19] were introduced as a new instrument, to cope with the insufficiency of international monetary reserves. In 1978 countries' obligation to maintain the gold equivalence of their currency was suppressed, and countries were left free to autonomously define their exchange policies. Finally, in 1992 the possibility was introduced to impose sanctions on Member States failing to comply with the Fund's conditions.[20]

In the second half of the 1990s the characteristics of the crisis also changed. The composition of international financing shifted from bank loans to non-bank financial channels, guided by the course of major stock exchange centers. New communication technologies allowing almost instantaneous financial transactions (transfers of funds) contributed to the crisis in liquidity that occurred in 1994 in Mexico and later in some Asian countries and other countries transitioning to a market economy (mainly Russia). As soon as a country became "at risk", the response of international investors became to instantaneously withdraw invested capitals. The ensuing crises were long-lasting and directly involved the financial authorities of the world's major economies and international economic organizations. This shift in the nature of the financial crisis led to the beginning of the debate on the reform of the international financial system.

With the transformation of the global scenario, both the IMF and the World Bank have partially modified their functions and priorities. Globally, the IMF has the new role of monitoring the macroeconomic outcomes of member countries in order to promptly identify the early signs of imbalance, provide consultancy and adopt instruments of conditional loans to avoid economic collapse in those countries (Missoni and Alesani 2014).

The financial crisis that started in the United States in 2007 and became global in the following year exposed these financial institutions to increasing requests for debt renegotiation and other forms of financial support. In response to these requests, with the support of creditor countries, the IMF has tripled its lending capabilities and revised its policies, introducing certain flexibility in credit lines towards countries with strong "fundamentals" (IMF 2018).

The IMF today maintains its role as a lender, including for more advanced economies. For example, in recent years the IMF collaborated with the European Union and the European Central Bank (the "Troika") in the so-called "rescue plans" of Greece, Ireland and Portugal. This new role is the one most closely related to global health issues and to the transformation of health systems, which no longer concern only the poorest countries.

6.4.2 Structure and functions of the International Monetary Fund

The representative organ of the IMF is the Board of Governors, where all the Member States are represented; it meets twice a year. The Governor of the Central Bank or the Minister of Economy generally leads national delegations. Decisions are in principle taken by simple majority, although in practice voting is avoided and decisions are adopted by consensus. In the IMF (as in the World Bank) the vote is weighted, i.e. Member States' voting rights are proportional to their contributions or "Quotas". This mechanism substantially differs from the OMOV principle (one member one vote), typical of most UN and other international organizations. Thus, in the Bretton Woods organizations, wealthy countries tend to be in control of the governing bodies.

The day-to-day work of the IMF is overseen by its 24-member Executive Board, which represents the entire membership and is guided by the International Monetary and Financial Committee, or IMFC, and supported by the IMF staff. The Managing

Director is the head of the IMF staff and Chair of the Executive Board and is assisted by four Deputy Managing Directors. The IMFC also has 24 members and advises the Board of Governors on the supervision and management of the international monetary and financial system.

6.4.3 Structure and functions of the World Bank

The World Bank Group currently includes five institutions, all with the status of United Nations specialized institutions. The "World Bank" is the name commonly used for the International Bank for Reconstruction and Development (IBRD) and the International Development Association (IDA), which together provide low-interest loans, zero-interest loans and grants to developing countries. The other three organizations are the International Finance Corporation (IFC), the Multilateral Investment Guarantee Agency (MIGA) and the International Center for Settlement of Investment Disputes (ICSID).[21]

The International Bank for Reconstruction and Development (IBRD) is the main organization of the group formed in Bretton Woods in 1944. Participation in the Bank is limited to states that are members of the International Monetary Fund, and

> the reason for the statutory prediction of this condition should be sought in the fact that the States were obliged to adhere to the strict economic parameters imposed by the Monetary Fund as an essential prerequisite for accessing to the funding of the Bank.
>
> (Megliani 2001: 167)

The World Bank describes itself "like a cooperative, made up of 189 member countries" (World Bank 2017);[22] however, it is rather like a limited company with its member countries as shareholders,[23] where the shares subscribed by each country vary according to the economic weight of the subscriber (one vote for each share of the Bank's capital stock held by the member).[24] Hence the weighted voting mechanism, as in the case of the IMF

> is not based on the principle of equality between members but intended to ensure the effectiveness of the political-economic orientation of the market, peculiar to this International Organization.
>
> (Megliani 2001: 167)

The representative body of the World Bank is the Board of Governors. It normally meets once a year; decisions are taken by majority vote, although consensus is often used. The Board may delegate its powers to the Executive Directors, except in the case of admission of new members, modification of capital stock, suspension of a member, decision on appeals from interpretations of the Agreement by the Directors, cooperation agreements with other international organizations, distribution of net income and suspension of the Bank's activity.

The 25 Executive Directors are responsible for the Bank's general operations. Five are appointed by the shareholders with the largest number of shares (USA, UK, France, Germany and Japan), the rest are elected by Governors without the right to a direct appointment of their representative. The appointed Directors' voting rights are equal to those of the state which appointed them, while elected Directors' voting rights are equal to the sum of the voting rights of the states that elected them. It should be noted that the Directors represent not only the interests of the Bank, but also the interests of the states that appointed or elected them. The President and the staff, on the other hand, respond exclusively to the Bank.

The President of the Bank, traditionally of US nationality according to an unwritten rule, is appointed by the Directors. He/she is in charge for five years, chairs the Board of Directors and ordinarily has no vote except a deciding vote in the case of an equally divided Board. He/she is also chief executive officer of the Organization and has control over the funding process.

In 1980 the Board of Governors of the World Bank established the Administrative Tribunal.[25] The Tribunal is the independent judicial forum of last resort for the resolution of cases submitted by members of the World Bank Group staff alleging non-observance of their contracts of employment or terms of appointment. The Tribunal's decisions are final and binding. The World Bank decided not to use the administrative courts already existing in the United Nations and the International Labor Organization (ILO).

The Bank also has two subsidiary bodies: the Advisory Board, consisting of experts selected by the Board of Governors among representatives of the banking, commercial and industrial sectors, tasked to express opinions on general political matters of the Bank; and the Lending Committee, with the function of recommending projects and reporting about loans granted by the Bank.

The World Bank's main purpose was originally to assist in the reconstruction and development of countries hit by the second world conflict, facilitating productive investment and reconversion of the war industry for peaceful purposes. Soon, however, the Bank shifted its attention to the needs of its developing country members, focusing primarily on large infrastructure projects such as dams, electrical grids, irrigation systems and roads.

In the 1970s, under the presidency of Robert McNamara, the World Bank's attention shifted to poverty eradication and to people-oriented development projects, rather than exclusively the construction of infrastructures. Later the World Bank's operations expanded, increasingly influencing macroeconomic policies and countries' institutional development, mainly through sectoral and structural adjustment loans. In the early 1980s the Bank intervened in highly indebted countries with Structural Adjustment Programs (SAP), which had dramatic social and environmental effects with dramatic impact on health and nutritional and educational levels for tens of millions of children in developing countries (Cornia *et al.* 1987).

In the following decades, the Bank introduced poverty reduction strategies and focused on issues of social development, including health care, education, communications, cultural heritage and good governance. The scope of World Bank Group–United Nations collaboration greatly expanded over the years, covering virtually every area related to sustainable development, with a view to ending poverty and promoting shared prosperity, working together on the Millennium Development Goals, the Post-2015 Development Agenda, and Financing for Development.

The International Development Association (IDA) was established in 1960. The purpose was to provide loans on favorable terms[26] to states that were born out of decolonization and without the requirements of reliability required by both the capital market and the World Bank itself. Another aim was to promote economic development and to raise the standard of living in less-developed areas. Participation in IDA is reserved only for members of the Bank and, as in the case of the Bank, there is a strong asymmetry in the weight of decision-making among the Member States, where "industrialized countries have many more shares than developing countries to exercise control over the organization" (Megliani 2001: 181). The structure of IDA is also perfectly similar to the Bank and in fact their governing organs often share the same members; this also explains why the IDA and the IBRD are commonly referred to as The World Bank.

6.4.3.1 World Bank health policies

Since 1970, World Bank's President McNamara had been advocating for the Bank to support health and nutrition programs. The 1975 Health Sector Policy Paper was one of the Bank's first efforts to engage in health policy issues. In 1974, the World Bank co-sponsored one of its most successful health programs, the Onchocerciasis Control Program (OCP), aiming to eradicate onchocerciasis (river blindness). The program was cosponsored by the United Nations Development Program (UNDP), the Food and Agriculture Organization and WHO, and also involved the private sector. The OCP gave the bank a boost in the health sector. In 1979, the bank established a Health, Nutrition and Population (HNP) department and defined the policy to allow funding in health projects. The 1980 World Development Report pointed out that malnutrition and ill health were two of the worst symptoms of poverty and that improving health and nutrition would be likely to accelerate economic growth. In 1980 a Health Sector Policy Paper was produced. The 1987 study Financing Health Services in Developing Countries: An Agenda for Reform, and the World Development Report, 1993 (see Chapter 4) were a hallmark in the World Bank's engagement in health and gave the World Bank new legitimacy in the sector. However, by far the most dramatic change in the Bank's role in global health has been its increased financial support for HNP through loans, credits and grants (Ruger 2005), which from 1980 to 2000 involved the application of market-based solutions and privatization of healthcare delivery, aligning with broader trends across the Bank's wider portfolio (Sridhar *et al.* 2017).

The current World Bank's mission statement is "End extreme poverty" and "promote a shared prosperity".[27] The focus on poverty reduction was the result of an attempt by the World Bank to analyze and review its past experience. James Wolfensohn, President of the World Bank from 1995 to 2005, highlighted the need to rethink the Bank's approach to development. He insisted on the critical need for economic growth and appropriate macroeconomic policies for reducing poverty but pointed out that growth alone would not be enough. An effective poverty reduction would require appropriate "pro-poor" institutions, *governance* and effective actions to cope with high levels of inequality in fields such as land and education. In Wolfensohn's view, effective social safety networks should also be put in place, and gender and racial discrimination issues properly addressed (Wolfensohn 2000).

In this context, the Bank defined its strategy by two *pillars* with the aim of contributing to the achievement of the Millennium Development Goals. The first pillar is based on the assumption that successful development is driven by the private sector, with a government that provides infrastructure, human capital and a proper legal and judicial system to create a favorable environment for entrepreneurship and economic activity. The second pillar focuses on creating economic and social integration opportunities for the poor through health, education and reduction of vulnerability to crises (World Bank 2001).

The 1997 edition of the Bank's HNP sectoral guidelines, despite asserting that "universal access is one of the most effective ways to provide health care for the poor" based on the experience in "developed" and middle-income countries, pointed out that "non-targeted approaches can also be wasteful" (World Bank 1997: 6) and concluded that

> in low-income countries, non-targeted approaches often have to be restricted to a very limited range of public health and food fortification programs, and a few essential health services, to be financially viable.
>
> (World Bank 1997: 6)

Regarding strategies to improve healthcare systems' performance, the Bank systematically pointed out the limits of the public sector, favoring a "more balanced public/private mix" and promoting the participation of NGOs, local communities and the private sector in the delivery of services. The Bank proposed a country-specific approach to reform, which needed to take into consideration each country's socioeconomic conditions. However, a single philosophy inspired the Bank's strategy: where the private sector was strong, the role of the public sector should be reduced; where the latter was predominant, the development of the private sector should be promoted (World Bank 1997).

In 2007 the HNP sectoral guidelines were updated for the following decade with the "Healthy Development: The World Bank Strategy for Health, Nutrition, and Population Results" in light of the important changes in the international architecture of development assistance for health. While in the previous decade the Bank was the main financier of HNP, by 2007 new multilateral organizations, global initiatives and philanthropies had assumed a prominent role in the health sector, with much of that new funding being earmarked toward the fight of just a few priority diseases, such as HIV/AIDS, malaria, tuberculosis and some vaccine-preventable diseases. Notably, they neglected other approaches such as health system strengthening at the country level, and to a certain extent maternal and child health, nutrition and population priorities. Thus, the new strategy made the case for

> sharpening the Bank focus on results on the ground; for concentrating Bank contributions on its comparative advantages, particularly in health system strengthening, health financing, and economics; for supporting government leadership and international community programs to achieve these results; and for exercising selectivity in engagement with global partners.
>
> (World Bank 2007: 11)

In this context, especially in the lower-income countries, the Bank identified five strategic directions for the following decade:

1. Renew Bank focus on HNP results.
2. Increase the Bank contribution to client-country efforts to strengthen and realize well-organized and sustainable health systems for HNP results.
3. Ensure synergy between health system strengthening and priority-disease interventions, particularly in LICs.
4. Strengthen Bank capacity to advise client countries on an intersectoral approach to HNP results.

5. Increase selectivity, improve strategic engagement and reach agreement with global partners on collaborative division of labor for the benefit of client countries.

(World Bank 2007: 31)

In the context of the new strategy, and particularly in relation to the creation of synergies between vertical and system-building interventions, in 2009 the Bank partnered with GAVI and the Global Fund to Fight AIDS, Tuberculosis and Malaria in the "Health Systems Funding Platform", a mechanism intended to increase coordination and streamlining of international resources for national health programs (Hafner and Shiffman 2013).

After almost two decades of undue policy influence, the Bank's renewed advocacy of country-owned and aligned development approaches appeared rather rhetorical:

> With such evident discrepancies occurring between the Bank's aid effectiveness rhetoric and its actual practices – and given the length of time over which they have been occurring, questions must be asked about the merit and appropriateness of having the Bank play such an influential role in the Platform's in-country HSS activities.
>
> (Brown et al. 2013)

In addition, the lack of formal agreements for any real partnership at country level raised doubts about the Bank's real interest in pursuing the principles of aid effectiveness, while hierarchical governance was highlighted as the persistent dominant development practice at the Bank (Brown et al. 2013).

The election in 2012 of World Bank President Dr Jim Kim, who was not, as usual, an economist but rather a global health practitioner, a medical doctor and an anthropologist who made his reputation providing medical care to poor people, and a former critic of the Bank, was considered an important sign of change. The Bank under Kim introduced new financing mechanisms to coordinate and focus funding streams from international donors, such as the Global Financing Facility (GFF), designed to bridge the funding gap for addressing preventable death and disease among children and women, and made new pushes on tobacco taxation, improving road safety, and a variety of nutrition initiatives. Kim also received widespread praise for his leadership in financing the Ebola response, leading to the establishment of a Pandemic Emergency Financing Facility to address the need for rapid response measures in the case of epidemics. Strengthening the core financing functions of countries' health systems became another important area of intervention in the push for universal health coverage. In this context, the Bank has been working with its private sector arm, the International Finance Corporation (IFC), to promote business involvement in health care, a highly debated initiative, including within the Bank. A 2014 Bank assessment found that "while its health financing efforts had increased the number of people in the insurance market, it did not always have a substantial effect on poor people" (Loewenberg 2015).

Indeed, "Kim's vision for the bank is to use its knowledge and capital to serve as an 'honest broker' between the interests of the global market system, emerging country governments, and people in poverty, to ensure that all sides benefit" (Sridhar et al. 2017). However, the Bank's mandate to create new markets may contrast with the fundamental concept at the heart of universal health coverage, that access to good quality health care is a human right (Tichenor and Sridhar 2017).[28]

Although the strategic HNP guidelines have not been updated since 2007, the goal of Universal Health Coverage by 2030 is highlighted in the Bank's public profile as part of the wider commitment by the World Bank Group (WBG) to help nations build healthier, more equitable societies and to improve fiscal performance and country competitiveness. To that purpose the World Bank provides financing, state-of-the-art analysis, and policy advice to improve service delivery and expand access to quality, affordable health care, working closely with donors, development partners, governments and the private sector. Main focus areas include ending preventable maternal and child mortality, reducing stunting and improved nutrition for infants and children, strengthening health systems and health financing, ensuring pandemic preparedness and response, promoting sexual and reproductive health and rights, and the prevention and treatment of communicable diseases (World Bank 2017).

Beyond its specific role in the context of global health policies, the World Bank remains the largest funding agent of Development Assistance to Health (DAH) within the UN system and the second largest funder overall (Sridhar *et al.* 2017). Unlike the WHO, the World Bank is able to influence decision-making at country level, through substantial financial incentives and engaging with Ministers of Finance and across sectors to reach health goals. Together with the Regional Development Banks and other international financial institutions, in particular the IMF, the World Bank plays a significant role in influencing macroeconomic policies and key health determinants.

6.5 UNAIDS

6.5.1 *Origins*

UNAIDS, the Joint United Nations Program on HIV/AIDS, was established in 1994 by the ECOSOC (United Nations Economic and Social Council) after a long and troubled gestation (UNAIDS 2008).

It was constituted as a joint program, co-funded by various entities of the United Nations system on the basis of the principles of "co-ownership, collaborative planning and execution, and an equitable sharing of responsibility" (ECOSOC 1994), to replace the WHO Global Program on AIDS that had led the global action against the epidemic until then.

Initially the subsidiary bodies and the UN specialized agencies that joined were UNDP, UNICEF, UNFPA, WHO, UNESCO and the World Bank. Later the group was joined by UNODC (1999), ILO (2001), WFP and UNHCR (2003) and UN Women (2012). UNAIDS remains the only cosponsored Joint Program in the United Nations system.

6.5.2 *Structure and functions*

UNAIDS was established to ensure coordination of actions for the control of HIV/AIDS within the UN system, in collaboration with civil society, national governments, the private sector, global institutions and people living with HIV/AIDS; the importance of UNAIDS's role increased with the spread of the pandemic and with the high priority given to HIV/AIDS in the global agenda.

UNAIDS's commitment is aimed at ensuring universal access to prevention, treatment and care for affected people; the ultimate goal is to stop and reverse the spread of HIV according to specific targets for each country. UNAIDS defines the global guidelines and it is one of the main sources of data on HIV/AIDS.

UNAIDS combines the resources of its Secretariat with the broad technical competencies and the experience of the 11 organizations that contribute to the funding of the program.

UNAIDS's budget represents about 1% of total global resources to fight the pandemic; however, UNAIDS keeps control of all global resources through the UNAIDS Unified Budget, Results and Accountability Framework (UBRAF). Besides ensuring the maximum coherence, coordination and impact of the pool resources, UNBRAF also plays an important role in the mobilization of contributions to support the Secretariat's activities.

The Executive Director of UNAIDS is appointed by the Secretary-General of the United Nations and reports to the Program Coordination Board (PCB).

The PCB is the executive body that supervises policies, strategies, financial aspects, monitoring and evaluation of UNAIDS. It is composed of representatives of 22 Member States elected for three-year periods and based on a regional distribution. In addition, representatives of all the cosponsoring organizations and five non-governmental organizations participate in the PCB. UNAIDS is the only United Nations entity with civil society represented on its governing body.

The Committee of Co-sponsoring Organizations meets regularly and works as PCB's standing committee, considering the most important issues and giving strategic direction to the program.

With the creation of the Global Fund to Fight AIDS, Tuberculosis and Malaria (GFATM) in 2002, the US President's Emergency Plan for AIDS Relief (PEPFAR) in 2003, UNITAID in 2005 and a growing number of NGOs and other private and public actors active in the fight against HIV/AIDS, the global scenario deeply changed, and UNAIDS needs to reposition itself to remain the driving force behind the pandemic response.

6.6 The World Trade Organization and other free trade regimes

6.6.1 *The origins*

The World Trade Organization (WTO) was established in Marrakesh at the end of the last round of multilateral negotiations under the General Agreement on Tariffs and Trade (GATT) (Uruguay Round 1986–1994). As already mentioned, the original project of the Bretton Woods International Conference provided for a system based on three universal multilateral economic institutions, of which the International Trade Organization (ITO) – aimed at promoting the liberalization of trade and the elimination of protectionist barriers – never started due to lack of ratification of the Settlement Agreement by a number of states concerned with the implications of restricting their national trade policies. Subsequently, part of the agreement gave rise to the GATT, which was concerned with the rules aimed at promoting trade liberalization through the reduction of customs duties. Subsequent rounds of multilateral negotiations further reduced tariffs and other protectionist barriers. The changes and the increasing complexity of GATT's system of rules also led to its progressive transformation into an organization. The WTO Agreement signed at Marrakesh at the end of the Uruguay Round contains a wide range of annexed agreements, including in Annex 1A the GATT itself, which remains the reference text for the basic principles of international trade disciplines, as well as several other agreements related to trade in goods (agriculture, technical barriers to trade, subsidies and anti-dumping, among others); in Annex 1B the General Agreement on Trade in Services (GATS); and in Annex 1C the Agreement on the Trade-Related Aspects of Intellectual Property Rights (TRIPS). It is worth noting that in the case of conflict between the provisions of the GATT and another Agreement contained in Annex 1A, the latter will prevail. Another important innovation, included in Annex 2, regulates the settlement of disputes among Member States: the introduction of the "reverse consensus", whereby a decision must be approved unless there is a consensus against it, makes the system more predictable and quasi-judicial. On the other hand, countries are not allowed to adhere to individual agreements; on the basis of the principle of a "single undertaking", Member States are bound by all the multilateral agreements reached in Marrakesh.

6.6.2 Structure and functions

The WTO, which is headquartered in Geneva, is an international organization with its own legal personality, with immunities and privileges identical to those of the specialized agencies of the United Nations. It does not have a constitutional link with the UN, and it is therefore one of the "related organizations" in the UN system. The WTO-UN relations are governed by the "Arrangements for Effective Cooperation with other Intergovernmental Organizations – Relations Between the WTO and the United Nations" signed on 15 November 1995. The WTO Director-General participates in the Chief Executive Board, the coordinating body within the UN system.

The tasks of the WTO do not include the implementation of initiatives, and its functions can be summarized in supporting and monitoring the compliance of the multilateral regulations enshrined in the trade agreements, and the promotion of free trade.

Specifically, the WTO's functions are to: administer trade agreements, act as a forum for commercial negotiations, settle trade disputes, monitor national trade policies, assist developing country members in matters concerning trade-related policies through technical assistance and training programs and cooperate with other international bodies.

Membership is subject to specific negotiations. Although protocols are signed by governments, "the goal is to help producers of goods and services, exporters, and importers conduct their business" (WTO 2017).

The WTO representative organ is the Ministerial Conference; it is composed of Member States' Trade Ministers and meets at least every two years. On that occasion, it can take decisions that have until today always taken the form of "declarations", defining goals and Member States' new commitments. When the Ministerial Conference is not in session, decisions may be taken by the General Council, which, depending on the agenda, has distinct denominations: it is referred to as the Dispute Settlement Body (DSB) when it deals with disputes between Member States, and the Trade Policy Review Body (TPRB) if the agenda relates to the evaluation of trade policies. The aforementioned collegiate bodies are supported by third-level bodies responsible for specific areas of work: the Council for Trade in Goods (Goods Council), the Council for Trade in Services (Services Council) and the Council for Trade-Related Aspects of Intellectual Property Rights (TRIPS Council).

The Secretariat, which deals with the day by day administration, is led by a Director-General, who also represents the WTO.

On a number of occasions, specific tasks are delegated to subsidiary bodies, such as committees and working groups also composed of representatives of Member States. In addition, there are Panels which are set up to settle disputes and which involve independent experts.

As a rule, the decisions of the collegiate bodies are taken by consensus. When this cannot be reached, and a vote is required, the "one country one vote" system is used, with formal equality among members, unlike the International Financial Institutions, where the voting right is weighted on the basis of members' financial contributions. However, the decision-making process based on consensus has its own weaknesses, and the importance of substantive informal procedures, with the implications in terms of transparency and predictability of decisions, cannot be overestimated. As mentioned above, to make the system more predictable in the decision-making process, the so-called "reverse consensus" was introduced, whereby the DSB must approve a decision unless there is a consensus against it.

Since the Seattle Conference (1999), the WTO has suffered several failures as a result of deep contrasts between the interests of emerging economies and those of the more advanced economies, especially the United States and the European Union. The Doha Round,[29] the negotiating process launched with the Fourth WTO Ministerial Conference held in Doha, Qatar in November 2001, aimed to significantly reform the international trade system by reducing barriers to trade and introducing new rules aimed at improving developing countries' commercial prospects in areas such as agriculture, services, access to the market of manufactured products, facilitation of international trade, and intellectual property rights (Narlikar 2005). Despite several attempts, the negotiations have been suffering a major stalemate since 2008.

Meanwhile, global trade equilibrium is radically and rapidly changing, and with it free trade negotiations have shifted towards bilateral and regional trade agreements, such as the Trans-Pacific Partnership (TPP) and the Transatlantic Trade and Investment Partnership (TTIP).

6.6.3 The WTO system of multilateral trade agreements: main health-related aspects

The WTO agreements with a more direct impact on health and health care are the following: Technical Barriers to Trade (TBT), Application of Sanitary and Phytosanitary Measures (SPS), Trade-Related Aspects of Intellectual Property Rights (TRIPS) and the General Agreement on Trade in Services (GATS).

All WTO agreements share two fundamental principles: the principle of the Most Favored Nation (MFN) and that of National Treatment (NT). These principles also apply to agreements of public health interest.

According to the MFN principle, Member States commit to not discriminating between their trading partners; in other words, Member States must offer to every WTO Member the same conditions they offer to their "most favored" partner, in terms of both imports and exports.

The NT principle states that once goods have cleared customs there can be no discrimination between national and imported goods. It must be noted, however, that from the beginning GATT's Article XX (General exceptions) established that

> Subject to the requirement that such measures are not applied in a manner which would constitute a means of arbitrary or unjustifiable discrimination between

countries where the same conditions prevail, or a disguised restriction on international trade, nothing in this Agreement shall be construed to prevent the adoption or enforcement by any contracting party of measures:
[…]
(b) necessary to protect human, animal or plant life or health.

(GATTS 1986: Article XX b)

In the WTO Agreements, there are clauses which allow for special measures to face public health challenges.

Under the TBT agreement, all member countries have the right to restrict trade for "legitimate objectives" such as the protection of human health and the life and health of plants and animals, environmental protection, national security and the prevention of deceptive practices. However, the objective of the TBT agreement is to prevent such restrictions from being "unnecessary" barriers to trade. In practice, any technical specification cannot be more restrictive than needed to achieve its legitimate aim. To this end, Member States are invited to refer to international standards in the identification of such technical standards and compliance verification procedures, although remaining free to define their own standards. In the latter case, however, they must be able to justify their choices if requested by any other member state.

The SPS agreement was designed to prevent Member States from using non-tariff barriers, such as sanitary or phytosanitary measures to protect their national agricultural production, given their obligation to reduce tariffs and subsidies to agriculture. The SPS Agreement contains specific rules that countries need to comply with if they want to restrict trade for purposes of food safety or protection from diseases transmitted via plants or animals (zoonoses). Also, in this case countries' sovereignty to determine the levels of health protection they deem appropriate is recognized, provided that the measures taken do not represent unnecessary, arbitrary, unjustifiable, or otherwise surreptitious, international trade restraints. The SPS agreement also encourages member countries to refer to international standards, guidelines and recommendations. If the adopted measures do not refer to such international standards, the Member State is required to produce scientific evidence of the actual existence of a health risk justifying such measures. On the other hand, the available scientific knowledge may not always be sufficient for an objective and comprehensive assessment of the risk for human, animal or plant health. In that case, the SPS agreement allows for the adoption of provisional measures based on information available with regard to the concerned product or process; however, it is up to the member state itself to look for any additional information and review the adopted measure within a reasonable time lapse. Such a temporary measure can be taken, for example, as an emergency response to an outbreak suspected to originate from imported products. The SPS agreement explicitly recognizes international reference standards developed by organizations such as the FAO / WHO Codex Alimentarius, the Office International des Epizootie (also known as the World Animal Health Organization) and the organizations operating within the International Plant Protection Convention (IPPC).

The TRIPS agreement requires Member States to introduce minimum standards for the protection and enforcement of intellectual property rights such as patents, trademarks and industrial designs and geographical indications. In accordance with Article 7 of the Agreement, the objective is to contribute to the promotion of technological innovation and to the transfer and dissemination of technology and in a manner conducive to social and economic welfare, and to a balance of rights and obligations.

(TRIPS 1994, art. 7)

The health sector is specifically concerned with patents – in particular related to biomedical products and technologies – for which TRIPS establishes a protection period of 20 years from registration (art. 33), with consequent restrictions on access to those products during that period (see below). The TRIPS agreement, however, envisages significant exceptions such as the possibility of limiting the exclusive rights of the patent owner on the basis of public health considerations. In particular, Article 8 introduces "flexibilities" recognizing the right of WTO member countries to

adopt measures necessary to protect public health and nutrition, and to promote the public interest in sectors of vital importance to their socio-economic and technological development provided that such measures are consistent with the provisions of this Agreement.

(TRIPS 1994, art. 8)

To avoid abuse of the above-mentioned right and to grant some protection to patent holders, the Members can use patents without the authorization of the right holder only if

prior to such use, the proposed user has made efforts to obtain authorization from the right holder on reasonable commercial terms and conditions and that such efforts have not been successful within a reasonable period of time.

(TRIPS 1994, art. 31b)

However, "in the case of a national emergency or other circumstances of extreme urgency or in cases of public non-commercial use" even that condition could be waived; nevertheless, the right holder "shall be notified as soon as reasonably practicable" (TRIPS 1994, art. 31b).

The interpretation of the extent to which these "flexibilities" hold was clarified at the Doha Ministerial Conference in November 2001, when it was established that protection of patents under the TRIPS agreement "does not and should not prevent Members from taking measures to protect public health" (WTO 2001). The Doha Declaration identified specific measures that governments could adopt to address public health needs such as "compulsory licenses" and "parallel imports".

A compulsory license is issued by a government to allow the use of a patented invention, and thus the national manufacturing of a product, without the consent of the patent holder.

With parallel imports, a country can circumvent buying from the patent owner by importing the needed product from a third country where the product is marketed by the patent owner (or trademark- or copyright-owner, etc.) or with the patent owner's permission.

Regarding compulsory licensing, however, even when facing emergencies TRIPS authorized its use "predominantly for the supply of the domestic market of the Member authorizing such use" (TRIPS 1994, art. 31f). It immediately became clear that countries with insufficient pharmaceutical manufacturing capacities would not be able to invoke compulsory licensing. Thus, it was decided to waive the limitation in the TRIPS agreement to predominantly supply the local market (art. 31f), allowing countries that could not secure access to needed medicines at affordable prices to import these medicines from a third country where they could be produced by local drug makers under a compulsory license. This provision was integrated in a new Article 31bis of the TRIPS Agreement giving full legal effect to the system (an in-depth analysis of TRIPs and access to drugs is provided in Chapter 11).

The General Agreement on Trade in Services (GATS) aims to establish a multilateral framework of principles and rules for trade in services with a view to the expansion of this sector under conditions of transparency and progressive liberalization. GATS identifies four possible ways of trading in services:

Cross-border supply is defined to cover services flows from the territory of one Member into the territory of another Member (e.g. diagnostic, therapeutic and counseling services provided via telecommunications or mail, i.e. telemedicine, e-health);

Consumption abroad refers to situations where a service consumer moves into another Member's territory to obtain a service (e.g. medical tourism);

Commercial presence implies that a service supplier of one Member establishes a territorial presence, including through ownership or lease of premises, in another Member's territory to provide a service (e.g. domestic subsidiaries of foreign health insurance companies, or clinics);

Presence of natural persons consists of physical persons of one Member entering the territory of another Member to supply a service (e.g. doctors or nurses).

In the case of the GATS, WTO members can choose which sectors and sub-sectors to open up to trade and to international competition.[30]

It must be emphasized that "services supplied in the exercise of governmental authority", i.e. "any service which is supplied neither on a commercial basis, nor in competition with one or more service suppliers", are excluded from the GATS (GATS, art. I.3). Medical services offered free of charge by public facilities clearly fall into this category; thus GATS provisions do not apply.

Starting from the third year after their entry into force, governments may revise their schedule of commitments in relation to sectors and sub-sectors. However, in the case that changes may have consequences to the detriment of another country, the commercial partners of the country which has proposed the revision may request compensatory adjustments (GATS, art. XXI).

The GATS also stipulates that Member States may take all measures necessary to "protect human, animal or plant life or health" (GATS 1986: Art. XIV). As a general principle, "subject to the requirement that such measures are not applied in a manner which would constitute a means of arbitrary or unjustifiable discrimination between countries where like conditions prevail, or a disguised restriction on trade in services".

6.6.4 Interagency collaboration on intellectual property rights and health

As described above, WTO Agreements may influence health and health policies. Thus, interagency collaboration between WTO and WHO is very important. In 2002 the two organizations undertook a joint study to examine the linkages between trade and health policies, so as to enable both trade and health officials to better understand and monitor the effect of these linkages. The study covered areas such as drugs and intellectual property rights, food safety, tobacco and many other issues which have been subject to intense debate (WHO, WTO 2002).

The Doha Declaration on the TRIPS Agreement and Public Health of 2001, which promoted TRIPS as part of the wider action to address public health challenges and clarified a number of public health-related flexibilities, can also be considered the beginning of the trilateral cooperation between WHO, WTO and the World Intellectual Property Organization (WIPO). The Doha Declaration was also a point of reference in negotiations on the WHO Global Strategy and Plan of Action on Public Health, Innovation and Intellectual Property.[31]

Since 2009, collaboration among WHO, WIPO and WTO has intensified with a marked increase in the sharing of knowledge to ensure coherence of the policies at the interface between intellectual property and public health, as part of increasing international efforts to improve the ability of the world's poor to have access to medicines and to ensure the availability of new and more effective medicines. The above-mentioned WHO Global Strategy, the WIPO Development Agenda and the WTO Declaration on the TRIPS agreement and public health all provide the broader framework for the trilateral cooperation.[32]

The trilateral cooperation is intended to contribute to enhancing the empirical and factual information basis for policy-makers and supporting them in addressing public health in relation to IP and trade.

In this context, WIPO provides neutral and fact-based information and links its technical capacities, such as in the field of patent information or IP infrastructure, to the health policy dialogue. The aim is to contribute to a better understanding of the role of the IP system and to support an inclusive and informed debate on the benefits and limitations of the IP system in meeting public health challenges.

The joint WHO-WTO-WIPO commitment produced a number of trilateral symposia on relevant issues, such as: Access to Medicines Pricing and Procurement Policies (2010); Patent Information and Freedom to Operate (2011); Medical Innovation and Business Models (2013); Innovation and Access to Medical Technologies in Middle-Income Countries (2014); Public Health, Intellectual Property, and TRIPS (2015); Antimicrobial resistance, appropriate use of antibiotics, access and innovation (2016); and how innovative technologies can promote health-related SDGs (2018).[33]

In 2013, the three agencies published a trilateral study on "Promoting Access to Medical Technologies and Innovation: Intersections between public health, intellectual property and trade", focusing on advancing medical and health technologies while ensuring they reach the people who need them (WHO, WIPO, WTO 2013).

6.6.5 *Free trade agreements negotiated outside the WTO*

As already mentioned, as a consequence of the stalling of WTO negotiations, attention has shifted towards the formulation of regional arrangements such as the North America Free Trade Agreement (NAFTA), Free Trade Area of the Americas (FTAA) or the latest Trans-Pacific Partnership (TPP) and Transatlantic Trade on Investments Partnership (TTIP). These negotiations are opposed by many civil society organizations and some political forces for many reasons, including their possible adverse effects on health and health services. While there are numerous indirect indications of possible adverse effects, for sure there is no evidence of positive effects on health. Identifiable health risks are mainly related to the weakening of legislation on the protection of the

120 *Global governance and health*

environment, agriculture and the food chain, and hence the reduced ability to protect the health of citizens and consumers. Several authors have also reported the potential adverse effects of market liberalization on health services, including privatization of services, quality standards, increased cost of medication and increased health inequalities (Cattaneo 2014). Recent systematic reviews on the impact of free trade agreements show a common association between implementing regional trade agreements (RTAs) or related trade and investment policies and higher consumption of processed foods and sugar-sweetened beverages, higher prevalence of cardiovascular diseases and higher BMIs (Barlow *et al.* 2017). Clearly trade policy-makers and negotiators tend to be accountable to economic and trade ministries, which are in turn accountable to economic and business interests and tend not to appreciate the health consequences of trade and trade policies (Jarman 2017).

Currently the global trade agenda is under attack from multiple sides. Often concerns have been related to the secrecy of the negotiations or the potential of the agreement to damage individual rights to privacy. In addition, there have been concerns about reduced availability of generic medicines, as in the case of the Anti-Counterfeiting Trade Agreement (ACTA) signed by the EU (European Commission), the US and eight other countries, but later rejected by the European parliament. In other cases, ratification only followed after modifications were introduced to address criticisms, as in the case of the Canada-EU Comprehensive Economic Trade Agreement (CETA), ratified in late 2016. The TTIP negotiations between the EU and the US faced negative public opinion, "including concerns raised in Germany about food safety regulations and fears in the UK that the agreement would accelerate privatization within the National Health Service, and the talks stalled in 2016 after the UK's Brexit vote and seem unlikely to be restarted in their current form" (Jarman 2017). President Trump decided to withdraw the US from the Trans-Pacific Partnership (TPP), thus blocking the agreement. Thus, while the WTO multilateral system is stalled, the current generation of free trade agreements is also suffering. For those seeking to positively influence health policy it may be an opportunity to revise trade governance in a way that the next generation of trade agreements may benefit health, or at least avoid any foreseeable negative impact (Jarman 2017).

In Chapter 11 we provide more insights into the effects of trade liberalization policies on health by considering some specific areas.

Notes

1. A condition often referred as the "veto" power of the permanent members.
2. A full list of UN documents on health crisis can be found at www.securitycouncilreport.org/un-documents/health-crises/.
3. The question was "In view of the health and environmental effects, would the use of nuclear weapons by a State in war or other armed conflict be a breach of its obligations under international law including the WHO Constitution?". On 8 July 1996, the Court found that it was not able to give the advisory opinion requested by the World Health Assembly. Indeed, the Court concluded that the responsibilities of the WHO were necessarily restricted to the sphere of "public health" and could not encroach on the responsibilities of other parts of the United Nations system. Such issues as the use of force, the regulation of armaments and disarmament were within the competence of the United Nations Organization and lay outside that of the specialized agencies (ICJ 1996).
4. The Trusteeship Council suspended operation on 1 November 1994, after Palau, the last of the Trust Territories, became independent. By a resolution adopted on 25 May 1994, the

Council amended its rules of procedure to drop the obligation to meet annually and agreed to meet as occasion required – by its decision or the decision of its President, or at the request of a majority of its members or the General Assembly or the Security Council.
5 International organizations (inter-governmental institutions and international NGOs alike) usually have a "three-tiered" structure with a representative body (i.e. the Assembly), an executive body (i.e. the Board) and a bureaucratic/operational body (i.e. the Secretariat) (Missoni and Alesani 2014).
6 Formerly the United Nations Fund for Population Activities, it began operations in 1969 as the United Nations Fund for Population Activities (the name was changed in 1987) under the administration of the United Nations Development Fund. In 1971 it was placed under the authority of the United Nations General Assembly.
7 Since then the 7th of April hasd been celebrated as World Health Day.
8 The admission of associated members is upon "application made on behalf of such territory or group of territories by the Member or other authority having responsibility for their international relations" (Art. 8, WHO Constitution). In the case of territories whose independence has not been recognized by the corresponding Member State, the territory (who considers itself an independent state, and whose independence may have been recognized bilaterally by other Member States) cannot attend the WHA and cannot establish autonomous relations with WHO. This is for example the case of Taiwan, whose independence is not recognized by the People's Republic of China, which considers Taiwan one of its provinces.
9 The merging of pre-existing international health organizations represented one of the most difficult issues at the San Francisco Conference, and on which it was more difficult to find agreement. Led by the United States, an entire section of the Conference insisted on keeping the Pan American Organization separate and autonomous, in association with the WHO, for which it would serve as the Regional Committee for the Americas. This influenced WHO regionalization with the creation of regional organizations. In fact at that point, the newly established Arab League healthcare organization asked for the same conditions; as a consequence it was decided that "The Pan American Sanitary Organization [renamed Pan American Health Organization in 1958 – Ed.] represented by the Pan American Sanitary Bureau and the Pan American Sanitary Conferences, and all other inter-governmental regional health organizations in existence prior to the date of signature of this Constitution, shall in due course be integrated with the Organization" (WHO 2014). The current six WHO regions were identified at the first WHA, which decided that regional organization would be established as soon as the majority of the members of that area had agreed. Following this decision, all regional organizations were constituted between 1948 and 1951. Among the pre-existing organizations, only PAHO remained as an autonomous organization and thus signed an association agreement with the WHO in 1949.
10 The US previously provided up to 25% of the total funds, but in recent years has asked for a reduction of its mandatory contributions.
11 The Regulations were reviewed and renamed International Health Regulations (IHR) the first time in 1969, and again in 2005 after a decade-long negotiation. The new agreement entered into force in 2007 and is binding for all the 194 Member States. Besides the WHO Constitution, the IHR are, together with the Framework Convention on Tobacco Control, the only legally binding international provision in global health governance.
12 Lee was compelled to sanction and recall the WHO representative in Thailand, who had published an editorial in *The Bangkok Post* drawing attention to the negative aspects of the bilateral Free Trade Agreement between the USA and Thailand, and had to trade the US support for "3 by 5" with the softening of his stand toward the food industry in the Global Strategy on diet, physical activity and health.
13 Lee refused to enter into any negotiations with staff representatives and issued a letter to every WHO staff member worldwide threatening to sack the employees who took part in the action. However, he did not carry out his threat.

122 *Global governance and health*

14 Summarized in: Convening for better health; Generating evidence on health trends and determinants; Providing advice for health and development; Coordinating health security, and Strengthening health systems and institutions.
15 With the dollar value set to one thirty-fifth (1/35) of an ounce of gold.
16 Keynes' proposal, on the other hand, provided the creation of a reserve currency (the Bancor) administered by a central bank. The value of the Bancor would be tied to the six most important products traded on the international market, including oil, so that it could always reflect its real purchase value. The value of all national divisions would thus be based on the value of world currency. The strict control of the movement of capital would not have allowed the accumulation of surplus or deficit. On the contrary, Keynes believed that the free movement of goods and capital would inevitably lead to inequalities and instability.
17 Organization of the Petroleum Exporting Countries.
18 For a more extensive analysis of these events in relation to global health, see Chapter 4.
19 For a more detailed description of the instrument, see www.imf.org/en/About/Factsheets/Sheets/2016/08/01/14/51/Special-Drawing-Right-SDR.
20 Sanctions include the progressive application of the following measures: state's inability to make further use of Fund's resources; suspension of voting rights; compulsory withdrawal from the IMF.
21 The International Financial Society (IFC) was set up in 1956. It is the largest global development institution focused exclusively on the private sector; it provides financing investment, supports capital mobilization in international financial markets and provides advisory services to businesses and governments.

   The Multilateral Investment Guarantee Agency (MIGA) was set up in 1988 to encourage foreign investment in the developing countries, by providing to investors and lenders political risk insurance (guarantees) – normally not available on the market – against losses caused by non-commercial risks such as expropriation, non-convertibility of currencies and restrictions on financial transfers, as well as civil wars and conflicts.

   The International Centre for Settlement of Investment Disputes (ICSID) was set up in 1966 and provides international facilities for conciliation and arbitration of investment disputes.
22 World Bank (2017) Organization. www.worldbank.org/en/about/leadership.
23 By definition in a cooperative each member contributes equity capital, and shares in the control of the firm on the basis of the one member, one vote principle (and not in proportion to his or her equity contribution).
24 In addition to share votes, basic votes are distributed among member countries; however, these are calculated so that the sum of all basic votes is equal to 5.55% of the sum of basic votes and share votes for all members. Thus, basic votes do not make any difference in the weighted system.
25 The IMF also formally established its own Administrative Tribunal in1994.
26 These are interest-free loans, with 10 years of grace and last between 35 and 40 years.
27 www.worldbank.org/en/who-we-are.
28 On 7th January 2019 Jim Yong Kim announced he will resign effective 1st February, more than three years ahead of the expiration of his term 2002.
29 Also known as the Doha Development Round or Doha Development Agenda.
30 In November 2017 only 60 out of the 164 WTO Member States had made commitments in the field of "8. Health related and social services", including (A) Hospital services, (B) Other Human Health Services, (C) Social Services and (D) other. The category does *not* include services classified under "1. Business services", included in the commitment of 107 Member States, and which include (A) Professional Services, such as (h) Medical and dental services, (i) Veterinary services, (j) Services provided by midwives, nurses, physiotherapists and paramedical personnel (WTO-World Bank 2017).
31 www.who.int/phi/implementation/phi_globstat_action/en/.
32 www.wipo.int/policy/en/global_health/trilateral_cooperation.html.
33 www.wipo.int/meetings/en/topic.jsp?group_id=311.

References

Barlow, P., et al., 2017. The health impact of trade and investment agreements: a quantitative systematic review and network co-citation analysis. *Globalization and Health*, 13(1), 13. http://doi.org/10.1186/s12992-017-0240-x.

Benkimoun, P., 2006. How Lee Jong-wook changed WHO. *The Lancet*, 367, 1806–1808.

Braveman, P., Starfield, B., Geiger, H.J., 2001. World health report 2000: how it removes equity from the agenda for public health monitoring and policy. *BMJ,* 323, 678–681.

Brown, T.M., Cueto, M., Fee, E., 2006. The World Health Organization and the transition from international to global public health. *American Journal of Public Health*, 96(1), 62–72.

Brown, S.S., Sen, K., Decoster, K., 2013. The health systems funding platform and World Bank legacy: the gap between rhetoric and reality. *Globalization and Health*, 9, 9.

Brundtland, G.H., 1998. *Speech to the Fifty-first World Health Assembly*. Geneva: World Health Organization. 13 May.

Cassels, A., Smith, I., Burci, G.L., 2014. Reforming WHO: the art of the possible. *Public Health*, 128(2), 202–204.

Cattaneo, A., 2014. Trattati bilaterali di libero commercio e salute. *Sistema Salute*, 58 (4), 431–439.

Chan, M., 2006. *Speech to the World Health Assembly*. Geneva: World Health Organization, 9 November.

Chan, M., 2008. *Address to the Sixty-first World Health Assembly*. Geneva: World Health Organization, 21 May.

Chan, M., 2010. *Introductory remarks at an informal consultation on the future of financing for WHO*, 12 January. Available from: www.who.int/dg/speeches/2010/financing_who_20100112/en/index.html.

Chan, M., 2013. WHO Director-General addresses the Sixty-sixth World Health Assembly, 20 May. Available from: https://www.who.int/dg/speeches/2013/world_health_assembly_20130520/en/.

Chow, J.C., 2010. *Is the WHO Becoming Irrelevant?* Foreign Policy, December 8. Available from: http://foreignpolicy.com/2010/12/09/is-the-who-becoming-irrelevant/.

Cornia, G.A., Jolly, R., Stewart, F. (Eds.), 1987. *Adjustment with a Human Face: Protecting the Vulnerable and Promoting Growth*. New York: Oxford University Press.

CSOs, 2016. *Civil Society Statement on the World Health Organization's Proposed Framework of Engagement with Non-State Actors* (FENSA). 69th World Health Assembly, May. Available from:www.babymilkaction.org/wp-content/uploads/2016/05/Civil-Society-Statement-60.pdf.

CSDH, 2008. *Closing the gap in a generation. Health equity through action on the social determinants of health. Final report of the Commission on Social Determinants of Health.* Geneva: World Health Organization.

Deacon, B, Ollila, E., Koivusalo, M., Stubbs, P., 2003. *Global Social Governance. Themes and Prospects.* Helsinki: Ministry of Foreign Affairs of Finland, Hakapaino Oy.

Eccleston-Turner, M., McArdle, S., 2017. Accountability, international law and the World Health Organization: a need for reform? *Global Health Governance*, XI(1), 27–39.

ECOSOC, 1994. Resolution 1994/24. Joint and co-sponsored United Nations programme on human immunodeficiency virus/acquired immunodeficiency syndrome (HIV/AIDS. Economic and Social Council, 44th plenary meeting, 26 July.

FCTC, 2003. *Framework Convention on Tobacco Control*. Geneva: Word Health Organization.

FCTC, 2017. Parties to the WHO Framework Convention on Tobacco Control, Word Health Organization. Available from: www.who.int/fctc/signatories_parties/en/.

Flynn, P., 2010. The handling of the H1N1 pandemic: more transparency needed, Parliamentary Assembly, Council of Europe, Social, Health and Family Affairs Committee, AS/Soc (2010)12, 23 March.

Ford, N., Piedagnél, J., 2003. WHO must continue its work on access to medicines in developing countries. *The Lancet*, 361, 3.

GATTS, 1986. *General Agreement on Tariffs and Trade*. Geneva, July. Available from: www.wto.org/english/docs_e/legal_e/26-gats_01_e.htm.

Ghebreyesus, T.A., 2018. *Together for a healthier world. Vision statement by the Director General.* World Health Organization. Available from: www.who.int/dg/vision/en/.

Global Health Watch, 2005. *Global Health Watch 2005–2006. An alternative world health report*, London: Zed Books Ltd.

Global Health Watch 2014. *Global Health Watch 4. An alternative world health report.* London: Zed Books.

Godlee, F., 1994. The World Health Organization: the regions—too much power, too little effect. *BMJ*, 309(6968), 1566–1570.

Gostin, L.O., Friedman, E.A., 2014. Ebola: a crisis in global health leadership. *The Lancet*, 384, 1323–1325

Hafner, T., Shiffman, J., 2013. The emergence of global attention to health systems strengthening. *Health Policy and Planning*, 28(1), 41–50.

Hawkes, N., 2011. "Irrelevant" WHO outpaced by younger rivals. *BMJ*, 343, d5012. doi:10.1136/bmj.d5012.

Huang, Y., Meltzer, G., 2016. Who have been the best WHO Director-Generals? Council on Foreign Relations, 25 November. Available from: www.cfr.org/blog/who-have-been-best-who-director-generals.

ICJ, 1996. Legality of the Use by a State of Nuclear Weapons in Armed Conflict (Request for Advisory Opinion by the World Health Organization). Communiqué n.96/22. The Hague: International Court of Justice, 8 July.

IHR, 2008. *International Health Regulations (2005)* (2nd edn.). Geneva: World Health Organization.

IMF, 2018. About the IMF. Available from: www.imf.org/external/about.htm.

Jarman, H., 2017. Trade policy governance: what health policymakers and advocates need to know. *Health Policy*. http://doi.org/10.1016/j.healthpol.2017.09.002.

Lee, K., 2009. *The World Health Organization*. Abingdon: Routledge.

Loewenberg, S., 2015. Special report. The World Bank under Jim Kim. *The Lancet*, 386(9991), 324–327.

Megliani, M., 2001. L'Organizzazione delle Nazioni Unite. In Draetta, U., Fumagalli Meraviglia, M. (Eds.), *Il diritto delle organizzazioni internazionali. Parte speciale*. Milan: Giuffré.

Missoni, E., 2006. *Critical analysis of WHO's role in promoting health*. Presented at the International Conference "The Ottawa and Bangkok Charters: from principles to action", SIASS, Firenze, 21–23 November.

Missoni, E., 2011. WHO reform: threats and opportunities. A healthier political functioning. *Bulletin of Medicus Mundi Switzerland*, 122, December.

Missoni, E., Alesani, D., 2014. *Management of International Institutions and NGOs. Framework, Practices and Challenges*. Abingdon: Routledge.

Motchane, J.L., 2002. Health for all or riches for some: WHO's responsible? *Le Monde diplomatique*, July.

Narlikar, A., 2005) *The World Trade Organization. A Very Short Introduction*. Oxford: Oxford University Press.

PHM, 2011. People's Health Movement. Comments on The future of financing for WHO. 64th World Health Assembly. Available from: www.ghwatch.org/who-watch/WHA64/PHM-Statement.

Richardson, J., Wildman, J., Robertson, I.K., 2001. A critique of the World Health Organisation's evaluation of health system performance. *Health Economics*, 12, 355–366.

Ruger, J.P. 2005. The changing role of the World Bank in global health. *American Journal of Public Health*, 95(1), 60–70.

Saloojee, Y., Dagli, E., 2000. Tobacco industry tactics for resisting public policy on health. *Bulletin of the World Health Organization*, 78(7), 902–910.

Sridhar, D., Winters, J., Strong, E., 2017. World Bank's financing, priorities, and lending structures for global health. *BMJ*, 358, j3339–4. http://doi.org/10.1136/bmj.j3339.

Smith, R., 1995. The WHO: change or die. *BMJ*, 310, 543–544.

Tichenor, M., Sridhar, D., 2017. Universal health coverage, health systems strengthening, and the World Bank. *BMJ*, j3347–5. http://doi.org/10.1136/bmj.j3347.
TRIPS, 2017. *Trade-Related Aspects of Intellectual Property Rights*. Annex 1C of the Marrakesh Agreement Establishing the World Trade Organization, signed in Marrakesh, Morocco, on 15 April 1994 (as amended on 23 January 2017). Available from: www.wto.org/english/docs_e/legal_e/31bis_trips_e.pdf. .
UN, 1945. *Charter of the United Nations*. Available from: www.un.org/en/charter-united-nations/index.html.
UN, 2000. Security Council, Resolution 1308, 17 July.
UN, 2011. Security Council, Resolution 1983, 7 June.
UN, 2014. Security Council, Resolution 2177, 18 September.
UN, 2018. Repositioning of the United Nations development system in the context of the quadrennial comprehensive policy review of operational activities for development of the United Nations system. Resolution adopted by the General Assembly on 31 May 2018. A/RES/72/279, 1 June.
UN, 2018a. Political declaration of the third high-level meeting of the General Assembly on the prevention and control of non-communicable diseases. Seventy-third session. Agenda item 119. Follow-up to the outcome of the Millennium Summit. A/73/L.2, 3 October.
UNAIDS, 2008. UNAIDS – The First Ten Years. Geneva: UNAIDS.
UNFPA, 2017. United Nations Population Fund. Available from: www.unfpa.org/about-us.
Walt, G., 1994. *Health Policy. An Introduction to Process and Power*. London: Zed Books.
Walt, G., 2004. WHO's World Health Report 2003. Shaping the future depends on strengthening health systems. *BMJ*, 328, 6.
WHO, 1986. The Ottawa Charter for Health Promotion. First International Conference on Health Promotion, Ottawa, 21 November 1986. Available from: www.who.int/healthpromotion/conferences/previous/ottawa/en/.
WHO, 2000. *World Health Report 2000*. Geneva: World Health Organization.
WHO, 2001. *Macroeconomics and Health: Investing in Health for Economic Development. Report of the Commission on Macroeconomics and Health*, chaired by Jeffrey D. Sachs. Geneva: World Health Organization.
WHO, 2004. *International migration of health personnel: a challenge for health systems in developing countries*. Fifty-seventh World health Assembly, A/57.19, 22 May. Geneva: World Health Organization.
WHO, 2008. *Financial Report and Audited Financial Statements for the period 1 January 2006–31 December 2007*, A61/20, 28 March. Geneva: World Health Organization.
WHO, 2008a. *World Health Report 2008. Primary Health Care. Now more than ever.* Geneva: World Health Organization.
WHO, 2010. *WHO Global Code of Practice on the International Recruitment of Health Personnel*. Sixty-third World Health Assembly. Agenda item 11.5, A63/16, 21 May. Geneva: World Health Organization.
WHO, 2011. *WHO. Voluntary Contributions by fund and by donor for the year ended 31 December 2010*. Sixty-fourth World Health Assembly. Provisional agenda item 17.1, A64/29 Add.1, 7 April. Geneva: World Health Organization.
WHO, 2011a. *WHO. Status of collection of assessed contributions, including Member States in arrears in the payment of their contributions to an extent that would justify invoking Article 7 of the Constitution. Report by the Secretariat*. Sixty-fourth World Health Assembly, A64/31, 21 April. Geneva: World Health Organization.
WHO, 2011b. *WHO. The future of financing for WHO. World Health Organization: reforms for a healthy future. Report by the Director-General*. Sixty-fourth World Health Assembly. A64/4 Provisional Agenda Item 11, 5 May. Geneva: World Health Organization.
WHO, 2014. Constitution of the World Health Organization. In *Basic Documents* (48th edn.). Geneva: World Health Organization.

WHO, 2016. *Framework of engagement with non-State actors.* 69th World Health Assembly WHA69.10 Agenda item 11.3, 28 May. Geneva: World Health Organization.

WHO, 2017. WHO's work with the United Nations. Prevention and control of noncommunicable diseases in the UN. Available from: http://www.who.int/un-collaboration/health/unga-ncds/en/.

WHO, 2017a. Commission on Social Determinants of Health, 2005–2008. World Health Organization. Available from: www.who.int/social_determinants/thecommission/en/.

WHO, 2017b. *Overview of WHO reform implementation. Report by the Director-General.* 70th World Health Assembly, A70/50 Provisional agenda item 23.1, 24 April. Geneva: World Health Organization.

WHO, 2017c. *Overview of WHO reform implementation. Leadership and management at WHO: evaluation of WHO reform, third stage.* 70th World Health Assembly, A70/50 Add.1 Provisional agenda item 23.1, 15 May. Geneva: World Health Organization.

WHO, WIPO, WTO, 2013. *Promoting Access to Medical Technologies and Innovation. Intersections between public health, intellectual property and trade.* Geneva: World Health Organization, World Intellectual Property Organization.

WHO, WTO, 2002. WTO *Agreements and public health. A joint study by the WHO and the WTO Secretariat.* World Health Organization-World Trade Organization: Geneva.

Williams A., 2001. Science or marketing at WHO? A commentary on 'World Health 2000'. *Health Economics,* 10: 93–100.

Wolfensohn J., 2000. Foreword. In Granzow S. (Ed.), *Our Dream: A World Free of Poverty.* Oxford: Oxford University Press.

World Bank, 1997. *Sector Strategy. Health, Nutrition, & Population.* The Human Development Network. Washington DC: The World Bank Group.

World Bank, 2001. *World Bank Group. Strategic Framework*, January 24.

World Bank, 2007. *Healthy development. The World Bank strategy for health, nutrition, & population results.* Washington DC: The World Bank.

World Bank, 2017. Health/Overview/Strategy. Last updated 19 June 2017. Available from: www.worldbank.org/en/topic/health/overview#2.

WTO, 2001. *Declaration on the TRIPS agreement and public health.* Adopted on 14 November 2001, Doha WTO Ministerial 2001: TRIPS. WT/MIN(01)/DEC/2 20 November. Available from: www.wto.org/english/thewto_e/minist_e/min01_e/mindecl_trips_e.htm.

WTO, 2017. *What is the WTO.* Available from: www.wto.org/english/thewto_e/whatis_e/whatis_e.htm.

Zeltner, T., Kessler, A.A., Martiny, A., Randera, F., 2000. *Tobacco Industry Strategies to Undermine Tobacco Control Activities at the World Health Organization.* WHO Committee of Experts. Geneva: World Health Organization, July.

Unless otherwise indicated, all websites were accessed on 9 August 2018.

7 Governments and their groupings

7.1 Introduction

Most economically advanced countries allocate a fraction (0.1–1%) of their gross national income (GNI) to Official Development Assistance (see Chapter 13) – hence, they are referred to as "donors". About 10% of the donated amount is channeled towards health. In the Dodgson and collaborators' global health governance map, one country was indisputably predominant: the United States of America (Dodgson *et al.* 2002). It can be argued that over the last decades important changes affected geopolitical equilibriums, modifying that single supremacy; however, these changes have not seemed to significantly influence global health governance.

As one example, in 2010 the People's Republic of China surpassed Japan and Germany in economic terms (i.e. GDP), becoming the second economy behind the United States;[1] yet, its GDP per capita still ranks among middle-income countries. In terms of the volume of the Official Development Assistance in Health (ODAH), several countries are still more influential than China, whose ODAH was calculated at 5.7 billion dollars in 2013, a level comparable to that of Australia that year (IHME 2017; Shajalal *et al.* 2017).[2]

Between 2000 and 2016, the United States allocated 148.8 billion dollars for ODAH – more than any other country by far, followed by the United Kingdom (38.5 billion), Germany (17.3 billion), France (16 billion), Japan (15.8 billion), Canada (12.6 billion), the Netherlands (10.6 billion), Norway (9,6 billion), Sweden (8.4 billion) and Australia (7.1 billion). In that period the sum of the funds allocated to ODAH from all national treasuries combined reached 326.7 billion dollars (IHME 2017).

Bilateral relations undoubtedly play a role in the field of global health governance. The largest amounts of resources budgeted as "global health" flow along the bilateral channel, including both operations and research. The United States is the most significant donor for Development Assistance for Health (DAH); its President's Emergency Plan for AIDS Relief (PEPFAR) launched in 2003 was the largest commitment ever by a single nation toward an international health initiative and represented 70% of all actors' resources for the fight against the disease. It has been argued that the program was designed primarily to serve US domestic interests and that "the US involvement in global health generally is motivated as much or more by concerns to protect national interest (or regime interest) than by humanitarian, human rights or security objectives" (MacLean and Brown 2009). The priority given to domestic interests obviously might also apply to many (if not all) other countries.

Analyzing the UK's engagement in global health, Herrick (2017) concluded that there is a clear trade-off between the achievement of results through targeting aid and programs to those countries which will deliver the best return on investment and those countries and regions of greatest need, thus highlighting "the strategic nature of the geopolitics underpinning the UK's global health investment" (Herrick 2017).

However, it is thought that the USA and the UK, the largest global health funders, might reduce their political and financial commitments, preferring to invest nationally, whereas Germany's global health contribution (both political and financial) is expected to grow in both the multilateral and the bilateral arena (Kickbusch et al. 2017).

The WHO formally remains the main multilateral forum for the determination of global policies in the health sector. Hence, it is not surprising that the funding of that organization, especially through earmarked voluntary contributions, represents a strategic factor in that context.

The UK, for example, thanks to generous voluntary contributions, is the second largest member state contributor to the WHO after the US (through both mandatory/ assessed and voluntary contributions). Therefore, the UK wields an influence on the processes and decisions of the WHO greater than Japan or Germany, whose economies, and therefore their assessed contributions to the WHO, are larger than those of the UK. Countries such as Norway or Sweden whose assessed contributions have a much lower economic weight on WHO's total budget show a strategic vision in global health and in the relationship with WHO by choosing to contribute to the organization with proportionally much higher voluntary contributions than all other member states. This increases the weight of those countries in the interaction with WHO, again surpassing much larger economies such as Japan or Germany (WHO 2017). Member states' overall financial contributions also have implications in the geographic distribution of WHO's technical and managerial staff, which according to the rule should mirror by 45% the amount of member states' contribution, another 45% should be equally distributed among member states and 10% according to their population. In practice, other factors certainly play a role in the geographic representation of WHO staff (see Figure 7.1) (WHO 2014).

Clearly, governments exercise political and economic influence on global health and its determinants through many other channels and domains of global governance, at both the multilateral and bilateral levels, including political and economic forums (summits, conferences, ad hoc meetings, etc.). Indeed, national policies in global health have recently been defined as policies that connect "a country's work on global health across more than one government policy sector, in which the health sector may not have a leading implementation role, with the aim to act in and on the global health governance system" (Jones et al. 2017).

Some of the issues influenced by policies decided in other sectors (such as trade and the environment) will be further analyzed in Chapter 11.

Finally, certain countries have joined on the basis of common socioeconomic characteristics or interests into more or less informal groups that have often included health issues in their wider agenda.

7.2 Groups of most influential countries: G8, G20 and BRICS

In addition to the role individual countries play within international institutions, where voting rights are sometimes weighted in consideration of their economic weight (this is

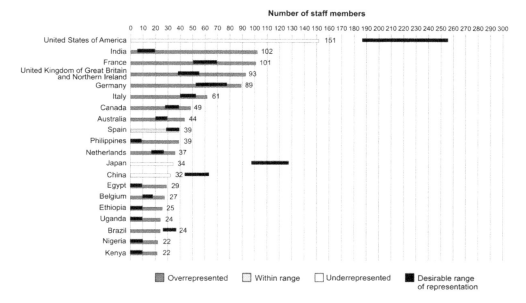

Figure 7.1 WHO Member States with the highest representation in the professional and higher categories.
Source: WHO, 2014. Human resources: annual report. Report by the Secretariat. Sixty-Seventh World Health Assembly A67/47.

specially the case for International Financial Institutions), over the years more or less informal groups have emerged. These new groupings have substantially changed global governance dynamics.

Here we will examine in particular the "Group of the big eight" (G8), the emerging role of the G20, and the BRICS (Brazil, Russia, India, China and South Africa)[3].

7.2.1 The G7/G8

7.2.1.1 The origins

The "Group of Eight" (G8) is an informal forum for consultation on major international economic and political issues, among the heads of the seven most industrialized countries in the world (Canada, France, Germany, Japan, UK, Italy and the United States) (G7), plus Russia (which joined in 1992, but only in relation to the political agenda). The President of the European Commission is also invited to participate in the forum.

The first meeting of the G6 was held in Rambouillet, France, in November 1975. Canada joined the following year at the San Juan summit in Puerto Rico, while the European Commission joined for the London assembly in 1977. The Soviet Union and then Russia have been involved in post-summit meetings since 1991. Since the 1994 summit (Naples, Italy), the G7 integrated Russia at each meeting constituting the so-called P8 (Political 8), but the lengthy process of its integration in the group was only completed in 2006, when Russia hosted the summit in St. Petersburg. However, in 2014 when Russia was again about to host the summit, as a result of the Russian role in the

130 *Global governance and health*

political crisis in Crimea (Ukraine) the other members of the group decided to meet in Brussels without Russia, and Russia was subsequently suspended from the group.

7.2.1.2 Structure and functions

The G7/G8 has maintained its informal character and has no secretariat, nor does it have formal rules and procedures. The presidency rotates yearly among the seven members, and is maintained for the entire calendar year. The country hosting the summit sets the agenda, acts as the group's spokesperson during that year, coordinates the working groups and accounts for the involvement of international institutions and non-state actors.

In preparation for each summit, the personal leaders' representatives – the so-called *sherpas*[4] – meet periodically for the development and the verification of the agenda. Numerous ministerial meetings are planned too (with ministers of finance, of the environment and of foreign affairs), where the subjects of specific competencies are examined in more depth. Occasionally the group sets up task forces or expert working groups on issues they consider of special relevance.

The G7/G8 summits have mainly been devoted to macroeconomic issues, international trade and relations with developing countries, as well as to issues related to economic relations between East and West, energy issues and terrorism. Since its foundation the agenda has extended considerably to issues such as employment, environment, international crime, aspects related to human rights and security, and – with increasing attention – health. The summit indirectly but powerfully influences the international community, its priorities and focus and in some cases launches its own initiatives.

The media give considerable attention to the G7/G8 summits, which over the years have become an opportunity for civil society organizations to attract public attention to the most relevant issues. Unfortunately, on many occasions peaceful demonstrations have developed into violent clashes, which reached dramatic levels during the Genoa G8 in 2001.

7.2.1.3 The influence on global health policies

Given the informal nature of the group, the G8's influence on the global agenda mainly depends on the issues on the summit's agenda, and on the strength and continuity with which the related initiatives are then sustained over time, in the broader context of their political objectives (Harman 2012).

Health was first included in the G8 agenda in 1996, in the Lyon summit. On that occasion health was instrumental in advocating an increase in public aid development, as some health indicators, such as maternal and child mortality, were proposed as a measure of progress towards more general goals. In Denver (1997), specific reference was made to infectious diseases (HIV/AIDS, malaria and tuberculosis) and specifically to the need to strengthen disease surveillance systems and support the development of a vaccine against HIV. In 1998, the Birmingham G8 communiqué mentioned the WHO Roll Back Malaria program and stressed the need to consider health in the broader context of development. Regarding HIV/AIDS, support for vaccine development was reiterated, together with a new emphasis on preventive programs, on the need to develop appropriate therapies and on the call for increased support to UNAIDS. In Cologne, in

1999, the focus shifted to debt relief. This would free resources to be invested in poverty reduction policies addressing social and health needs.

Health has become more relevant in the G7/G8's agenda since the 2000 summit held in Okinawa, which "marked a turning point both for the governance of global health and for the G8 in regards to the shift from providing financial support for the UN agencies to the creation of new institutional arrangements to channel and spend money" (Harman 2012: 69).

At Okinawa the final communiqué stated: "Good health contributes directly to economic growth whilst poor health drives poverty" (G8 2000). Clearly the accent was on the economic goal, rather than on health as a priority in itself, indicating a systems view in search of a response strategy:

> Only through sustained action and coherent international co-operation to fully mobilize new and existing medical, technical and financial resources, can we strengthen health delivery systems and reach beyond traditional approaches to break the vicious cycle of disease and poverty.
>
> (G8 2000)

However, in the following lines the communiqué contradicted the systemic approach, turning its attention to disease control, specifically of HIV/AIDS, malaria and tuberculosis, due to the negative impact of those diseases on the economic development of affected countries. The G8 committed to work on "strengthened" partnership with "governments, the World Health Organization (WHO) and other international organizations, industry (notably pharmaceutical companies), academic institutions, NGOs and other relevant actors in civil society" (G8 2000) to reduce by 2010 the number of HIV-positive people, tuberculosis mortality and prevalence, and the incidence of malaria.[5] The proposed partnership aimed at mobilizing additional resources, prioritizing the development of equitable and effective health systems, expanded immunization, nutrition and micro-nutrients and the prevention and treatment of infectious diseases, promoting political leadership, supporting innovative partnerships, including with NGOs, the private sector and multilateral organizations, working to make existing cost-effective treatments and preventive measures more universally available and affordable in developing countries, addressing access to medicines in developing countries, and assessing obstacles being faced by developing countries in that regard, and strengthening cooperation in the area of basic research and development on new drugs, vaccines and other international public health goods. A conference would be convened later that year in Japan to agree on a new strategy and define the operations of the "new partnership", progress would be assessed the following year at the Genoa Summit, and the G8 would work with the UN to organize in 2001 a conference on strategies to facilitate access to AIDS treatment and care (G8 2000).

An indefinite idea of partnership – fluctuating between a generic concept of shared commitment on common objectives, and one or more specific future joint ventures between actors with very different interests – was now part of the G8 agenda (Berlinguer and Missoni 2001).

At the beginning of the following year, in preparation for the Genoa summit, the Italian G8 Presidency circulated a technical proposal with a comprehensive health agenda. A few months later, arguably under the influence of the financial ministers, the agenda was first narrowed to the creation of a "Genoa Trust Fund for health care" (G8

132 *Global governance and health*

Presidency 2001), and then further modified to give birth to the "Global Fund to Fight AIDS, Tuberculosis and Malaria" at the Genoa Summit in July, thus perpetuating the tendency towards disease-oriented selective approaches (Missoni 2004) (see Chapter 4, Box 4.3).

In the following years the G8 summits' communiqué almost regularly included a section dedicated to health. The group's support of the Global Fund and call for its long-term funding were repeatedly reiterated, and additional issues were addressed, on some occasions launching new initiatives and financial mechanisms for health. In Kanasnakis (Canada) renewed commitment for the fight against AIDS in Africa was expressed in the context of the G8's support of the New Partnership for Africa's Development (NEPAD) and a call was made for additional efforts to eradicate polio by 2005.

In Evian (France) in June 2003, a G8 Health Action Plan was issued. It included themes such as improved access to health services in poor countries (including medicines at affordable prices), vaccine development and the mobilization of new funds for polio eradication. Inspired by the recent SARS outbreak, the G8 also made a call for international cooperation in response to epidemics.

In 2004, at the Sea Island summit (USA), a call was made to fill the financial gap toward the eradication of polio, and support was expressed for the establishment of a global HIV vaccine company, namely "a consortium to accelerate the development of an HIV vaccine, globally improving coordination, sharing of information and collaboration" (Klausner and Fauci 2003).

In 2005, in Gleneagles (UK), "building on the valuable G8 Global HIV/AIDS vaccine enterprise", the group committed to take forward work

> on market incentives, as a complement to basic research, through such mechanisms as Public Private Partnerships and Advance Purchase Commitments to encourage development of vaccines, microbicides and drugs for AIDS, malaria, tuberculosis and other neglected diseases.
>
> (G8 2005)

Among the proposed mechanisms there was the International Finance Facility (IFF), based on British experience and announced the previous year as a joint UK and France commitment. The initiative was joined in 2005 by Italy, Spain and Sweden with an initial total commitment of nearly US$ 4 billion to support and scale up the work of GAVI (IFFIm 2018). At the G8 meeting in the UK, the Italian Minister of Economy and Finance presented the Advanced Market Commitments for Vaccines as a new tool in the fight against disease (Cali and Missoni 2014). In Gleneagles the agreement was also reached to write off the entire external debt owed by 18 highly indebted poor countries to the World Bank, the International Monetary Fund and the African Development Fund. The measure would ostensibly save 10 million lives a year, and ensure access to free primary health care for all and promote universal access to AIDS treatment by 2010.

In 2006, in St. Petersburg (Russia), the emphasis was once again on infectious diseases. The group was concerned with a pandemic of human and avian influenza and the possible impact on world economy, and called for support for the WHO Global Outbreak Alert and Response Network. Other issues were also mentioned such as access to health services, health systems' weakness, lack of resources and the emigration of qualified health workers (G8 2006).

In 2007, in Heiligendamm (Germany), focus was on supporting "growth and responsibility" in Africa. The fight against HIV/AIDS, tuberculosis and malaria was framed in the context of renewed commitment to develop fair and sustainable mechanisms for the financing of healthcare systems, according to principles of the Paris Declaration on Aid Effectiveness (OECD/DAC 2005). At the summit the first G8 Health Review was presented on the group's commitments and achievements.

In 2008 – 30 years after the Alma Ata Declaration – the attention was focused again on health systems' functioning and the importance of primary health care (WHO 2008). The Toyako Framework for Action, a report prepared by G8 health experts and integrated into the Leaders' Declaration (G8 2008), highlighted the need for strengthening of health systems to comprehensively address health challenges, whereby disease-specific approaches and strengthening of health systems should be mutually reinforcing, focused on a human security perspective based on protection and empowerment of individuals and communities, and advocated a longer-term perspective extending beyond the 2015 MDGs' deadline as well as the effective utilization of resources consistent with the principles of the Paris Declaration on aid effectiveness (G8 Health Experts 2008; Reich and Takemi 2009).

In continuity with that renewed attention, the following year, in L'Aquila (Italy) the G8 proposed "an integral and integrated approach for the achievement of the Millennium goals related to health, universal health services access, with particular regard to PHC" and recognized "health as an objective of all policies" (G8 2009; Missoni 2009).

A new initiative was launched the following year in Canada. The Muskoka Initiative, named after the town where the summit took place, committed new funding to contributing to the reduction of maternal, neonatal and child mortality in developing countries (5 billion US dollars, to be disbursed by 2015) (G8 2010). While the G8 had recognized the need to verify and report progress since 2006, only in 2009 did they decide to adopt a specific monitoring mechanism. An accountability report on G8 Commitments to Health and Food Security reporting the state of delivery and results with regard to health and nutritional initiatives was presented the following year at the Deauville meeting in France (G8 2011).

In 2012 in Camp David (USA) the agenda included the protection of intellectual property for pharmaceutical products and the fight against counterfeiting. In 2013 in Lough Erne (UK) the G8 stated its support for the New Alliance for Food Security and Nutrition, a public-private alliance jointly launched the year before by the United States, the African Union Commission and the World Economic Forum (WEF),[6] as well as for the Global Nutrition for Growth Compact – another alliance initiated by the governments of the United Kingdom and Brazil and the British Children Investment Fund Foundation.

The 2014 summit was planned to be held in Russia; however, as a result of the Russian interference in the political crisis in Crimea (Ukraine), Russia was left out and the G7 met in Brussels (Belgium). The summit was also marked by the dramatic spread of the Ebola epidemic, which led the G7 to reaffirm the importance of the WHO International Health Regulations (IHR), and to declare their commitment to support its implementation in affected African countries, including through the Global Health Security Agenda, an initiative launched by the United States Department of Health, and other multilateral initiatives (G7 2014).

In 2015 The G7 Summit held in Elmau (Germany) echoed the full global agenda of that year: the UN Climate Conference in Paris COP 21, the UN summit in New York to set the future universal global sustainable development post-2015 agenda, and the Third International Conference on Financing for Development in Addis Ababa to support the implementation of that agenda. Although almost under control, the Ebola epidemic was still high on the health agenda at the Elmau summit, and was one of the three sections about health in the final declaration, together with concerns about resistance to antibiotics, and "neglected tropical diseases". As on previous occasions, the statement was also used to express support for a number of initiatives launched by institutional actors external to the group, such as the new public-private partnership called the Global Financing Facility for every woman and every child, proposed during the 69th session of the UN General Assembly in September that year and with the purpose of raising funds on the financial market, as well as the World Bank's development of a Pandemic Emergency Financing Facility (G7 2015).

The G7 summit held in Ise-Shima (Japan) was the first after the historic adoption of the 2030 Agenda, and the G7 declared itself to be "fully committed to implementing the health-related Sustainable Development Goals (SDGs)". Three specific areas of commitment were identified in the annex G7 Ise-Shima Vision for Global Health recalled in the declaration: (a) reinforcing of the Global Health Architecture to strengthen response to public health emergencies, specifically reaffirming "the WHO's central role in that architecture"; (b) attaining of UHC with strong health systems and better preparedness, emphasizing "the need for a strengthened international framework to coordinate the efforts and expertise of all relevant stakeholders [...] including disease-specific efforts"; and (c) antimicrobial resistance (AMR), with a commitment "to make collective efforts for strengthening and actively implementing a multi-sectoral One Health Approach, taking into account the sectors including human and animal health, agriculture, food and the environment" (G7 2016).

In 2017, in Taormina (Italy), the G7 leaders' final communiqué devoted only the last and very generic paragraph to health (G7 2017), leaving it to G7 Health Ministers to follow up in a later meeting that year. That meeting mostly reiterated generic commitments and support for external initiatives. Remarkably, in line with the One Health Approach outlined in Ise-Shima the previous year, a new intersectoral perspective was emerging. Challenges to global health were identified beyond the healthcare and the health sector "including conflict and crisis, social inequalities, rapid globalization and urbanization, environmental-related factors, and increased movement or displacement of people" (G7 Health Ministers 2017). Environmental factors, gender perspectives in health policies and antimicrobial resistance received special attention. The intention of the United States to exercise its right to withdraw from the Paris Agreement (COP 21) was acknowledged and opposed by the "strong commitment" of all the other partners to swiftly implement it (G7 Health Ministers 2017).

As shown, the G7/G8 has played and continues to play an important role in promoting the inclusion of specific issues in the global health agenda.

> Issues of global health have been effectively snowballed within the G8's wider agenda, from basic importance within the summit communiqués, to commitments to pre-existing UN agencies, to the formation and support for institutions independent of the UN.
>
> (Harman 2012: 70)

Indeed, in some cases the summits were an opportunity to launch the constitution of new organizations, as in the paradigmatic case of the Global Fund to Fight AIDS, Tuberculosis and Malaria, but much more often they provided support for specific initiatives, especially if proposed by the hosting country, or other multilateral institutions and public-private organizations.

Despite some effort in following through with the commitments made, several authors still point out an excess of rhetoric and a lack of transparency and true accountability (Buse 2015). Some have claimed that often the "new" funds earmarked to cope with global health issues are "recycled forms of debt relief" (Harman 2012: 70). Despite a certain weight placed in recent years in support of health systems, the focus has mostly been on specific themes and vertical initiatives, excluding fundamental issues such as those linked to the socioeconomic determinants of health (Harman 2012), a trend that may change with the One Health Approach introduced in 2016.

An additional criticism of the G8 has been that health came onto the G8 agenda at a time of harsh criticism of the group, and the inclusion of health has been key to the repositioning the G8 as a "forum for discussion as to how to solve the world's common problems". These authors suggest that "health is not fundamental to the G8's agenda", and will always remain in the background of the group's focus on the global political economy (Harman 2012).

7.2.2 The G20

The first meeting of financial ministers and bank governors of the 19 countries with the largest economies plus the European Union took place in December 1999 in Berlin (Germany) in response to the financial crisis originating in Asia, but which had already hit the Western countries. Since then the G20 system, which includes 80% of the world's economy and two-thirds of the world's population, has grown rapidly, expanding its working agenda to include security issues, corruption, good governance and use of chemical weapons in Syria (in 2013). As a consequence of the 2007–2008 financial crisis the G20, attended by heads of government during this year, considerably expanded its horizons by discussing several other global governance issues.

In Brisbane (Australia) in 2014, the response to the Ebola virus outbreak was included in the G20 agenda. The issue was mentioned in the final official statement, while, in a separate statement on social, humanitarian and economic impacts of the epidemic, support was expressed for the work of WHO and an appeal was made to governments and international financial institutions to provide assistance. The statement also stressed the importance of the strengthening of healthcare systems to improve their capacity to respond to epidemics. That single-page document contained specific, measurable, politically binding and long-term commitments (concerned with the prevention of future crises rather than just with the containment of the ongoing one) rarely seen previously in the relevant documents of the G7/G8 summits. Some authors argued that this approach could indicate that the G20 were ready to play a direct role in the global health landscape (Kirton 2014). Nevertheless health was still mentioned as a determinant of the global economic scenario, as two years later, when in their 2016 "G20 Action Plan on the 2030 Agenda for Sustainable Development", the G20 summit recognized health as a "necessary component for socio-economic stability" and "a key aspect of sustainable development". Significantly, it asserted the "need for an improved and coordinated approach to strengthening health systems, thereby contributing to universal health coverage" (G20

2016). In 2017, under the Germany G20 presidency, health received higher attention. For the first time, a G20 Health Ministers' Meeting was held and new emphasis was put on moving towards universal health coverage. The Hamburg Update of the G20 Action Plan included a number of "concrete collective actions" of the group. With reference to the SDG3, three areas were mentioned: support the leadership and coordination of WHO for health crises management, in line with the countries' obligations under the International Health Regulations; contribute to health systems strengthening with the aim to develop resilient health systems; and the implementation of National Action Plans against Antimicrobial Resistance applying the One Health approach, introduced the previous year at the G7 summit (G20 2017). Despite this, the emphasis remains on the response to epidemics and ability to control the spread of infectious diseases, while a comprehensive approach to health still appears to be lacking.

7.2.3 The BRICS

The BRICS nations (Brazil, Russia, India, China and South Africa) are part of the G20; however, this group of countries has an autonomous role and a different profile. Their financial contribution to global health was estimated at around a total of 5.6 billion US dollars in 2010 (Fan *et al.* 2014; Blanchet *et al.* 2014). Undoubtedly the BRICS have attempted to build strategic coordination in areas of global governance. In health they have been looking for some level of coordinated strategic relationship with the WHO (Gautier *et al.* 2014; Acharya *et al.* 2014). On the other hand, even if the Ministers of Health of these five countries now regularly meet to share vision and concerns, their joint statements and communiqués do not seem to have a great impact on influencing global health policies and it is still unclear whether the BRICS share sufficient problems and interests to lead a coherent collective action. Gill and Benatar (2017) openly dismiss "the idea that [the BRICS] are significantly influencing global health as a unified political bloc, despite evidence of some cooperation on finance and in health, with one or two BRICS countries supporting specific health initiatives".

Although a group of countries with growing economic weight may play a greater role in the field of macroeconomic policies, it is not immediately clear why this would also translate into a leading role in health policies (McKee *et al.* 2014).

Synthesizing the role of major economies and their groupings, one can agree with Gill and Benatar's (2017) remark that "global governance frameworks are still dominated by the wealthier sections of society and the ruling strata of the United States and its G-7 allies, in a framework that now incorporates their counterparts in the G-20, including the BRICS, which do not threaten the frameworks of market-based neoliberal governance".

Notes

1 http://data.worldbank.org/data-catalog/GDP-ranking-table.
2 At the 2018 Seventh Forum on China-Africa Cooperation (FOCAC), the Chinese President Xi Jinping pledged a new aid plan for US$ 60 billion. In that context China pledged to launch a healthcare initiative with the decision "to upgrade 50 medical and health aid programs for Africa, particularly flagship projects such as the headquarters of the African Center for Disease Control and Prevention and China-Africa Friendship Hospitals. Exchange and information cooperation will be carried out on public health. Cooperation programs will be launched on

the prevention and control of emerging and re-emerging communicable diseases, schistosomiasis, HIV/AIDS and malaria. China will train more medical specialists for Africa and continue to send medical teams that better meet Africa's needs. More mobile medical services will be provided to patients for the treatment of cataract, heart disease and dental defects". The Chinese plan is made particularly attractive to African countries by the "five-no" approach claimed by Chinese authorities, i.e. "no interference in African countries' pursuit of development paths that fit their national conditions; no interference in African countries' internal affairs; no imposition of our will on African countries; no attachment of political strings to assistance to Africa; and no seeking of selfish political gains in investment and financing cooperation with Africa". Available from: www.xinhuanet.com/english/2018-09/03/c_129946189.htm (accessed 4 September 2018).

3 The acronym BRIC was coined in 2001 by Jim O'Neill, a senior official of the Goldman Sachs, to indicate four emerging national economies (Brazil, Russian Federation, India and China). The acronym later became BRICS to include South Africa (Mckee et al., 2014).

4 Besides the *sherpa*, there are two *vice-sherpa*, one tasked with political issues, mainly referring to the Ministry of Foreign Affairs, and the other in charge of economic matters, referring to the Ministry of the Economy.

5 Later those objectives would be included in the Millennium Development Goal n.6 with targets to be achieved by 2015.

6 The World Economic Forum (WEF) is a Swiss foundation, which presents itself as the international organization for public-private cooperation. Founded in 1971 by the Swiss entrepreneur Klaus Schwab, it annually convenes political and economic leaders in Davos (Switzerland).

References

Acharya S., et al., 2014. BRICS and global health. *Bulletin of the World Health Organization*, 92(6), 386–386A.

Berlinguer, G., Missoni, E., 2001. Anche la salute é 'globale. *Politica Internazionale*, (1/2), 273–284.

Blanchet, N., Thomas, M., Atun, R., Jamison, D., Knaul, F., Hecht, A.R., 2014. *Global collective action in health: The WDR+20 landscape of core and supportive functions*. World Institute for Development Economics Research.

Buse, K., 2015. G7 health commitments: greater specificity for greater accountability. *The Lancet*, 386(9994), 650.

Cali, M.L., Missoni, E., 2014. La finanza innovativa. La partecipazione italiana a IFFIm e AMC. *Sistema Salute*, 58(4), 440–452.

Dodgson, R., Lee, K., Drager, N., 2002. *Global Health Governance. A conceptual review*. Discussion Paper n. 1, London and Geneva: Centre on Global Change & Health, London School of Hygiene & Tropical Medicine – Dept of Health & Development and World Health Organization.

Fan, V.Y., Grépin, K.A., Shen, G.C., Chen L., 2014. Tracking the flow of health aid from BRICS countries. *Bulletin of the World Health Organization*, 92(6), 457–458.

Gill, S., Benatar, S.R., 2017. History, structure and agency in global health governance. Comment on "Global health governance challenges 2016 – are we ready?" *International Journal of Health Policy and Management*, 6(4), 237–241.

G7, 2014. G7 Brussels Summit Declaration. Brussels, 5 June. Available from: www.g8.utoronto.ca/summit/2014brussels/declaration.html.

G7, 2015. Leaders' Declaration G7 Summit, 7–8 June. Available from: www.bundesregierung.de/Content/EN/_Anlagen/G7/2015-06-08-g7-abschluss-eng_en.pdf.

G7, 2016. G7 Ise-Shima Leaders' Declaration. Ise-Shima, Japan, 27 May. Available from: www.g8.utoronto.ca/summit/2016shima/ise-shima-declaration-en.html#health.

G7, 2017. G7 Taormina Leaders' Communiqué. Taormina, Italy, 27 May. Available from: www.g8.utoronto.ca/summit/2017taormina/communique.html.

G7 Health Ministers, 2017. G7 Milan Health Ministers' Communiqué, 5–6 November. Available from: www.g7italy.it/sites/default/files/documents/FINAL_G7_Health_Communiquè_Milan_2017_0.pdf.

G8, 2000. G8 communiqué Okinawa 2000, 23 July 2000.

G8, 2005. The Gleneagles Communiqué. Available from: www.g8.utoronto.ca/summit/2005gleneagles/communique.pdf.

G8, 2006. G8 Documents (St. Petersburg, 2006). Fight against infectious diseases. Available from: www.g8.utoronto.ca/summit/2006stpetersburg/infdis.html.

G8, 2008. G8 Hokkaido Toyako Summit Leaders Declaration. Hokkaido Toyako, 8 July. Available from: www.mofa.go.jp/policy/economy/summit/2008/doc/doc080714__en.html.

G8, 2009. G8 Leaders Declaration. Responsible leadership for a sustainable future. L'Aquila. Available from: www.g8.utoronto.ca/summit/2009laquila/2009-declaration.html.

G8, 2010. G8 Muskoka Initiative. Recovery and new Beginnings. Muskoka, Canada, June. Available from: www.mofa.go.jp/policy/economy/summit/2010/pdfs/declaration_1006.pdf.

G8, 2011. Deauville accountability report. G8 Commitments on Health and Food Security: state of delivery and results, Deauville, France. Available from: www.g8.utoronto.ca/summit/2011deauville/accountability.html.

G8 Health Experts, 2008. Toyako Framework for Action on Global Health – Report of the G8 Health Experts Group. 8 July. Available from: www.mofa.go.jp/policy/economy/summit/2008/doc/pdf/0708_09_en.pdf.

G8 Presidency, 2001. Genova Trust Fund for Health Care, April. Available from: www.eduardomissoni.net/CV/dimissioniG8/genovafund.doc.

G20, 2016. G20 Action Plan on 2030 Agenda for Sustainable Development. Hangzhou.

G20, 2017. Hamburg Update: Taking forward the G20 Action Plan on the 2030 Agenda for Sustainable Development.

Gautier, L., *et al.*, 2014. Reforming the World Health Organization: what in influence do the BRICS wield? *Contemporary Politics.* Available from: http://dx.doi.org/10.1080/13569775.2014.907987.

Harman, S., 2012. *Global Health Governance.* Abingdon: Routledge.

Herrick, C., 2017. The strategic geographies of global health partnerships. *Health & Place*, 45, 152–159.

IFFIm, 2018. Origins of IFFIm. Available from: www.iffim.org/about/origins-of-iffim/.

IHME, 2017. *Financing Global Health 2016.* Seattle, WA: Institute for Health Metrics and Evaluation.

Jones, C.M., Clavier, C., Potvin, L., 2017. Are national policies on global health in fact national policies on global health governance? A comparison of policy designs from Norway and Switzerland. *BMJ Global Health*, 2, e000120.

Kickbusch, I., *et al.*, 2017. Germany's expanding role in global health. *The Lancet,* 390, 898–912.

Kirton, J., 2014. The G20 Discovers Global Health at Brisbane, University of Toronto, G20 Information Centre, 15 November. Available from: www.g20.utoronto.ca/analysis/141115-kirton-ebola.html.

Klausner, R.D., *et al.*, 2003. The need for a global HIV vaccine enterprise. *Science*, 300, 2036.

MacLean, S.J., Brown, S.A., 2009. Introduction. The social determinants of global health: confronting inequities. In:MacLean, S.J., Brown, S.A., Fourie, P. (Eds.), *Health for Some. The Political Economy of Global Health Governance.* International Political Economy Series. New York: Palgrave MacMillan.

McKee, M., *et al.*, 2014. BRICS' role in global health and the promotion of universal health coverage: the debate continues. *Bulletin of the World Health Organization*, 92(6), 452–453.

Missoni, E., 2004. Il Fondo globale per la lotta all'HIV-AIDS, tubercolosi e malaria. In Missoni, E. (Ed.), *Osservatorio sulla Salute Globale. Rapporto 2004 Salute e Globalizzazione*. Milan: Feltrinelli.

Missoni, E., 2009. 2009 was not a 'dead year' for G8's health agenda. *The Lancet*, 19, 374(9707), 2053–2054.
Reich, M., Takemi, K., 2009. G8 and strengthening health systems: follow-up to the Toyako summit. *The Lancet*, 373, 508–515.
Shajalal, M., *et al.*, 2017. China's engagement with development assistance for health in Africa. *Global Health Research and Policy*, 2, 24.
WHO, 2008. World Health Report 2008. *Primary Health Care. Now More Than Ever*. Geneva: World Health Organization.
WHO, 2014. Human resources: annual report. Report by the Secretariat. Sixty-Seventh World Health Assembly A67/47. Geneva: World Health Organization.
WHO, 2017. Mid Term Programmatic and Financial Report for 2016–2017, Seventieth World health Assembly A70/40, Provisional Agenda Item 20.1. Geneva: World Health Organization.
Unless otherwise indicated, all websites were accessed on 9 August 2018.

8 Non-state actors

8.1 The origins

One of the characteristics of globalization is the inherent shift from "international" to "global" governance, characterized by the growing transnational role of non-state actors (NSAs). This is also true for health-related global governance, which shifted over the twentieth century from single-issue concerns and support of national regulation, towards dealing with transnational issues, bringing in new rules, systems and competencies in international public health regulation, giving a greater profile to non-state actors in health (Loewenson 2003).

Traditionally scholars divide society into three sectors: the public sector, the market and civil society (in the economic field often also referred to as the "third sector"). In practice the borders between the three sectors have become more and more blurred, especially between market and civil society. On the one hand, hybrid public-private actors emerged and, on the other hand, private organizations with very distinct characteristics and interests have often been confounded under the same category. Traditional non-profits, transnationally operating development Non Governmental Organizations (NGOs), and more or less structured networks and social movements, philanthropies and NGOs clearly associated with businesses have often been indistinctly grouped under concepts such as private sector (which technically includes profits and non-profits), third sector or even civil society (Missoni and Alesani 2014).

The collaboration with "professional groups and such other organizations as may be deemed appropriate" was already included among the objectives of the World Health Organization (WHO) listed in its Constitution (WHO 1948). This option was not available to pre-existing international health organizations, such as the Office International de l' Hygiène Publique established in 1907 (Fidler 2001).

In recent years, in the context of the WHO reform process the relationship between the Organization and NSAs was harshly debated due to the risk of conflicts of interest and undue interference by the diversity of actors interacting with WHO and representing often highly contrasting interests (Richter 2014).

After 17 months of negotiations, in 2016 the World Health Assembly endorsed the WHO Framework of Engagement with Non-State Actors (FENSA) (WHO 2016, 2017) (see Chapter 6), which manages to clearly distinguish and classify the different entities (see Box 6.3). We will adopt that classification and in the following sections we will take a closer look at these actors and their role in global health.

BOX 8.1 Non-state actors

(a) **Non-governmental organizations** are non-profit entities that operate independently of governments. They are usually membership-based, with non-profit entities or individuals as members exercising voting rights in relation to the policies of the non-governmental organization, or are otherwise constituted with non-profit, public-interest goals. They are free from concerns which are primarily of a private, commercial or profit-making nature. They could include, for example, grassroots community organizations, civil society groups and networks, faith-based organizations, professional groups, disease-specific groups and patient groups.

(b) **Private sector entities** are commercial enterprises, that is to say businesses that are intended to make a profit for their owners. The term also refers to entities that represent, or are governed or controlled by, private sector entities. This group includes (but is not limited to) business associations representing commercial enterprises, entities not "at arm's length" from their commercial sponsors, and partially or fully state-owned commercial enterprises acting like private sector entities.

(c) **International business associations** are private sector entities that do not intend to make a profit for themselves but represent the interests of their members, which are commercial enterprises and/or national or other business associations. They have the authority to speak for their members through their authorized representatives. Their members exercise voting rights in relation to the policies of the international business association.

(d) **Philanthropic foundations** are non-profit entities whose assets are provided by donors and whose income is spent on socially useful purposes. They shall be clearly independent from any private sector entity in their governance and decision-making.

(e) **Academic institutions** are entities engaged in the pursuit and dissemination of knowledge through research, education and training.

Source: WHO, 2016.

8.2 Transnational private business sector entities and their relevance in influencing policies affecting global health

Transnational companies (TNCs) and businesses have always more or less transparently put pressure on national governments in order to expand their markets. Individually or through various forms of business associations (see Box 8.1, b and c), these private entities have progressively extended their influence on international policy-making, both by lobbying national policy-makers and by directly interacting with the relevant international institutions.

In the health sector, the contribution of the biomedical industry to research and development cannot be denied. Nevertheless, being naturally oriented towards profit maximization, in general the healthcare-related industry has pushed for health sector commercialization, increasing consumption of biomedical products and technologies often without evidence of their cost-effectiveness or neglecting iatrogenic risks. A more comprehensive economic assessment of the impact of transnational pharmaceutical companies' marketing strategies on the health sector should also consider other elements such as the negative impact on local pharmaceutical production, the dependence on unsecured supplies and the introduction and push for the prescription of second-choice or higher-cost drugs in contrast with public policies promoting generic and essential drugs.

Other industries with an evident direct impact on health (tobacco, food, agro-industry, etc.) have often denied their responsibility and actively interfered with public regulation.

In the last decades of the twentieth century, to adapt their competitiveness to the new globalized context TNCs reviewed their organizational and governance models. With the aim of enhancing their public profile and creating consensus around their brands, they moved from a traditional approach where management responds exclusively to the shareholders, to a model which takes into account a wider "network" of stakeholders, including governments, pressure groups, research institutes and, more in general, public opinion and the multiple and diverse expressions of the civil society. In this regard, interest grew considerably around corporate social responsibility (CSR), i.e. the engagement of companies in actions that promote some social good, beyond the interests of the firm and in addition to social or environmental requirements prescribed by the law.

Besides the need to show "moral and social responsibility", Logan (1993: 8–10) identified two other reasons for companies to engage in social promotion: the possibility to influence the social and political environment in which their economic activity takes place, and the direct promotion of their commercial interests.

Private entities' influence has been favored, since the 1980s, by the emergence of increasingly structured partnerships between the corporate sector and multilateral public actors, according to the strategies promoted by the Bretton Woods Institutions (Buse and Walt 2000).

In the health sector, TNCs often supported those partnerships through their corporate philanthropic foundations, or through direct funding and/or in-kind donations to United Nations' programs and initiatives. A few examples: the Mectizan Donation Program, through which the pharmaceutical company Merck would donate the drug Ivermectin in any needed amount until the eradication of onchocerciasis (river blindness) in a number of African countries; Glaxo Wellcome's Malarone[1] Donation Program in Africa; Pfizer's donation of Zithromax (azithromycin) for the fight against trachoma; and SmithKline Beecham's donation of Albendazole to contribute to the elimination of lymphatic filariasis.

Although donations may be vital in the fight against diseases, all these initiatives provide businesses with substantial returns on investment in terms of image and international positioning, and necessarily respond to well-planned market strategies.[2] Indeed, in many countries, and especially in the US, tax deductions favor donations, which in the end are financed by taxpayers.

In the opinion of representatives of the sector, at the end of the 1990s contributions already went beyond mere financial support:

> Since 1998, the industry has contributed US$1.9 billion in donations of products to developing countries through partnerships. In addition, we are engaged in

many initiatives that provide education, infrastructure, and technical assistance to developing countries.

(Bale 2002)

Based on the most recent analyses conducted by the Institute for Health Metrics and Evaluation, corporate donations increased almost five times from a total value of 160 million in 2000 to 770 million dollars in 2017 (IHME 2018).

However, these figures are very limited when compared with those of the global healthcare market. The pharmaceutical market itself was worth 1.135 trillion dollars in 2017 and has a forecasted compound annual growth rate (CGAR) between 3% and 6% through to 2022 (IQVIA 2018). The global market, on the other hand, is extremely poorly distributed, with more than 80% of pharmaceutical expenditure concentrated in only ten countries. Furthermore, the largest pharmaceutical and biotechnology industries (generically referred to as Big Pharma) exert strong influence on governments (with huge expenses for lobbying) and their positions in global negotiations. Moreover, financing of universities, professional and patient organizations, conferences and vocational training programs falls under the modalities through which the biomedical industry ensures recognition to academics and influences policy-makers, often without declaring obvious risks of conflict of interest (Global Health Watch 2011).

The influence of private insurances and healthcare providers has also grown in recent years, exerting considerable pressure on the developing countries' emerging markets. Private insurance in low-income countries is used mainly by the better-off part of the population and if it is not well regulated has the potential to jeopardize public assistance policies (Birn *et al.* 2009). Transnational management consulting companies are increasingly involved in global policy-making. For example, in the United Kingdom health service privatization is linked to a sort of "revolving door" that connects large private companies and transnational consulting firms with public authorities: (1) private consultants who take up public functions, building relationships that serve the interests of the private sector, and (2) former civil servants who join private businesses after being in leading public sector positions (Global Health Watch 2017). This "revolving door" also affects many global health initiatives and institutions, eliciting issues of accountability and conflicts of interest. Consulting companies such as Pricewaterhouse Coopers (PwC), Boston Consulting Group (BCG), KPMG, McKinsey and others have become closely associated with global health organizations, including WHO, World Food Program (WFP), UNITAID and the Stop TB partnership. They are fundamental local and global partners of the Global Fund to Fight AIDS, Tuberculosis and Malaria, and have contributed significantly to the development of GAVI's strategies (Global Health Watch 2014, 2017). Initially providing managerial advice, consulting companies soon moved to offering strategic guidance. Leading with "value for money" metrics, they assume from the start that there is a market-based solution to every problem. Using consulting approaches based on an industrial model, they choose to solve issues "through problem-fixing and 'efficiency' gains, combined with a focus on immediate results", thus tending "to collapse health and human development into a technical exercise" (Global Health Watch 2017: 284).

The private sector often seeks to influence any relevant public statutory regulation which might impact on its profitability. In the case of the relations with WHO, although the corporate sector contributes only 3% to WHO's extra-budgetary funds (WHO 2018), the relationship with the Organization could be used to influence its decisions aiming to regulate the market against their interests. Since its adoption FENSA has regulated WHO's engagement with private sector entities by type of interaction. FENSA states that

> When engaging with private sector entities, it should be borne in mind that WHO's activities affect the commercial sector in broader ways through, among others, its public health guidance, its recommendations on normative standards, or other work that might indirectly or directly influence product costs, market demand, or profitability of specific goods and services.
>
> (WHO 2016)

Strategies used to oppose public regulation include delaying the introduction of international legal instruments (e.g. conventions, codes, agreements, resolutions), blocking the adoption of international instruments, influencing the content of international instruments, challenging the credibility/validity of international instruments, undermining the legitimacy and capacity of international organizations charged with negotiating international instruments and challenging the competence of a UN body to develop norms in a particular domain. Sometimes covert strategies are also used by industry to influence international regulations. For example, industry-funded self-denominated "scientific organizations" enter into scientific debates on norms and standards without disclosing their close links with industry (Buse and Lee 2005).

Historical examples of TNCs' resistance toward WHO's regulatory initiatives are their opposition to the introduction of the WHO/UNICEF International Code of Marketing of Breast-milk Substitutes, and to the launch of the WHO Essential Drugs program in the 1980s. More recently, tobacco companies spared no effort to derail the Framework Convention on Tobacco Control (FCTC), which entered into force in 2005, and the transnational food industry (Big Food) strongly opposed WHO's Global Strategy on Diet, Physical Activity and Health (DPHAS) aimed at regulating the production, marketing and consumption of sugar content in foods and beverages (Missoni 2015).

In the attempt to preempt public regulation and dilute impetus for public action, industry often opts for self-regulation, i.e. setting and enforcing its own rules and policies for operating within a specific domain. Global private standards may also be adopted when industry perceives that they are needed due to weak or non-existent public regulation of the market.

Industry self-regulation may consist of the adoption of private market standards and norms, or be related to social standards, rules and norms.

Market standards range from advertising and public relations codes of conduct (a set of standards that companies set themselves) to standards governing the threads on screws used within medical equipment. Self-regulation with regard to social standards consists of voluntarily adopting and observing specific practices, including CSR initiatives, on the basis of public or social concern (raised by consumers, including public boycotts, shareholder activism, etc.) rather than in consideration of the functioning of the market per se. Self-regulation may also respond to threat of impending public regulation which may be more onerous, or be strategically adopted to gain competitive advantage against competitor firms which cannot or will not uphold the standards. In any case, all voluntary self-regulatory initiatives are developed to ultimately improve firms' financial performance (Buse and Lee 2005).

Finally, co-regulation represents a bargain between public authorities and the private sector. In this case "the public and private actors negotiate on an agreed set of policy or regulatory objectives which are results-oriented. Subsequently, the private sector takes responsibility for implementation of the provisions" (Buse and Lee 2005). Global public-private partnership initiatives are considered a form of co-regulation. They allow the transnational industry to interact closely with governments, multilateral and bilateral institutions and other global players, providing additional opportunities to influence policies and strategies that affect public health (see Chapter 9).

8.3 Civil society organizations and their relevance in influencing policies affecting global health

Organizations which are considered an expression of civil society represent an extremely wide and diverse number of subjects (in terms of origins, values, methods of intervention, etc.). Different terms, such as civil society organizations, non-profits, private voluntary organizations, grassroots organizations, Third Sector organizations and others have been used almost synonymously, giving rise to a jungle of different acronyms.[3]

In the domain of international studies and practices, and specifically in the area of global health, it has become very fashionable to refer to "civil society" and its organizations.

The term civil society has had different meanings in different contexts and different historical moments. In contemporary language, in a sociopolitical context civil society is understood as the

> sphere of relations among individuals, groups and social classes, which develop outside of power dynamics that characterize state institutions. In other words, civil society is represented as the arena of economic, ideological, social or religious conflicts that the state ought to resolve either by mediation or by suppression; as the base from which questions arise to which the political system is called upon to respond; as the domain of various forms of mobilization, association and organization of the social forces that move towards the achievement of political power.
> (Bobbio 2004)

However, in general political parties and other actors which are directly involved in the power of the state and in the economic production that they try to control and manage tend not to be considered part of civil society (Steiner and Alston 2000).

In this context, non-profit organizations, led by values of sociopolitical commitment and adopting participatory management structures and promoting social cohesion and the spirit of cooperation, can be viewed as the "infrastructure" of civil society (Barbetta and Maggio 2008). They are often referred to as "Civil Society Organizations" (CSOs); however, due to the diversity of their values and very different kind of interests that they may pursue, boundaries of the category tend to be blurred. Indeed,

> CSOs are broadly understood to be non-state, not-for-profit, voluntary organizations. In reality, however, there may be state or market links to CSOs that blur the borders between the non-state and not-for-profit aspects of these organizations. States or the private for-profit sector may play a key role in the

establishment of some CSOs or provide significant funding, calling into question their independence from the state and private sectors.

(WHO 2001)

In the field of economics, the space between the State and the Market is traditionally defined as Third Sector, a loose category encompassing all organizations operating between state and private firms and which are, in principle, privately run and do not pursue profit-oriented goals. Law, power of compulsion and formal codification of legitimacy are the main tools of the first sector (state); exchange, rational calculation of competitive economics and market drive the second (private for-profit business). Income does not usually motivate participation in the Third Sector, and resources are mobilized by the ability to seek and attract them voluntarily while value-driven action and commitment hold the organizations together (Lewis 2007).

Although the definition of NGO was consolidated (see below), from the mid-1990s onwards, the UNDP and the World Bank have preferred to use the term CSO rather than NGOs in UN documents, reflecting a desire to engage with a wider range of groups, with the implication that NGOs are only a part of civil society, and sometimes unduly grouping both non-profits and the private sector commercial organizations into the same category (Missoni and Alesani 2014).

The term NGO was used for the first time in official documents in the adoption of the United Nations Charter, in 1945, where it was formally introduced under Article 71 in relation to the activity of ECOSOC. The relationship between NGOs and ECOSOC is currently regulated under ECOSOC Resolution 1996/31, allowing international, regional and national NGOs to obtain consultative status with ECOSOC only if they comply with a number of criteria, including, among others, that the NGO's aims and purposes are in conformity with the spirit, purposes and principles of the Charter of the United Nations, that the organization is independent from any government, that it has established headquarters and an organizational structure, that it follows democratic decision-making and representation processes, and that it derives its own resources mainly from the contributions of its affiliates (ECOSOC 1996). Among the criteria, there is no reference to the "international" (or transnational) character of NGOs. It should also be noted that by requiring a representative structure and democratic decision-making mechanisms, ECOSOC criteria in fact exclude the possibility of conferring consultative status on Foundations, which by definition are not membership-based organizations (Missoni and Alesani 2014).

To define International NGOs, the Union of International Associations (UIA) provides specific criteria regarding aims, members, structure, finance and relations with other organizations. The aims must be genuinely international in character, with the intention to support operations in at least three countries. Membership must be open to any appropriately qualified individual or entity in the organization's area of operations. Closed groups are excluded. Voting power guidelines must ensure that no one national group can control the organization. According to UIA's criteria, just accepting foreigners as members does not qualify a national organization as an INGO. Religious orders or communities governed on a hierarchical basis, as well as informal social movements are equally excluded (Missoni and Alesani 2014).

Although not included among International NGOs according to the UIA definition, many national NGOs operate transnationally, specifically development NGOs which have or are eligible to the consultative status with ECOSOC. Many of them play an important role in global health, especially through humanitarian and development assistance in health (DAH) (see Chapter 13).

The International Committee of the Red Cross (ICRC) and the International Federation of the Red Cross and the Red Crescent Societies (IFRC), sometimes referred to as humanitarian NGOs, actually have a particular status deriving from the Geneva Conventions (Box 8.2)

BOX 8.2 The Red Cross and Red Crescent Movement: governance and membership

The International Conference of the Red Cross and the Red Crescent

The International Conference is the "supreme deliberative body of the Movement" where "States Parties to the Geneva Conventions exercise their responsibilities under the Conventions and in support of the work of the Movement". It provides a non-political forum for dialogue on humanitarian issues.

"The International Conference contributes to the unity of the Movement, to the achievement of its mission in full respect of the Fundamental Principles, and to the respect for and development of international humanitarian law ..." (Article 10).

The International Conference brings together the States Parties to the Geneva Conventions of 1949 and the International Red Cross and Red Crescent Movement.

A range of regional and international organizations, the United Nations and several of its specialized agencies, non-governmental organizations, academic institutions and others, may participate as observers to the International Conference.

In addition to formal decisions (resolutions) of the Conference, participants also make commitments in the form of pledges.

Members of the Conference

(1) The International Red Cross and Red Crescent Movement
The International Red Cross and Red Crescent Movement is the largest humanitarian network in the world. Its mission is to alleviate human suffering, protect life and health, and uphold human dignity especially during armed conflicts and other emergencies. It is present in every country and supported by millions of volunteers.

The components of the Movement are:

(a) **190 National Red Cross and Red Crescent Societies**
The 190 National Red Cross and Red Crescent Societies are recognized and act as auxiliaries to their national authorities in the humanitarian field. They provide a range of services including disaster relief, and health and social programs. In wartime they assist the civilian population and support the medical services of the armed forces.

(b) **The International Committee of the Red Cross (ICRC)**
The International Committee of the Red Cross (ICRC) is an impartial, neutral and independent organization whose exclusively humanitarian mission is to protect the lives and dignity of victims of armed conflict and other situations of violence and to provide them with assistance. The ICRC also endeavors to prevent suffering by promoting and strengthening humanitarian law and universal humanitarian principles.

Established in 1863, the ICRC is at the origin of the Geneva Conventions and the International Red Cross and Red Crescent Movement. It directs and coordinates the international activities conducted by the Movement in armed conflicts and other situations of violence. ICRC enjoys a specific legal status and specific privileges and immunities under both international and domestic law.

(c) **The International Federation of Red Cross and Red Crescent Societies (IFRC)**
The International Federation of Red Cross and Red Crescent Societies (IFRC) was founded in 1919. It is a membership organization established by and composed of National Societies.

The general objective of the International Federation is to inspire, encourage, facilitate and promote at all times all forms of humanitarian activities carried out by National Societies with a view to preventing and alleviating human suffering and thereby contributing to the maintenance and promotion of human dignity and peace in the world.

Its strategic aims are to: save lives, protect livelihoods, and strengthen recovery from disasters and crises; enable healthy and safe living; and promote social inclusion and a culture of non-violence and peace.

The **Council of delegates** is a forum for matters concerning the Red Cross as such, outside the discussions with States. The Council of Delegates is convened by the **Standing Commission** of the Red Cross and Red Crescent and co-organized by the International Committee of the Red Cross and the International Federation of Red Cross and Red Crescent Societies.

(2) States Parties to the Geneva Conventions
Switzerland, as depository State of the Geneva Conventions of 1949 and their Additional Protocols, maintains the list of the States Parties to the Geneva Conventions.

The Standing Commission

The Standing Commission of the Red Cross and Red Crescent acts as the trustee of the International Conference between conferences. The International Conference is co-organized by the International Committee of the Red Cross and the International Federation of Red Cross and Red Crescent Societies.

> The Swiss government appoints a Commissioner of the Conference, who is at the disposal of the Standing Commission and the co-organizers to support preparation of the Conference. The Commissioner contributes in particular to aspects of a political or strategic nature.

It must also be stressed that both the UIA and the ECOSOC definition allow for entities very different in structure and goals to be referred to as NGOs.

For example, the mission, interests and structure of the International Federation of Pharmaceutical Manufacturers and Associations (IFPMA), which represents the research-based pharmaceutical industry, differ substantially from those of the Nobel laureate Doctors Without Borders/Médecins Sans Frontiéres (MSF), which is an international movement made up of 19 national associations providing worldwide independent, impartial assistance to people whose survival is threatened by conflicts or catastrophes; nevertheless, both are technically NGOs.

This has led many NGOs to insist on the need to make a clear distinction between public-interest NGOs (PINGOs) and NGOs serving global business interests (i.e. business-interest NGOs, BINGOs) (Missoni and Alesani 2014). The issue was intensively debated in recent years in the context of the WHO reform process, when the relationship between the Organization and non-state actors (NSAs) was introduced in the agenda and very diverse actors interacting with WHO were indiscriminately grouped in the same category, despite the highly contrasting interests they represent. The WHO Framework of Engagement with Non-State Actors (FENSA) adopted in 2016 (WHO 2016, 2017) (see Chapter 6) clearly defined NGOs as:

> non-profit entities that operate independently of governments […] usually membership-based, with non-profit entities or individuals as members exercising voting rights in relation to the policies of the nongovernmental organization, or […] otherwise constituted with non-profit, public-interest goals. They are free from concerns which are primarily of a private, commercial or profit-making nature.
>
> (WHO 2016)

Extending the category to:

> grassroots community organizations, civil society groups and networks, faith-based organizations, professional groups, disease-specific groups, and patient groups.
>
> (WHO 2016)

Within development assistance for health, national and international NGOs have historically focused on health service delivery. In the last decades of the last century NGOs have proliferated and have also progressively enhanced their role in global social governance. The exponential growth of NGOs[4] (in particular development NGOs) responded to a certain extent to the affirmation of the neoliberal model with a reduced role of the state in providing health and social services. In the 1990s, non-governmental development organizations moved into a mainstream position in development policy. Indeed, they became important partners to donors and intergovernmental organizations, and played an increasing role in the international arena, moving from the promotion and provision of services to participation in the development of the global agenda.

Although international NGOs were somehow recognized as representatives of the "international civil society" conferring on them to a certain extent the right to participate in the formulation of global policies, increased attention was given to the legitimacy of their involvement and the need to ensure their transparency (Harman 2012). According to several critical voices, the legitimacy conferred on a certain international non-governmental sector may have been a response to the need of multilateral organizations – in particular of the United Nations system – to regain their own legitimacy in a time of confidence crisis[5] (Anderson 2000).

From a theoretical standpoint, several reasons motivate the involvement of the CSO organizations in health-related global governance. On the one side, the increasing interconnectedness and growth of information networks have helped to share knowledge and build shared frameworks on policy issues; on the other side, over the last decades the world experienced social disintegration and widening inequality and poverty. This complex and contradictory environment gave rise to new issues, processes and actors in global health governance, including a new role for social movements. There was also some attempt to establish a civic presence at the global level, as in the case of the People's Health Movement (Loewenson 2003).

The enhanced profile of CSOs rests on a number of considerations, such as their transnational character, which better reflects a common good that transcends the individual interests of states; the need for both a vertical subsidiarity linking global advocacy and local action as well as a horizontal one widening the mix of public-private actors involved, including CSOs; the perception of CSOs as a force of a more human-centered development, thus counterbalancing powerful commercial interests within current processes of globalization, and reinforcing the public-interest roles of states against the growing influence of markets, and increased pressure from CSOs for greater access to policy-making (Loewenson 2003).

Nowadays, the programs for international conferences and summits almost always include parallel sessions and forums with the participation of thousands of CSOs and even governments often include NGO representatives in their delegations. Also, the process which led to the adoption of the "2030 Agenda for sustainable development" (UN 2015) saw a broad involvement of CSOs.

During the first World Health Assembly in 1948, WHO established the principles that would regulate its relations with NGOs; the principles were revised in 1987. In 2001 the WHO launched the Civil Society Initiative, with the aim of promoting greater collaboration, as well as a more effective dialogue with NGOs and CSOs. As a result of that initiative a reform was proposed in 2003, but was rejected. In 2002 there were 189 NGOs which had an "official relationship" with the Organization, but at least 240 other non-governmental organizations also maintained some kind of relationship with the WHO at headquarters level, and it was estimated that up to several hundred NGOs collaborated with the Organization at the regional and national levels (Lanord 2002). Traditionally, in admitting NGOs to participate in the Civil Society Initiative, the Executive Board of the WHO interpreted the eligibility criteria broadly, including professional groups, disease-specific NGOs, international business associations and civil society groups. Though FENSA clearly distinguishes among NSAs, the latest list of 214 NSAs still lists together organizations whose nature and interests widely differ, such as the Bill & Melinda Gates Foundation, Medicus Mundi and the International Federation of Pharmaceutical Manufacturers and Associations (IFPMA) (WHO 2018a).

At the international level, many NGOs deal with health issues, some exclusively (e.g. Médecins Sans Frontières), and others within a more general engagement in development issues (e.g. Oxfam or Save the Children). Most of them were born as technical or humanitarian assistance organizations; however, the larger ones especially have increasingly taken on an important advocacy role.

While NGO involvement in international policy dates back to the nineteenth-century antislavery movements, the focus on transnational issues greatly increased over the last decades, with growth in scale, numbers and cross-border networking and communication among the NGOs involved (Loewenson 2003).

NGOs' direct or indirect influence on health-related global governance follows multiple pathways. These include initiatives to legitimize policies, mobilize constituencies, resources and actions around policies, monitor their implementation, contribute technical expertise to policy development, make global and international policy processes more publicly accessible through disseminating information and widen public accountability around these policies (Loewenson 2003).

Lee (2010) points out that:

> Traditionally, CSOs have played a supplementary role where government institutions have been weak or nonexistent, where there are gaps in funding and resources, or where neglected issues or constituencies require advocacy. Perhaps most visibly, CSOs are accepted as playing a critical watchdog role, ensuring that formally mandated governmental institutions fulfil their responsibilities appropriately, and keeping a watchful eye on corporate actors exerting undue influence or engaging in health harming activities.
>
> (Lee 2010)

CSOs have intervened in global policies related to women's health, ethical standards in humanitarian relief, tobacco control, food quality and safety, pharmaceuticals and access to treatment for HIV/AIDS (Loewenson 2003).Their essential role has been highlighted in achieving success in the negotiation, adoption and implementation of a number of global health governance instruments such as the International Code on the Marketing of Breast-milk Substitutes, the Framework Convention (FCTC) and the 2005 International Health Regulations (IHR), "fulfilling an unusually wide range of functions traditionally dominated by governments" (Lee 2010). In the field of disease surveillance, NGOs have played a supplementary role when state institutions did not promptly report to WHO, as was the case with the Ebola epidemic in West Africa in 2014.

CSO concerns around business interests in global policy have also led them to closely observe the nature of WHO relations with the private sector. A number of them have called for a greater involvement of developing countries' governments and CSOs in decisions on WHO's involvement in public-private partnerships, and have engaged in monitoring and evaluating WHO's work with commercial enterprises.

The global influence of CSOs gradually increased through the creation of more or less structured coalitions and networks of associations, often centered on a focal organization and acting as transnational movements. Some examples include the International Baby Food Action Network (IBFAN),[6] active in the promotion of breastfeeding and defense of the International Code on the Marketing of Breast-milk Substitutes; the People's Health Movement (PHM), demanding greater equity in global health policies; Health Action International (HAI), influencing policies on treatment access and pharmaceutical pricing; and Oxfam and Médecins Sans Frontières (MSF), which intervened in the WTO's Agreement on Trade-Related Aspects of Intellectual Property Rights (TRIPS) (Loewenson 2003).

By definition transnational social movements are very loosely structured spontaneous collectivities that bring together individuals, groups and organizations with a common cause, sharing the awareness of a common destiny and building concerted action, but with loose associations among their participants and without having one overall formal organization. However, given the increase in global interconnectedness as well as the impressive breakthroughs in communication technologies in recent years, social movements have progressively organized as networks, polycentric and flexible, increasingly generating and instantly sharing information, to create synergic action (Missoni and Alesani 2014). Transnational advocacy networks tend to become highly inclusive groupings that exclude only commercial groups, though they may include governmental elements. In particular, these networks may include (1) both national and international non-governmental research and advocacy organizations; (2) local social movements; (3) foundations; (4) the media; (5) churches, trade unions, consumer and intellectuals organizations; (6) parts of regional and international intergovernmental organizations; and (7) parts of the executive and/or members of governments (Steiner and Alston 2000).

According to Loewenson (2003), CSOs' visibility, the scale and resource (technical, financial, social) of their contributions, and their capacity to support state public-interest lobbies all influence their impact on global health policy processes and outcomes. CSOs that have proactively collaborated with sympathetic states and UN agencies have been effective in achieving policy impact. CSO coalitions that have been inclusive, proactive and flexible have been able to respond better to changing conditions influencing policy processes. If greater involvement in programs and services provides CSOs with additional credibility and legitimacy to contribute to health policy, then larger and better-resourced CSOs in the global North may gain greater access to funding and power than those in less advanced countries. This has motivated criticism of the inclusion of CSOs in policy processes, though this criticism has not adequately evaluated the nature of the CSOs involved. If large transnational CSOs, said to pay more attention to their membership than to the people in the South they ought to be servicing, lose sight of accountability mechanisms, mandates or competencies, then well-organized, internet-connected and often northern-based CSOs would have a disproportionate role in global health policy. This would reinforce more liberalized approaches to health and limit a southern-based, critical understanding of the determinants of social crises, impeding any challenges to the status quo (Loewenson 2003).

The action of civil society groups and organizations often involves opinion leaders who support its dissemination to the widest possible audience, and therefore should also be based on technical and scientific information coming from independent sources. Leveraging highly knowledgeable resources within academia and civil society worldwide who are sympathetic to their cause, CSO networks have also built their own monitoring, reporting and dissemination tools.

Since 2005, Global Health Watch has been gathering the work of many experts and researchers. It probably represents the most important worldwide experience of a collaborative attempt to build and report alternative knowledge on global health dynamics. The initiative originated in 2003 from the shared feeling by a number of CSOs and networks (PHM, the Global Equity Gauge Alliance and Medact) that

> the WHO reports were inadequate; that there was no report that monitored the performance of global health institutions; and, that the dominant neo-liberal discourse in public health policy also needed to be challenged by a more people-centered approach that highlights social justice.
> (Global Health Watch 2018)

A wide network of organizations committed to democratizing global health governance through initiatives aiming to shift the balance of forces which shape high-level decision-making also joined together to form WHO Watch, a project conceived to focus on issues in the WHO governing bodies' agenda and to act as another resource for advocacy and mobilization in global health governance. The project is also an example of how CSOs may form alliances and provide support to WHO delegations from smaller and weaker countries which lack autonomous resources to cover the wide range of issues that are discussed at WHO. The project leverages a specific set of resources which are particular to CSOs and represent one their greater strengths: volunteers. Indeed, WHO Watch mobilizes young health activists from around the world (particularly from LMICs) who come to Geneva in January and May of each year to monitor, document, analyze and advocate issues being discussed at the Executive Board and the WHA. Preliminary orientation workshops also represent a very interesting educational and professionalizing experience bringing together experts and junior professionals.

8.4 Global philanthropy and its relevance in influencing policies affecting global health

Several authors use the term *foundation* as a synonym for *philanthropic organization*. It may be difficult to differentiate foundations from other non-profits/CSOs/NGOs, and the term itself is often used as a synonym of fund, trust or endowment. At the national level, legislation often classifies them as NGOs without differentiating them from membership-based organizations. Indeed, the fundamental difference between Foundations and NGOs/CSOs is that foundations are established with an endowment and are board-driven. Revenues from the investment of the endowment in the market and from other assets provide them with operational and grant-making resources. Like other non-profits, foundations cannot distribute profits and must necessarily reinvest the economic surplus of their activity (if any) in activities characterizing their mission.

Private philanthropic foundations have increasingly become important players on the international development scene, with the USA having a history of philanthropic giving dating back to the 1910s when the Carnegie Endowment for International Peace and the Rockefeller Foundation were established. Today, the world's largest foundation is the Bill & Melinda Gates Foundation, with an increasing influence on global policies, especially in global health (Box 8.3)

BOX 8.3 The Bill & Melinda Gates Foundation

"Guided by the belief that every life has equal value, the Bill & Melinda Gates Foundation works to help all people lead healthy, productive lives. In developing countries, it focuses on improving people's health and giving them the chance to lift themselves out of hunger and extreme poverty. In the United States, it seeks to ensure that all people – especially those with the fewest resources – have access to the opportunities they need to succeed in school and life."

The Foundation is based in Seattle (Washington), USA.

History and structure

The Bill & Melinda Gates Foundation (BMGF) was set up in 2000 and incorporated the existing William H. Gates Foundation, established in 1994.

In 2006, Warren Buffet pledged more than US$ 30 billion to the BMGF, through shares of Berkshire Hathaway (to be paid in annual installments).

In order to separate the program work from the investment of the Foundation's assets, in 2006 the Foundation was re-designed into a two-trust structure:

- the Bill & Melinda Gates Foundation: it conducts all operations and grant-making work and is the entity from which all grants are made. Bill and Melinda Gates and Warren Buffet are the trustees for the foundation;
- the Bill & Melinda Gates Foundation Asset Trust: it holds the endowment, including the annual installments of Warren Buffett's gift, and manages the investment assets that provide proceeds to the BMGF to pursue its charitable goals. Bill and Melinda are the trustees. The endowment is managed by a team of outside investment managers.
- Warren has no involvement in the investment of the endowment through the Foundation Trust, including decisions that might be made regarding Berkshire Hathaway Inc. stock.

Both entities are tax-exempt private foundations that are structured as a charitable trust. Each entity has a distinct purpose, as explained below.

Grantmaking areas

Global Development Program

Promoting family health, vaccine delivery, emergency relief, and access to computers and the Internet in developing countries.

Global Growth & Opportunity Program

Aiming at catalyzing sustainable transformative change in the face of inequities and market failures, to realize the potential of untapped markets, and to see the economic and social benefits of including everyone.

Global Health Program

Seeking innovative, ambitious and scalable solutions to address health problems that have a major impact in developing countries.

Global Policy & Advocacy

Building strategic relationships with governments, private philanthropists, media organizations, public policy experts, and other key partners that are critical to the success of the foundation's mission.

United States Program

Works on education, libraries and access to the Internet, and emergency relief in the US; it also provides community grants and local efforts in the Pacific Northwest.

Financials

Foundation Trust Endowment: US$ 42.975 billion (2017)
   Total 2017 Program expenses: US$ 5.867 billion
   Total grant payments since inception (through December 2016): US$ 41.3 billion

"Because Bill, Melinda, and Warren believe the right approach is to focus the foundation's work in the 21st century, we will spend all of our resources within 20 years after Bill's and Melinda's deaths. In addition, Warren has stipulated that the proceeds from the Berkshire Hathaway shares he still owns upon his death are to be used for philanthropic purposes within 10 years after his estate has been settled."

Source: https://www.gatesfoundation.org.

Today, there are more than 200,000 foundations in the world (over 86,000 in the USA, an estimated 85,000 in Western Europe, 35,000 in Eastern Europe and a growing number in the global South, with some 10,000 foundations in Mexico, nearly 2000 in China and at least 1000 in Brazil), and numbers are bound to increase following the Bill Gates- and Warren Buffet-initiated "Giving Pledge" (2010) that led 183 (as of 2018)[7] of the world's wealthiest individuals to commit to spending a substantial part of their wealth in "giving back" for philanthropic causes (Martens and Seitz 2015).

It has been highlighted that increasing philanthropic funding is directly correlated to wealth accumulation and regressive tax measures; "Philanthropy may be growing, but only in the context of rampant inequality" (Martens and Seitz 2015).

Taking into consideration definitions from a variety of sources including the OECD/DAC and the World Bank, a private foundation (distinguished from a public one, governed with public funds and through public bodies) can be characterized by: (a) being non-governmental, (b) being non-profit, (c) possessing a principal fund of its own, (d) being managed by its own trustees and directors and (e) promoting social, educational, charitable, religious or other activities serving the common welfare, either by making grants to third parties or by operating their own programs and projects (Missoni and Alesani 2014).

Due to their non-profit-distributing nature, foundations are almost everywhere exempt from paying taxes. Also, contributions to foundations benefit from tax deductions, which are an important incentive for wealthy people and companies to start their own foundation (Global Health Watch 2017).

Foundations, however, differ in type, mission, funding, strategic priorities and approaches, geographic scope and overall influence. Some work mainly at global level, others at regional, and still others at national or local level.

Based on their origins, foundations acting at a global level may be classified into three main categories: (a) independent family foundations, established through the endowment of a wealthy individual or family group, (b) corporate foundations, whose assets derive from private companies and are often the expression of the Corporate Social Responsibility strategy of the originating company, and (c) as the legal form of public-private partnerships. This third group refers to a number of "hybrid" transnational organizations resulting from public-private partnerships that are often legally incorporated as foundations (described further in Chapter 9).

As already mentioned, due to the lack of a democratic decision-making structure (by definition foundations are established on the basis of an economic asset, and not on membership, as in the case of associations, and are managed by an independent board of directors), foundations are not eligible to gain consultative status with ECOSOC.

According to FENSA:

> Philanthropic foundations are non-profit entities whose assets are provided by donors and whose income is spent on socially useful purposes. They shall be clearly independent from any private sector entity in their governance and decision-making.
> (WHO 2016)

Thus, WHO regards corporate foundations as part of the private sector (businesses).

Independent foundations initiated by wealthy individuals or their family members (Rockefeller Foundation, Wellcome Trust, Ford Foundation, UN Foundation, Aga Khan Foundation, etc.) have often played – and continue to play – an important role in financing and influencing health care in different countries, as well as WHO and other international institutions. However, with the advent – in 2000 – of the Bill & Melinda Gates Foundation (see Box 8.3) the order of magnitude of the financial contributions of "philanthro-capitalism" (Birn 2014) shifted from millions to billions of dollars.

With a capital of more than 40 billion dollars,[8] invested in the stock market, and with donations of US$ 5 billion a year (of which approximately one-third goes to health activities) (KPMG 2018), in 2017 the Gates Foundation was, after the United States and the United Kingdom, the largest single donor (i.e. not a partnership among several actors) of initiatives in global health (8.7% of total Development Assistance in Health) (IHME 2018). The Gates Foundation, whose aim in global health is "to harness advances in science and technology to save lives in developing countries",[9] is also the second largest contributor to WHO (WHO 2018) and one of the largest contributors to a number of global public-private partnerships. Out of 23 global health partnerships that Buse and Harmer (2007) analyzed, seven relied entirely on Gates Foundation funding and in another nine the Gates Foundation was the largest single donor (Buse and Harmer 2007). In particular, the Gates Foundation sits on the board of directors of the two major GPPPs: the Global Fund to Fight AIDS, Tuberculosis and Malaria and GAVI, the Vaccine Alliance, which it initiated. The Gates Foundation, among many other philanthropies, applies a corporate, business model to its initiatives, a model that typically tends to have a narrow biomedical focus and relies on technical solutions to solve health problems, with investment in the discovery, development and delivery of existing and new vaccines being one of the top priorities, reflecting the Foundation's preference for interventions with quick, measurable and visible solutions. The Gates Foundation's support for vertical interventions has been undermining, directly or indirectly, more holistic approaches to health and health systems. Although the Gates Foundation has attracted professionals from universities, the World Bank and other International Institutions, the existence of a "revolving door" between the Gates Foundation and pharmaceutical corporations and direct support for the biotechnological industry has also been pointed out with some concern. Finally, personal relationships and privileged access to political elites contribute to the Gates Foundation's global influence (Martens and Seitz 2015).

Thus, the influence on global health policies by the Gates Foundation (and earlier, the Rockefeller Foundation) goes beyond direct grant-making and there has been wide criticism regarding their power to distort global priorities (McCoy *et al.* 2009; Birn 2014; Martens and Seitz 2015).

Besides concerns about its influence on global policies through its heavy omnipresence in international organizations, the contradiction between the Foundation's health mission and its investments has also been highlighted. Indeed, the fact that the Gates Foundation's funds derive from the proceeds of its investment in companies like Coca-Cola, McDonald's, Exxon, Monsanto and others whose products and methods of production and marketing are known to directly or indirectly damage health has been put under severe scrutiny from an ethical, conflict of interest and accountability point of view (McCoy *et al.* 2009; Stuckler *et al.* 2011).

> When the Gates Foundation is heavily invested in Coca-Cola and simultaneously works to orient developing country farmers towards production for Coca-Cola instead of alternative development strategies, such an approach has potential consequences for grant-receiving communities and their health.
>
> (Stuckler *et al.* 2011)

Although in general foundations "shall be clearly independent from any private sector entity in their governance and decision-making" (WHO 2016), corporate foundations are generally visibly branded according to the name of the parent company and are normally established as part of the corporate social responsibility (CSR) strategy of the company, which is necessarily linked to their wider market positioning strategy. Tax deductions are indeed an important incentive to establish a corporate foundation.

In many cases the corporate foundations that operate in the global health sector are linked to pharmaceutical companies; however, companies such as ExxonMobil, Shell and Nestlé active in sectors other than health, but with significant global impact on health, have also established foundations. Often, corporate foundations operate in the same geographic areas of operation as their parent company, thus also favoring their positioning on the local market and mitigating any resistance to their investments and productive activities (Birn *et al.* 2009).

Notes

1 A second-choice anti-malarial composed of atovaquone and proguanil.
2 Pharmaceutical companies are not philanthropic organizations and it would be misleading to consider their drug donations as an act of generosity. For example when Ivermectin (an old antiparasitic drug developed by Merck for veterinary use, marketed as Mectizan, whose patent had expired) was discovered to be very effective in the treatment of human onchocerciasis, Merck's first attempt was to sell the drug at market prices or at slightly lower prices, then the company tried to induce the WHO and the United States Congress to buy and distribute it in

countries where the disease is endemic, and only after the failures of these first approaches did it decide to donate the drug. Even in this way, however, Merck would have drawn a substantial strategic advantage through the WHO's indirect advertising and through the dumping on any other transnational or local company that could have undertaken the production of the drug, since it was no longer protected from patent (Birn *et al.* 2009).
3. Some examples in English: INGO (International NGOs); CSOs (Civil Society Organizations); PVOs (Private Voluntary Organizations); GROs (Grass-root Organizations); QUANGO (Quasi-Autonomous NGOs GONGOs (Government Organized NGOs); DONGOs (Donor Organized NGOs); DNGDOs (Domestic Non-Governmental Development Organizations); BINGOs (Business-Interest NGOs); PINGOs (Public-Interest NGOs).
4. Referring only to NGOs in connection with the UN, in 1946 there were 41 registered NGOs; today more than 5000 enjoy consultative status with the United Nations (http://csonet.org/).
5. As we will see later on in relation to public-private partnerships, opening doors to the commercial private sector was also seen by the United Nations as a way to regain consent.
6. International Baby Food Action Network.
7. A commitment to philanthropy. https://givingpledge.org/Home.aspx .
8. US$ 42.9 billions in 2017 – as a benchmark, the assets of the Wellcome Trust were US$ 17.3 billions and those of the Rockefeller Foundation were US$ 3.9 billions (2016). See: www.gatesfoundation.org/~/media/GFO/Who-We-Are/Financials/F_749874_17_GatesFoundation_FS--FINAL.PDF?la=en; and https://assets.rockefellerfoundation.org/app/uploads/20171107102708/The-Rockefeller-Foundation-Financial-Statement-2015–2016.pdf; https://wellcome.ac.uk/about-us/investments.
9. www.gatesfoundation.org/What-We-Do.

References

Anderson, K., 2000. The Ottawa Convention Banning Landmines, the role of international Non-Governmental Organizations and the Idea of International Civil Society. *European Journal of International Law*, 11, 91–120.

Bale, H., 2002. International Federation of Pharmaceutical Manufacturers Associations. The Lancet, 360, 953.

Barbetta, G.P., Maggio, F., 2008. *Nonprofit*. Bologna: Il Mulino.

Birn, A.-E., 2014. Philanthrocapitalism, past and present: The Rockefeller Foundation, the Gates Foundation, and the setting(s) of the international/global health agenda. *Hypothesis*, 12(1).

Birn, A.-E., Pillay, Y., Holtz, T.H., 2009. *Textbook of International Health. Global Health in a Dynamic World* (3rd edn.). Oxford: Oxford University Press.

Bobbio, N., 2004. Vedi alle voci 'pacifismo' e 'società civile'. *Corriere della Sera*, 29 March, 25.

Buse, K., Harmer, A., 2007. Seven habits of highly effective global public–private health partnerships: Practice and potential. *Social Science & Medicine*, 64(2), 259–271.

Buse, K., Lee, K., 2005. Business and Global Health Governance, Discussion Paper n. 5. Geneva: World Health Organization.

Buse, K., Walt, G., 2000. Global public-private partnerships: part I – a new development in health? *Bulletin of the World Health Organization*, 78(4), 549–561.

ECOSOC, 1996. Consultative Relationship between the United Nations and Non-Governmental Organizations. UN document: 1996/311, 49th plenary meeting, 25 July.

Fidler, D.P., 2001. The globalization of public health: the first 100 years of international health diplomacy. *Bulletin of the World Health Organization*, 79(9), 845.

Global Health Watch, 2011. *Global Health Watch 3. An alternative world health report*. London: Zed books.

Global Health Watch, 2014. *Global Health Watch 4. An alternative world health report*. London: Zed books.

Global Health Watch, 2017. *Global Health Watch 5. An alternative world health report*. London: Zed books.

Global Health Watch, 2018. About the GHW. Available from: https://ghwatch.org/about.
Harman, S., 2012. *Global Health Governance*. Abingdon: Routledge.
IHME, 2018. *Financing Global Health 2017: Funding Universal Health Coverage and the Unfinished HIV/AIDS Agenda*. Seattle, WA: Institute of Health Metrics and Evaluation.
IQVIA, 2018. *2018 and Beyond: Outlook and Turning Points*. Institute Report, IQVIA Institute for human data science, March 13.
KPMG, 2018. Bill & Melinda Gates Foundation Consolidated Financial Statements December 31, 2017 and 2016. Available from: www.gatesfoundation.org/~/media/GFO/Who-We-Are/Financials/F_749874_17_GatesFoundation_FS--FINAL.PDF?la=en.
Lanord, C., 2002. *A study of WHO's Official relations system with Nongovernmental Organizations*. WHO Civil Society Initiative, June, CSI/2002/WP4.
Lee, K., 2010. Civil society organizations and the functions of global health governance: what role within intergovernmental organizations? *Global Health Governance*, III(2), 1–20.
Lewis, D., 2007. *The Management of Non-Governmental Development Organizations*. Abingdon: Routledge.
Loewenson, R., 2003. *Civil society influence on global health policy. CSI/2003/B14*. Geneva: World Health Organization.
Logan, D., 1993. *Transnational Giving. An Introduction to the Corporate Citizenship Activity of International Companies Operating in Europe*. London: Directory of Social Change for Corporate Community Investment in Europe.
Martens, J., Seitz, K., 2015. *Philanthropic Power and Development. Who shapes the agenda?* Berlin: Misereor, GPF, Brot für di Welt.
McCoy, D., et al., 2009. The Bill & Melinda Gates Foundation's grant-making programme for global health. *The Lancet*, 373(9675), 1645–1653.
Missoni, E., 2015. Degrowth and health: local action should be linked to global policies and governance for health. *Sustainability Science*, 10(3), 439–450.
Missoni, E., Alesani, D., 2014. *Management of International Institutions and NGOs. Frameworks, Practices and Challenges*. Abingdon: Routledge.
Richter, J., 2014. Time to turn the tide: WHO's engagement with non-state actors and the politics of stakeholder governance and conflicts of interest. *BMJ*, 348, g3351–g3351.
Steiner, H.J., Alston, P., 2000. *International Human Rights in Context – Law, Politics, Morals*. Oxford: Oxford University Press.
Stuckler, D., Basu, S., McKee, M., 2011. Global health philanthropy and institutional relationships: how should conflicts of interest be addressed? *PLoS Medicine*, 8(4), e1001020.
UN, 2015. *Transforming our world: the 2030 agenda for sustainable development*. United Nations: New York, 25 September. Available from: https://sustainabledevelopment.un.org/post2015/transformingourworld/publication.
WHO, 1948. Constitution of the World Health Organization. Available from: http://apps.who.int/gb/bd/PDF/bd47/EN/constitution-en.pdf?ua=1.
WHO, 2001. *Strategic Alliances. The role of civil society in health*. Discussion Paper N. 1, December, CSI/2001/DP1. Geneva: World Health Organization.
WHO, 2016. *Framework of engagement with non-State actors*. Sixty-Ninth World Health Assembly WHA69.10 Agenda item 11.3, 28 May 2016. Geneva: World Health Organization.
WHO, 2017. *Overview of WHO reform implementation*. Seventieth World Health Assembly A70/50 Add.1, Provisional agenda item 23.1, 15 May 2017. Geneva: World Health Organization.
WHO, 2018. *WHO Results Report. Programme Budget 2016–2017*. A71/28 Seventy-First World Health Assembly Provisional agenda item 15.1, May 2018. Geneva: World Health Organization.
WHO, 2018a. English/French list of 214 non-State actors in official relations with WHO reflecting decisions of the 142th session of the Executive Board, January. Available from: www.who.int/about/collaborations/non-state-actors/non-state-actors-list.pdf?ua=1.
Unless otherwise indicated, all websites were accessed on 9 August 2018.

9 Global action networks and transnational hybrid organizations[1]

9.1 The origins

The creation of alliances and associations of various natures among non-state actors (NSAs) and traditional bilateral and multilateral development actors has characterized the transformation of the international development cooperation scenario during the 1990s, modifying previous roles and balances. Global public-private partnerships (GPPPs) are the result of a gradual mystification of the idea of partnership, a concept evocative of widely shared and respected values (joint commitment and pursuit of shared development goals),[2] to a multi-stakeholder organizational model, arguably more efficient and effective.

The idea of "partnership" was conceptualized in the mid-1940s as a precursor to the coming peace between nations (Buse and Harmer 2009). However, it was toward the end of the past century that this "feel good" evocative concept became one of the trendiest words in the international development community (Missoni 2006). Repeatedly, declarations and commitments published at the conclusion of international events included the launch of new partnerships.

The notion of partnership for development is not new. The Pearson Commission (1969) focused on partnerships between donors and recipient countries and considered the "specification of reciprocal rights and obligations" between partners and the "establishment of clear objectives that are beneficial to both parties to be essential requirements" (Pearson 1969).

In the 1970s, amidst calls for a New International Economic Order (NIEO), the position of the UN vs. transnational corporations (TNCs) was very clear. The UN engaged in normative work to regulate and monitor the activities of TNCs through the United Nations Centre on Transnational Corporations (UNCTC) and provided developing countries with advice about how to deal with TNCs that were perceived to be responsible for key aspects of underdevelopment and to exert undue influence over many third-world states. During the 1980s, there were several attempts to ensure international regulation of specific products. Successful examples were the 1981 WHO/UNICEF International Code of Marketing of Breast-milk Substitutes, the 1985 FAO Code of Conduct on the Distribution and Use of Pesticides and the 1988 WHO Ethical Criteria for Medicinal Drug Promotion (Utting 2000).

By the late 1970s and early 1980s, neoliberal ideologies had influenced public policy and attitudes toward private sector relations with the World Bank and the IMF, championing a greater role for the latter. Increasing Official Development Aid (ODA) funds were channeled through NGOs. By the end of the 1980s, formal, sometimes challenging consultations with UN agencies, as well as conflict-ridden relations that had characterized their relations with industry, gave way to tentative explorations of ways to link up NGOs, industry and the public sector. The new *"entente* between private-for-profit (corporate) and public sectors in particular" (Buse and Walt 2000) was also a result of changes in the international scene. An ideological shift took place from "freeing" the market to "modifying" the market. Following the new prevailing socio-political orthodoxy, a form of neo-corporatism was conceptualized in which a variety of stakeholders, including private sector representatives, were now believed to have a legitimate say in public policy-making (Buse and Walt 2000).

By the turn of the last century, OECD indicated the "partnership model" as a new framework for development cooperation. The "partnership model" offered greater clarity regarding the roles of partners but insisted on local "ownership" as a guiding principle. Identified development goals would be reached only through "concerted actions developed through a process of dialogue and agreement in a true spirit of partnership". A multi-stakeholder approach to development was considered essential for success, as well as "an individual approach that recognize[d] diversity among countries and societies and that respect[ed] local ownership of the development process" (DAC 1996).

International institutions faced mounting criticism of bureaucratization, ineffectiveness and lack of transparency by governments. States, particularly the large donor countries, used such criticism to justify budget arrears and aid fatigue as well as the imposition of a policy of "zero real budget growth", progressively limiting UN autonomy, paired with a shift toward earmarked voluntary contributions. This situation pushed the UN institutions to identify new and more effective institutional mechanisms and ways to increase their financial resources.

Partnership with businesses was possibly seen as a way for major multi-lateral institutions to regain a central position in global policy-making and to access new funding sources and greater legitimacy. The axiom was that in an interdependent world the collaboration between public institutions and businesses would lead to win-win interactions; this provided a rather "forceful justification" for the creation of public-private partnerships (Buse and Walt 2000). The idea was that partnering with civil society and business had "turned into a necessity for the United Nations in order to 'get the job done'" (Witte and Reinicke 2005).

On the other hand, in the face of economic globalization, businesses looked at the UN in a new light. The private sector was also compelled to make considerable concessions and to reconsider traditional corporate strategies under the pressure of civil society group actions in industrialized countries. Partnering with International Institutions could help to improve the image of transnational companies, increase their influence in the global arena, and obtain direct financial benefits (tax breaks, market development, penetration and manipulation) (Buse and Walt 2000).

Addressing the World Economic Forum (WEF) in Davos on 31 January 1999, Annan invited the business community to join the United Nations to "initiate a global compact of shared values and principles, which will give a human face to the global market" (Annan 1999). The Global Compact was officially launched at UN Headquarters in New York, on 26 July 2000, and soon became one of the most visible public-private institutions. The Global Compact is a coalition of UN agencies, governments, companies, labor organizations and civil society organizations that have pledged to promote and implement ten Global Compact Principles on human rights, labor, the environment and anti-corruption, derived from UN conventions (Andonova 2005).

The Rockefeller foundation played a pivotal role in the development of global health partnerships. In 1994, little more than a decade after HIV was identified as the cause of AIDS, the Rockefeller Foundation convened a meeting in Bellagio (Italy) with representatives of both intergovernmental organizations and non-state actors to explore possible paths to develop HIV vaccines. The meeting led to the foundation of the International AIDS Vaccine Initiative (IAVI), one of the first partnerships to incentivize "pro-poor-product development". Between 1994 and 2000 the Rockefeller Foundation provided seed-funds for the start of other partnerships such as the Global Alliance for TB Drug Development (TB Alliance), the International Partnership for Micorbicides and the Pediatric Dengue Vaccine Initiative (Moran 2018).

The Rockefeller Foundation was soon joined by the then emerging global health player, the Bill & Melinda Gates Foundation. The Gates Foundation convened major players in global immunization and challenged them to give concrete responses to the reduced international attention to children's immunization. The key UN agencies, leaders of the vaccine industry, representatives of bilateral aid agencies and major foundations met, in March 1999, at Bellagio in northern Italy, to respond to the challenge. Rather than establish a new international organization, participants agreed to work together through a new partnership: the Global Alliance for Vaccines and Immunizations (GAVI). In November 1999, the Gates Foundation pledged US$ 750 million over five years to GAVI. Two months later, in January 2000, GAVI was formally launched at the World Economic Forum in Davos, Switzerland.[3]

The new alliance soon became the most quoted example of a new organizational model, i.e., the Global Public-Private Partnership (GPPP), an independent organization including national governments, public health and research institutions, technical agencies, philanthropists, the industry, the UN and its specialized agencies (Missoni 2004).

In June 2000 the UN, OECD, IMF and WB jointly presented the report "A Better World for All" aimed at assessing progress toward poverty reduction and to outline a common vision. Obstacles to the desired "development effort to pursue faster, sustainable growth strategies that favor the poor" were identified:

> Weak governance. Bad policies. Human rights abuses. Conflicts, natural disasters and other external shocks. The spread of HIV/AIDS. The failure to address inequities in income, education and access to health care, and the inequalities between men and women .... Limits on developing countries' access to global markets, the burden of debt, the decline in development aid and, sometimes, inconsistencies in donor policies (...).
>
> (UN *et al.* 2000)

In the report, the proposed response to these failures was to form "strategic partnerships that capitalize on each partner's intrinsic strengths, reflect shared goals and objectives and build on existing achievements" (UN *et al.* 2000).

In the discourse of international meetings sponsored by, or with the participation of, UN agencies and other international and bilateral public actors, the rhetoric of partnership became dominant, with the concept progressively focusing on the need to create joint public-private ventures.

The Millennium Declaration, which the United Nations General Assembly adopted in September 2000, pledged development of "strong partnerships with the private sector and civil society organizations in pursuit of development and poverty eradication", and "a global Partnership for development" was listed as its eighth Millennium Development Goal (UN 2000).

Thus, behind easily shared "evocative" principles and values, the idea of global partnership was turning into a new operational and organizational approach.

The GAVI model elicited early and increasing concerns, especially regarding excessive emphasis on high-tech vaccines, lack of sustainability and transparency, and heavy reliance on private sector funding (Hardon 2001; Yamey 2001; Boseley 2002; Brugha et al. 2002), that the then executive director of GAVI dismissed as "complete nonsense" (Godal 2002). Nevertheless, although the need for new formal structures was challenged by several experts, in 2001 the G8 Genoa Summit established the Global Fund to Fight HIV/AIDS, Tuberculosis and Malaria (GFATM), adopting the same model.

Just a few years later, many independent authors questiond GPPPs' appropriateness, efficiency and sustainability (Poore 2004; Agatre Okuonzi 2004; Missoni 2004a), while GPPPs' advocates claimed the strategic importance of the new approach would contribute to strengthen horizontal and more integrated approaches (Nantulya 2004; Møgedal 2004). After 15 years the debate is still open. Partnerships and global initiatives have contributed to catalyzing the increase of financial resources for health, but there is no doubt that GPPPs have also contributed to the increase in the complexity of global health governance and to the marketization of public policies (Ruckert and Labonté 2014).

Most recently the "Agenda 2030" has devoted the 17th Sustainable Development Goal (SDG) to "the global partnership".[4] Among the specific targets, new emphasis is put on "Multi-stakeholder partnerships" including the need to "Encourage and promote effective public, public-private and civil society partnerships, building on the experience and resourcing strategies of partnerships" (UN 2015).

9.2 Definition, functions and structure

A number of different words, all eliciting a sense of common purpose or joint activity, have been used interchangeably with partnership: alliance, association, collaboration, compact, dialogue, forum, all referring to more or less structured interactions between public and private actors. Thus, partnership has become an extremely flexible concept. It embraces a range of actors inspired by very different motivations and objectives and involves very different types of relationships between partners (Utting and Zammit 2006).

Using a very inclusive approach and focusing on interconnectedness and the partnering goal, rather than on the dynamics and structure of the collaboration between different social sectors, Waddell (2011) has introduced the concept of Global Action Network (GAN). This definition de facto includes any globally networked action, thus all kind of global health initiatives (another widely used inclusive term), which do not necessarily involve both public and private actors.

Buse and Walt (2000) made explicit the essential public-private nature of GPPPs defining health GPPP as:

> a collaborative relationship which transcends national boundaries and brings together at least three parties, among them a corporation (and/or industry association) and an intergovernmental organization, so as to achieve a shared health-creating goal on the basis of a mutually agreed division of labor.
>
> (Buse and Walt 2000)

Later, Buse and Harmer (2009) suggested separately analyzing "relatively institutionalized initiatives, established to address global [health] problems, in which public and for-profit private sector organizations have a voice in collective decision-making" (Buse and Harmer 2009).

Indeed, more formal organizational settings need to be distinguished from several global "partnerships" that do not grant both public and private representation at the board level.

We prefer to adopt a both sociopolitical and managerial approach to define formally established GPPPs. In sociological terms GPPPs are hybrids, i.e. a mix of state, market and civil society; they are transnational as they are configured beyond the traditional domain of international, i.e. inter-governmental relations, and are structured organizations. Thus, we define Transnational Hybrid Organizations (THOs) as:

> regional or global independent organizations (i.e. with their own statute, legal personality, membership, governance structure, and resources) that include states in their membership, represented by governmental institutions and/or International Institutions, and at least one private transnational for-profit and/or non-profit, single- country and/or multi-country organization, with all components having representation and voice in the collective decision making.
> (Missoni and Alesani 2014: 78)

Exceptionally, the formal nature of THOs may stem from an international agreement. This is notably the case for the International Conference of the Red Cross and Red Crescent[5] (see Chapter 8) and the International Labour Organization (ILO)[6] (see Chapter 6). Most commonly, the legal basis of THOs' independence is the result of the incorporation of the GPPP as a private organization according to national legislation of the country where it is based, as in the case of GAVI and GFATM, which are incorporated as private foundations under Swiss law. These *GPPP organizations*, by definition, lack legal personality under international law, although states may grant immunity to these partnerships from the jurisdiction of domestic courts and other privileges (see GAVI and GFATM below).

However, global public-private partnerships also include *GPPP initiatives* (which may sometimes evolve into organizations, thus into THOs). These can be further subdivided into:

- Partnerships that associate public sector and NSAs in an initiative/program which is hosted by an II, an INGO or a company possibly with their own budgets, autonomous decision-making bodies and procedures, and specifically assigned staff (contracted by the hosting organization or seconded by partners), but without becoming incorporated as a new self-standing organization; i.e. these partnerships do not have legal status, domestically or internationally, and instead operate through the legal entity of an international organization acting as its host. The host organization also provides the partnership with immunity from the jurisdiction of domestic courts.
- II's specific initiatives in which the international organization interacts with NSAs without establishing a joint decision-making body.

Finally there are global partnerships and networks associating only private actors (profit and non-profit), which by definition are not GPPPs. All the above-mentioned categories are instead included in Waddell's wide GAN concept (see Figure 9.1).

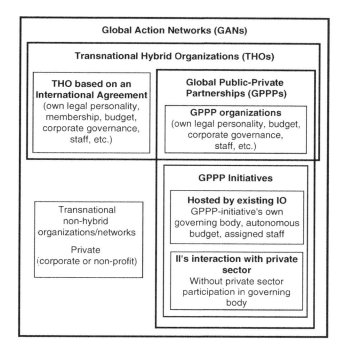

Figure 9.1 Classification of THOs, GPPPs and other global networks.
Source: Missoni and Alesani 2014.

9.2.1 Governance

Almost by definition, there cannot be one single reference organizational model for hybrids. The purpose, membership and the process leading to theirs establishment determine their organizational parameters. In most cases, with notable exceptions of hybrid organizations created through an international agreement (such as ILO or the International Conference of the Red Cross and Red Crescent), transnational hybrids established as GPPPs are not membership-based, thus have no representative body (general assembly), and are board-driven. Their organizational settings, whether UN-hosted initiatives, public-private interactions or independent organizations, vary significantly and are strictly related to the nature and diversity of their participants, and the level of inclusiveness.

By the very nature of THOs, each organization has its unique governance architecture. In the absence of a general assembly, conference or similar elective body bringing together the representatives of all members, governing boards are not elected, but established through the different constituencies that they express. Often a board's architecture is designed to ensure the representation and voice of specific stakeholders' constituencies (social sectors, interests, geographic regions, etc.), but in several cases co-optation of board members is the rule.

Most GPPPs have some kind of executive board for decision-making that is accountable to their partners, and a broader stakeholder forum that enables the partnership's different constituencies to participate and express their views. The GFATM and

GAVI are good examples of GPPP organizations that bring together governments, representatives of the corporate sector, global philanthropy, NGOs and even grassroots organizations. However, members of the board may not always be granted equal voting. In the GFATM, for example, both WHO and the World Bank have no voting rights (see below).

GPPP organizations operate in a hybrid governance framework that vests significant decision-making power in private actors (Moran 2018). Based on a sample of 23 health GPPPs, Buse and Harmer (2007) have observed that too often boards lack representation for a number of stakeholder groups. In the author's sample, low- and lower-middle-income countries were under-represented in governing bodies, and NGOs were least represented, whilst the corporate sector enjoyed disproportionate representation. The authors also argued that the high representation of the corporate sector was at odds with its financial contributions, while IIs' representation was modest. It is a reality that favors the role of private interests in decision-making and the subsequent processes of policy-making (Ruckert and Labonté 2014).

In some cases, certain stakeholders are technically represented on the board, but inadequate mechanisms exist to enable members to properly represent their constituencies and for them to evaluate the performance of their representatives (Buse and Tanaka 2011).

The board often will establish committees in the areas of finance, budget, nomination, and others commonly associated with organizations. In some cases technical or advisory panels are appointed (such as the Technical Review Panel in charge of evaluation of proposals submitted to the GFATM, or the Stop TB Working Groups concerned with specific areas of activity of that partnership).

9.2.2 Management and strategy

The management of THOs is commonly called the "Secretariat", borrowing the term from traditional IIs. Often in the first phases of a THO's development the intention and the promise is to keep the managerial structure lean. A THO's size generally grows with time and its budget. Size, in fact, has been found to be another critical success factor. Large secretariats may not be feasible or desirable, yet their size and structure should be a deliberate strategic consideration of any THO, bearing in mind the consequences of under-resourcing in achieving goals (Buse and Tanaka 2011).

The "businesslike partnership" and strong emphasis on adoptng private sector approaches is a common and defining feature of GPPP organizations (Moran 2018). But lack of strategic considerations can also lead to inefficiencies, which in turn require growing secretariats. The GFATM was originally thought of as a fundraising and financing institution, but ended up as a new grant-maker, often duplicating tasks and procedures at both the global and country levels (Missoni and Pacileo 2008).

As THOs' portfolios, areas of work and networks grow, professional management structures and strategies become increasingly critical to optimize their performance, monitoring capacity and accountability (Buse and Tanaka 2011).

The founding period of any new organizational model is one of experimentation and intense learning (Waddell 2011). This may justify the otherwise worrying statement of Richard Feachem, the then Executive Director of the GFATM, who, taking the helm of the initiative, emphatically declared:

As the Global Fund goes forward, together with all of you here, we tread into the unknown and into the darkness. No one has gone where we are going. The only light is the light of our imaginations ....

(Feachem 2002)

In their independent evaluation of several global health partnerships, Buse and Tanaka (2011) found that lack of clear and common vision for future operations and weak strategic planning were common features. They quoted William Foege's[7] statement that "An effective coalition is able to define what the last mile looks like", concluding that a clear vision is strictly linked to effectiveness (Buse and Tanaka 2011)

9.2.3 Financing

Among other reasons, the motivation for the creation of public-private alliances has been based on the assumption that the new model would attract private resources. However, THOs' funding still comes mostly from the public sector, while corporate partner financial contributions remain generally modest as private partners' initial commitments often do not live up to expectations (Buse and Harmer 2009).

Global innovative funding instruments (GIFIs) beyond partners' direct contributions have also been put in place to ensure needed resources for GPPP organizations and initiatives, such as bonds backed by government guarantees (e.g. GAVI's International Financial Facility for Immunization, IFFIM) (see below); levies on airline tickets, used by UNITAID to support purchase of drugs against HIV/AIDS, malaria and tuberculosis; and (PRODUCT) RED, whereby companies contribute to GFATM with a share of their profits on goods marketed under that trademark (Sandor *et al.* 2009) (see also Chapter 13).

9.3 Global public-private partnerships' influence on global policies for health

One of the preconditions to promote stronger collaboration between the public and the private sectors was based on the idea that "While neither the public nor the private sector alone can eliminate health inequities, focused partnerships involving both sectors have the potential to contribute to their reduction"[8] (IPPPH 2004). One might wonder how organizations with different values, interests and worldviews can collaborate to address and resolve key issues in public health (Reich 2000). Carol Bellamy, former Executive Director of the UNICEF, categorically argued that "it is dangerous to assume that the goals of the private sector are somehow synonymous with those of the United Nations, because most emphatically they are not" (Bellamy 1999).

According to some, only private enterprises can provide research, technology and development skills to address future information, environmental and global health challenges in the coming decades (Tesner 2000). In addition, the private sector itself claims the importance of its role in identifying solutions to global health problems. The pharmaceutical industry, for example, considers itself in a leading position to address the issue of limited access to essential medicines (Bale 2002).

In establishing a GPPP, all participating entities must accept the precondition of the compatibility between their respective objectives and the institutional responsibilities. Some have argued, for example, that in partnering with the business sector, public institutions must first accept the profit-making principle that motivates private enterprises (Muraskin 2000). Both the absence of a clear framework of norms and principles within which partnership agreements could be developed as well as the trivialization of the conflicts of interest arising from the participation of for-profit private partners pose a further challenge to ethics. At least in the long term, for-profit partners will demand some economic return (Nishtar 2004; Caines 2006). Even if driven by corporate social responsibility (CSR) strategies, companies must respond primarily to the expectations of their shareholders for return on investments (RoI).

The convergence of different and sometimes contrasting interests naturally entails risks, which must be kept under control, trying to maximize the health benefits of the new formula. Widdus (2003), among the pioneers of the public-private alliances, defined GPPP as a "social experiment" not free of risks, praising its aim and postponing judgment to a future evaluation based on evidence:

> The rationale for public-private collaboration in health work is not simply to capture money from profit-making enterprises on the one hand or facilitate the intrusion of business into the public policy setting on the other. True partnership is really about combining different skills, expertise and other resources – ideally in a framework of defined responsibilities, roles, accountability and transparency – to achieve a common goal that is unattainable by independent action.
>
> (Widdus 2003)

Every GPPP, like any organization that claims to operate for the public interest, must adequately address aspects such as whom it represents, to whom and how it is accountable, the presence of conflicts of interest and transparency. Also, due to the participation of the public health authority (WHO) in GPPPs, it is difficult to establish who can objectively evaluate the effective fulfillment of these requirements and the success of the formula, and with what criteria (Reich 2000).

As collaborations with the private sector were taking shape, the WHO – which has a responsibility to lead health activities at the global level – felt the need to set essential ethical principles, among which are the preservation of its reputation and values, as well as the clear contribution of partnerships in improving public health (WHO 2000). However, some groups have considered those guidelines insufficient to limit potential conflicts of interest inherent in the collaboration between WHO and commercial private entities (HAI 1999). With the advent of the GPPPs and the direct involvement of the WHO in many of them, the problem concerning interference between private and public interests within the Organization was brought up again. As part of the reform process undertaken in recent years, WHO's relationship with NSA came under severe scrutiny, with many observers fearing that overly general openness to the commercial sector could further weaken the WHO (Richter 2014). As mentioned above (see Chapter 8), the debate resulted in the Framework Engagement with Non-State Actors (FENSA) and somehow a clearer distinction among the different entities that may enter into collaboration with WHO (WHO 2016).

Buse and Walt (2000) pointed out the risks that GPPPs could pose to the United Nations (UN) governance system, fearing in particular that the new partnering arrangements could undermine the UN's characteristics of credibility, impartiality and integrity. In particular, the universality of multilateral institutions could be "diluted" due to the imbalances between participating organizations and institutions. Similarly, the risk was envisaged that the the neutrality of multilateral action could be jeopardized, due to GPPPs prioritizing interventions in countries that can guarantee greater success (and visibility) rather than those where the need is greater. The two authors conceived the possibility that GPPPs would take on the "profitable" activities, leaving it up to the United Nations to tackle the most complex and challenging problems (such as support for health systems and the training of human resources) for which it is harder to raise resources. In addition, GPPPs could weaken systems of multilateral governance, through the transferral of control and authority vested in UN governing bodies to those of GPPPs, where the private sector could have greater influence on strategies, resources and activities (Buse and Walt 2000).

Yamey (2002), editor of the *British Medical Journal* at that time, raised similar concerns:

> As the architecture of global health changes, its governance is shifting away from WHO and towards donors. The World Health Assembly may be slow and bureaucratic, but it has the advantages of representative legitimacy [...] and accountability to countries themselves. The new global health initiatives are outside of the assembly's governance and accountable primarily to their donors – private foundations and rich governments. These initiatives are arguably weakening the UN's influence on how global health funds are spent, by choosing which health interventions to fund (mainly communicable disease control), which strategies to use (predominantly vertical programmes), and which countries should receive support.
>
> (Yamey 2002)

On the other hand, and paradoxically, Gro Brundtland (Director-General of the WHO at the time) reportedly argued that the involvement of the United Nations and in particular the WHO in organizations such as GAVI and GFATM serves to give credibility to the new GPPPs (Yamey 2002). Thereby, GPPP organizations can be used by "big players" to circumvent the WHO itself, thus weakening its role and effort to address the priorities of global public health policies (Bartsch 2007).

THOs and other more or less structured global public-private interactions have undoubtedly contributed to increased awareness on a number of issues of social relevance, putting them firmly on the global political agenda. They have contributed to generating additional resources for specific actions, and towards the development of new biomedical products, although concerns have been raised about the sustainability of the introduction of new products and technologies. Global initiatives also have the merit of having increased free or low-cost access to certain drugs and vaccines, and having contributed to the strengthening of some components of health systems, for example with therapeutic standards and norms, along with technical management and financial strategies (Buse and Harmer 2007; Ruckert and Labonte 2014).

Undoubtedly, GPPPs have also contributed to an extraordinary and unprecedented rise in public and private resources directed toward pressing health challenges:

> But because the efforts this money is paying for are largely uncoordinated and directed mostly at specific high-profile diseases – rather than at public health in general – there is a grave danger that the current age of generosity could not only fall short of expectations but actually make things worse on the ground.
>
> (Garrett 2007)

170 *Global governance and health*

The creation of an ad hoc partnership to face specific challenges revitalized the selective approach that prevented the strategy envisaged in the Alma Ata Declaration from being implemented. Over the years we assisted in the "balkanization" of global health with overlapping and duplication of efforts, losses in the efficiency of interventions, and the emergence of parallel funding channels, management and assistance systems. Fragmentation occurs at both the global and the national level. Global partnerships do not take local systems' structural weaknesses into consideration; rather, at times, they risk making things worse. Incompatibilities have been highlighted between well-resourced vertical programs and under-resourced and weak public systems. The volume of funding channelled through GPPPs is often very high compared to public governmental health budgets of host countries. Beyond the possibility that they influence their macroeconomic stability, they certainly tend to determine the priorities and spending of those countries. New procedures to access funds for countries already suffering from lack of human, logistic and infrastructural resources have added further burden and layers of complexity to an already fragmented system. GPPPs compete among themselves and with other institutions to attract resources. Competitive recruiting of (often scarce) personnel for their projects takes them away from other sectors of the local health system (Yamey 2002; Dare 2003; Bartsch 2007; Italian Global Health Watch 2008; Ruckert and Labonte 2014). This harshly contrasts with the wide consensus on the principles of aid effectiveness, such as alignment and harmonization.

At the country level, the main concern seems to be related to the way single GPPPs operate. For example, the GFATM, the GAVI, Stop TB and Roll Back Malaria (RBM) differ considerably in their modus operandi: the first two function mainly as financing agencies, while Stop TB and RBM aim to coordinate interventions in their respective areas of interest in addition to providing technical assistance (Caines 2006).

In order to benefit from each global initiative, countries must invest heavily in following a variety of procedures (planning exercises, applications, reports, templates, timing, etc.) that are specific to each global initiative. Many GPPPs have set up specific national coordination mechanisms to guide and manage their activities (such as GFATM's Country Coordination Mechanism [CCM], or GAVI's Inter-agency Coordinating Committee [ICC]), whose functions and composition often overlap.

Finally, there is a gap in responsibility under international law in relation to GPPPs acts, arising from the absence of legal personality under international law. It has been suggested that "once a partnership is granted immunity, it will, similar to an international organization, be confronted with arguments that this immunity breaches the right of access to a court, if alternative means of dispute resolution are not available and effective". Thus, from a legal standpoint a lacuna of responsibility emerges (Clarke 2012).

9.4 The GAVI Alliance

The GAVI Alliance was launched in 2000 driven by some initial funding (US$ 750 million) from the Gates Foundation, which is still among the main donors.

GAVI served as an example of a GPPP model for later initiatives, including beyond the healthcare sector. GAVI was hosted by UNICEF until 2009, when it was established as a foundation under Swiss law and as a Public Charity in the United States.

Through a Headquarters Agreement, and further legislative acts, the Swiss authorities guaranteed GAVI autonomy and freedom of action, as well as privileges and immunities in Switzerland. GAVI was the first "international institution" to receive recognition under this piece of Swiss legislation (Clarke 2012).

GAVI's mission is to improve access to new and under-used vaccines[9] for children living in the world's poorest countries.

During the initial phase of GAVI's activity, it became increasingly clear that parallel investment was needed in health systems and delivery systems to deliver immunization and other health services in a sustainable manner, and the strengthening health systems goal was added in 2007. However, critics have highlighted that GAVI's main emphasis as regards strengthening of health systems is on equipment, while maintaining a persistent disconnection between immunization and the broader health system agenda (Global Health Watch 2017).

In June 2014, the GAVI Board approved a new five-year strategy, based on four strategic goals: accelerate equitable uptake and coverage of vaccines, increase effectiveness and efficiency of immunization delivery as an integrated part of strengthened health systems, improve sustainability of national immunization programmes and shape markets for vaccines and other immunization products.

GAVI's board, which is responsible for giving strategic direction and policy-making, is composed of 29 members. In addition to the Gates Foundation, the other members are representatives of five developed and five developing countries' governments; of three international institutions, i.e. WHO, the World Bank and UNICEF; one representative of the civil society organizations; two representatives of the vaccine industry (one from developing countries and one from industrialized countries); one representative from research and technical institutes; nine independent individuals in their personal capacity; and the CEO.

GAVI is financed through both public (79%) and private (21%) funding. This comes mainly from direct contributions, which include grants and agreements from donor governments and non-state actors (foundations, corporations and NGOs).

The Gates Foundation, which provided GAVI's initial capital, has repeatedly reaffirmed its support of the partnership, reaching a total commitment of US$ 4.1 billion, equivalent to 18.4% of all donors' contributions (as of 31 March 2018).[10]

Besides direct contributions, GAVI's funding model draws heavily on private sector thinking, which has led GAVI to become the channel for innovative financing mechanisms, which represent 24% of the total funding, in particular the International Financing Facility for Immunizations (IFFIm) and the Advance Market Commitment (AMC).

The IFFIm issues bonds guaranteed by the long-term commitment of participating donor governments[11] and by the World Bank as its Treasury Manager. Bonds are sold on the capital market, making big capitals readiliy available (front-load financing) for GAVI's activities.[12]

AMCs are also based on donors' long-term commitments,[13] for example for the pre-purchase of anti-pneumococcal vaccine, a product with limited demand on the market. The commitment to purchase the product "in advance on the market" was meant to incentivize pharmaceutical industries to invest in research and development for neglected diseases that primarily affect low-income countries.[14] However, the way that GAVI's AMC was applied was harshly criticized by CSOs for being "clearly designed to benefit four multinational giants in vaccine development and manufacturing", which had already developed the pneumococcal vaccines and "were looking for lucrative markets (which AMC provided)" (Global Health Watch 2017).

An additional mechanism was launched in 2016, Innovation for Uptake, Scale and Equity in Immunization (INFUSE). The new initiative aims at incubating tried and tested innovations that have potential to improve vaccine delivery. INFUSE aims at securing the necessary capital for businesses that offer new technology but struggle for the necessary funding, and at providing governments with the expertise required to select appropriate, cost-effective solutions. The mechanism connects selected businesses and innovators with GAVI's partners able to help take their solutions to scale.[15]

GAVI funding has clearly had a major impact on new and under-used vaccine introductions in many low- and middle-income countries. Indeed "GAVI-eligible countries have been significantly more likely to introduce new vaccines (90%) than GAVI-ineligible middle-income countries (65%)" (SAGE 2017). On the downside, routine immunization coverage also stalled over recent years in GAVI-eligible countries.[16]

Today GAVI influences the market of a vast group of vaccines by negotiating supply contracts with a large number of global suppliers and helping to keep prices down. GAVI has had some undeniable successes in negotiating lower prices; however, its tiered-pricing[17] policy has been criticized as it

> allows pharmaceutical companies to maintain market monopoly by blocking generic competition, preventing use of TRIPS flexibilities and maximising profits by selling at different prices to different market segments [*it also*] helps to skirt criticism of overpricing in low income country markets.
>
> (Global health Watch 2017)

In addition, GAVI's tiered-pricing policies have also been criticized for being "voluntary, arbitrary, ad hoc and conditional", while its pricing decisions would lack transparency (Global health Watch 2017).

9.5 The Global Fund to Fight AIDS, Tuberculosis and Malaria

The GAVI Alliance served as a model for the establishment of the Global Fund to Fight AIDS, Tuberculosis and Malaria (GFATM), which is now one of the main actors of global health governance, with yearly disbursements of about US$ 4 billion, and cumulative disbursements since its establishment of US$ 38 billion.[18]

The GFATM is by far the largest GPPP organization; it was launched by the Genoa G8 in 2001 (see Chapter 4, Box 4.3) and established from the beginning as a private foundation under Swiss law, with an agreement with the World Bank for the constitution of a trust fund for fundraising purposes and an "administrative service agreement" with the WHO, implying that all the staff of the Global Fund were WHO employees, but not responding to the WHO command line. WHO acted as its secretariat until 2009, when the agreement was suspended, and the GFATM became administratively autonomous, with its own policies, norms and procedures.

As a private foundation, GFATM and its staff can obtain privileges and immunities normally granted to intergovernmental organizations only by special single-country legal arrangements. As with GAVI, Switzerland recognized the GFATM international juridical personality and legal capacity "in Switzerland" (Clarke 2012). Similar immunities and privileges were granted to GFATM in the United States, which also designated GFATM an "International institution". Later 15 recipient countries signed a "Privileges and Immunities agreement" (P&I Agreement) with the GFATM, and it was reported that "coercive measures of making the recipient countries sign the P&I Agreement as a precondition to secure funding were applied" (Global Health Watch 2017).

> The purpose of the Global Fund is to attract, manage and disburse additional resources through a new public-private partnership that will make a sustainable and significant contribution to the reduction of infections, illness and death, thereby mitigating the impact caused by HIV/AIDS, tuberculosis (TB) and malaria in countries in need, and contributing to poverty reduction as part of the Millennium Development Goals.
>
> (GFATM 2012)

Designed as a financing and fundraising mechanism, the Global Fund does not implement programs directly. The GFATM framework document states that the organization bases its work "on programs that reflect national ownership and respect country-led formulation and implementation processes"; however, it conditions choices and methods of implementation. Proposals must respond to its specific criteria, such as "respecting country-level public-private formulation and implementation processes" (GFATM 2012). Indeed, "partnership" is another guiding principle and proposals must come from a Country Coordinating Mechanism (CCM) with broad representation of public and private entities. Under certain circumstances submissions from individual organizations would be eligible to submit proposals directly; however, this option is open only to non-governmental organizations, and not to public authorities (GFATM 2012). Other guiding principles of GFATM's action are performance-based funding (i.e. programs need to have proven, effective and time-bound results in order to receive continued funding) and "transparency".

Although the scope of GFATM was limited to the three diseases, over the years it widened. Not only the three diseases should be addressed "in ways that will contribute to strengthening health systems" (GFATM 2012), but GFATM's latest strategy (2017–2022) includes as a strategic objective the building of resilient and sustainable systems for health (RSSH) (GFATM 2018).

The GFATM was intended to be a "lean" organization, but evolved into a rather complex one. The Board includes 20 voting members and eight non-voting members.

Voting members include seven representatives from developing countries, eight representatives from donor countries, and five representatives from civil society and the private sector (one representative of a NGO from a developing country, one representative of an NGO from a developed country, one representative of the private business sector, one representative of a private foundation, and one representative of an NGO who is a person living with HIV/AIDS or from a community living with tuberculosis or malaria). The non-voting members include the Board Chair and Vice-Chair, one representative from the WHO, one representative from UNAIDS, one representative from the World Bank, which is the trustee of the Global Fund, one representative from the Partners constituency,[19] one representative of the public donors which are not part of a voting donor constituency but have each pledged a contribution of at least US$ 10 million in the current replenishment cycle, and the Executive Director of the Global Fund.

The decision-making process of GFATM is peculiar. Although the Board aims at making all decisions by consensus, when this cannot be reached a double-qualified majority will apply for a motion to be passed. The board will be divided into two voting blocks with equal representation by "donors" and "implementers": the first encompassing the eight donor seats, one private sector seat and one private foundation seat, and the second encompassing the seven developing country seats, the two NGO seats, and the representative of an NGO who is a person living with HIV/AIDS or from a community living with tuberculosis or malaria. In order to pass, motions require a two-thirds majority of those present from both blocks (GFATM 2017).

A second independent body, the Technical Review Panel, is made up of health, development and finance experts. The Technical Review Panel evaluates the technical merit of all requests for funding.

Oversight and assurance are also provided by the Office of the Inspector General, an independent body reporting directly to the Board that works to ensure that the Global Fund invests in the most effective way possible and to reduce the risk of misused funds.

Finally, a Partnership Forum forms part of GFATM's governance structure. It convenes a broad range of stakeholders, giving them the opportunity to contribute critical input, suggestions and views about the strategy that guides the GFATM.

At country level, each implementing country must establish a national committee, or Country Coordinating Mechanism (CCM), to submit requests for funding on behalf of the entire country, and to oversee implementation once the request has become a signed grant. The CCMs include representatives of every sector involved in the response to the three diseases. A Principal Recipient (PR) is also identified in each country. The PR is responsible for implementing grants, including coordination of other, smaller organizations, known as sub-recipients. PRs take on the financial as well as the programmatic responsibilities of the grant. Finally, as the GFATM has no local offices, or staff, Local Fund Agents (LFAs) "serve as eyes and ears on the ground". LFAs are independent consultants, mostly international management and auditing firms, who assess implementation and data. Currently there are 143 LFAs in 151 countries.[20]

Despite the tenet at the base of its constitution "to attract, manage and disburse *additional* resources", the GFATM was not able to attract more than 5% of its resources from the private sector, private foundations (with the Gates Foundation accounting for 4%) and innovative financing initiatives, and approximately 95% of total funding still comes from traditional official development aid (see Figure 9.2).[21] Notwithstanding, the private sector plays an influential role in the decision-making process.

The GFATM also works to develop alternative funding mechanisms. Among these the Product Red concept was started in 2006 by the rock star Bono, together with Bobby Shriver of the ONE campaign, of which RED is a division[22], and GFATM was the recipient of Product Red's raised funds. According to the Product Red business model, each partner company creates a product with the Product Red logo, and in return for the opportunity to increase revenue through the Product Red license, up to 50% of the profits gained by each partner are donated to the GFATM, which receives 100% of the funds raised with this mechanism.

A second mechanism used by the GFATM to raise funds is Debt2Health. This is a debt swap to raise funds for health: donors grant debt relief in exchange for a commitment by the beneficiary country to invest an agreed counterpart amount in its national health programs, through an approved GFATM grant.[23]

Finally, GFATM also looks for direct corporate engagemeent. At the 2018 World Economic Forum, the GFATM announced three new arguably "healthy" partnerships with the Swiss Bank Lombard Odier, the world's second largest beer brewer Heineken, and Unilever, a transnational holding with a wide range of junk food brands. All

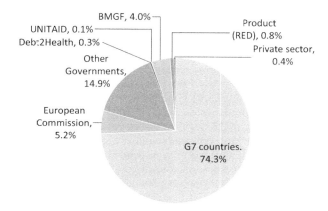

Figure 9.2 Contributors to the GFTAM – 2001–2016.
Source: authors' elaboration of GFATM data.

three initiatives inevitably raise issues regarding conflicts between private interests and GFAM's public responsibility toward populations' health (Legge 2018).

According to is own report, the GFATM "supports programs that have saved more than 22 million lives as of 2016".[24] This notable achievement is obviously not the result of GFATM financing alone, but the cumulative result of all actors globally committed in the fight for health in general and against the three diseases in particular. Among more specific merits attributed to the GFATM is that of helping to reduce prices of antiretroviral drugs and mosquito nets in low- and middle-income countries, inter alia by making transparent the prices and the sale conditions of the products purchased. As for other THOs and GPPPs in general, many critical issues have been pointed out. The influence of the private sector "on activities which are public funded and which essentially take place in the public sphere" and "the threat to the hitherto nation state driven system of global governance for health" are recurrent concerns (Global Health Watch 2017). The overlap of several of the GFATM activities (monitoring, surveillance, data collection, etc.) with the WHO mandate is part of the same health governance-related concerns (Blanchet *et al.* 2014).

Notes

1 This chapter is largely based on: Missoni, E., 2014. Transnational hybrid organizations, global public-private partnerships and networks. In Missoni, E. Alesani, D., Management of International Institutions and NGOs. Frameworks, practices and challenges. Abingdon: Routledge, 77–102.
2 As in the case of other fashionable and inspiring concepts – such as development (Rist 1996), and globalization (Petras and Veltmeyer 2001) – the same word may be subject to many different interpretations, with an undefined use eventually becoming instrumental to ideology (for development and globalization see Chapter 2)
3 www.gavi.org/about/mission/history/.
4 "Strengthen the means of implementation and revitalize the global partnership for sustainable development."
5 Established with the Geneva Protocols.

6 The League of Nations established the ILO as one of its agencies following the Treaty of Versailles ending World War I. With the establishment of the United Nations, in 1945 the ILO adopted a new Constitution, becoming a Specialized Agency of the UN. The hybrid nature of ILO is due to its tripartite governing structure representing governments, employers and workers.
7 William H. Foege is an American epidemiologist who is credited with devising the global strategy that led to the eradication of smallpox in the late 1970s. He is currently senior fellow in the Global Health Program of the Bill & Melinda Gates Foundation.
8 This text was be found on the website of the Initiative on Public-Private Partnerships for Health (www.ippph.org) on our last direct access on 23 August 2004 (see Missoni, E., Pacileo, G. 2005. Elementi di salute globale. Globalizzazione, politiche sanitarie e salute umana (1st edn.). Milano: Franco Angeli); since then the initiative has been suspended and the site is no longer directly accessible, but it is still partially accessible on specialized archiving platforms. https://web.archive.org/web/20050526154500/; www.ippph.org:80/index.cfm?page=/ippph/partnerships/name&typobj=0&thechoice=view&s_criteria=names&crit_id=0.
9 i.e. vaccines against rotavirus, pneumococcus, meningitis A, pentavalent vaccine, hepatitis B, pertussis, polio, yellow fever and second dose of the measles vaccine.
10 www.gavi.org/funding/donor-profiles/bmgf/.
11 Australia, France, Italy, the Netherlands, Norway, South Africa, Spain, Sweden and the UK. Brazil has pledged to become IFFIm's 10th donor.
12 www.gavi.org/funding/iffim/.
13 Donors participating in AMC are : Italy, UK, Canada, Russia, Norway and the Bill & Melinda Gates Foundation.
14 www.gavi.org/funding/pneumococcal-amc/.
15 www.gavi.org/infuse/about/.
16 www.gavi.org/progress-report/.
17 Tiered-pricing (also known as differential pricing and market segmentation) is a business strategy of charging different prices for the same product in different markets.
18 www.theglobalfund.org/en/financials/.
19 In May 2009 the Global Fund Board decided to create an additional non-voting seat on the Board to represent the constituency of key partners whose mission is directly related to the Global Fund (the "Partners Constituency") and who at the time were not represented on the Board. The initial membership of the Partners Constituency was the Stop TB Partnership, Roll Back Malaria and UNITAID.
20 www.theglobalfund.org/media/3247/lfa_selected_list_en.pdf?u=636637836230000000.
21 www.theglobalfund.org/en/financials/.
22 www.one.org/us/.
23 To date four Debt2Health agreements plus one framework agreement have been signed. They involve Germany and Australia as creditor countries and Indonesia, Pakistan and Côte d'Ivoire on the beneficiary side. Overall, they involve Euro 163.6 m. Half of that amount, Euro 81.8m, is paid to the Global Fund to be invested in the contracting beneficiary countries through the standard Global Fund processes and systems. The other half was unconditionally written off by the creditor countries. http://iif.un.org/content/debt2health.
24 www.theglobalfund.org/en/impact/.

References

Agatre Okuonzi, S., 2004. The Global Fund: preparing for the Messiah? *Health Policy and Planning*, 19(1), 55–56.

Andonova, L.B., 2005. International institutions. In *The Rise of Public-Private Partnerships in Global Governance*, Conference on the Human Dimensions of Global Environmental Change, Berlin, 2–3 December.

Annan, K., 1999. Secretary-General proposes global compact on human rights, labour, environment, in address to World Economic Forum in Davos. UN Press Release, 1 February.

Bale, H., 2002. International Federation of Pharmaceutical Manufacturers Associations. *The Lancet*, 360, 953.

Bartsch, S., 2007. Accountability of global public-private partnerships in health. *Sixth Pan-European Conference on International Relations*, University of Turin, Italy, 14 September.

Bellamy, C., 1999. Interview with J. Ann Zammit, The South Centre, 9 December 1999. UNICEF: Bellamy warns against partnership with private sector. UN Wire, 23 April.

Blanchet, N., et al., 2014. *Global collective action in health: The WDR+20 landscape of core and supportive functions*. World Institute for Development Economics Research.

Boseley, S., 2002. Charity attacks vaccine alliance. *The Guardian*, 16 January.

Brugha, R., Starling, M., Walt, G., 2002. GAVI, the first steps: lessons for Gobal Fund. *The Lancet*, 359, 435–438.

Buse, K., Harmer, A., 2007. Seven habits of highly effective global public–private health partnerships: practice and potential. *Social Science & Medicine*, 64(2), 259–271.

Buse, K., Harmer, A., 2009. Global health partnerships: the Mosh Pit of global health governance. In Buse, K., Hein, W., Drager, N. (Eds.), *Making Sense of Global Health Governance. A Policy Perspective*. Basingstoke: Palgrave MacMillan.

Buse, K., Tanaka, S., 2011. Global public-private health partnerships: lessons learned from ten years of experience and evaluations. *International Dental Journal*, 61(Suppl. 2), 2–10.

Buse, K., Walt, G., 2000. Global public-private partnerships: part I – a new development in health? *Bulletin of the World Health Organization*, 78(4), 549–561.

Buse, K., Walt, G., 2000a. Global public-private partnerships: part II – what are the health issues for global governance? *Bulletin of the World Health Organization*, 78(5), 699–709.

Caines, K., 2006. *Best practice principles for global health partnership activities at country level. High level Forum on the Millennium Development Goals: Selected Papers, 2003–2005*. Geneva: WHO, 104–20.

Clarke, L.C., 2012. *Responsibility of hybrid public-private bodies under international law: A case study of global health public-private partnerships*. Amsterdam: AUvA-DARE, University of Amsterdam.

DAC, 1996. *Shaping the 21st Century: The Contribution of Development Co-operation*. Paris: OECD.

Dare, L., 2003. WHO and the challenges of the next decade. *The Lancet*, 361, 170–171.

Feachem, R., 2002. Speech at the XIV International AIDS Conference, Barcelona Senior Lecture, 9 July. Available from: www.globalfundatm.org/journalists/speeches/speech_Feachem090702.html.

Garrett, L., 2007. The challenge of global health. *Foreign Affairs*, January-February, 14–38.

GFATM, 2012. *The Framework Document*. Geneva: The Global Fund to fight against HIV/Aids, Tuberculosis and Malaria. www.theglobalfund.org/media/6019/core_globalfund_framework_en.pdf?u=636650179950000000.

GFATM, 2017. Bylaws of the Global Fund To Fight Aids, Tuberculosis & Malaria. Approved by the Board on 28 January 2016 (GF/B34/EDP07) and amended by the Board on 14 November 2017 (GF/B38/DP05). www.theglobalfund.org/media/6007/core_globalfund_bylaws_en.pdf?u=636637835370000000.

GFATM, 2018. *The Global Fund Strategy 2017–2022. Investing to end epidemics*. Geneva: The Global Fund to fight against HIV/Aids, Tuberculosis and Malaria. www.theglobalfund.org/media/2531/core_globalfundstrategy2017-2022_strategy_en.pdf?u=636486807150000000.

Global Health Watch, 2017. *Global Health Watch 5. An Alternative World Health Report*. London: Zed Books.

Godal, T., 2002. GAVI, the first steps: lessons for the Global Fund. *The Lancet*, 360, 175–176.

HAI, 1999. *Comments on WHO Guidelines on Interaction with Commercial Enterprises* (Preliminary version July 1999). Amsterdam: Health Action International, 22 December.

Hardon, A., 2001. Immunization for all? A critical look at the first GAVI partners meeting. *HAI Europe*, 6(1).

IPPPH, 2004. Mission of the International Partnership for Public-Private Partnerships. https://web.archive.org/web/20040806234242/www.ippph.org:80/index.cfm?page=/ippph/about/mission.

Italian Global Health Watch, 2008. From Alma Ata to the Global Fund: the history of international health policy. *Social Medicine*, 3(1), 34–46.

Legge, D., Labonte, R., Sanders, D., 2018. Managing the conflicts between private interests and public responsibility. *BMJ* blog 08.02.2018. https://blogs.bmj.com/bmj/2018/02/08/managing-the-conflicts-between-private-interests-and-public-responsibility/.

Missoni, E., 2004. La Global Alliance for Vaccines and Immunizations come prototipo. In Missoni, E. (Ed.), *Osservatorio Italiano sulla Salute Globale. Rapporto 2004 Salute e Globalizzazione*. Milano: Feltrinelli, 217–220.

Missoni, E., 2004a. Il Fondo globale per la lotta all'Hiv-Aids, tubercolosi e malaria. In Missoni, E. (Ed.), *Osservatorio sulla Salute Globale. Rapporto 2004 Salute e Globalizzazione*. Milano: Feltrinelli, 221–232.

Missoni, E., 2006. Global public-private partnerships and global health governance. Paper presented at the Geneva Health Forum 2006, 31 August. Available from: http://ghf.g2hp.net/2012/10/28/global-public-private-partnerships-and-global-health-governance/.

Missoni, E., Alesani, D., 2014. *Management of International Institutions and NGOs. Framework, practices and challenges*. Abingdon: Routledge.

Missoni, E., Pacileo, G., 2008. Global public-private partnerships. In *Global Health and Development Assistance Rights, Ideologies and Deceit*. 3rd Report of the Italian Global Health Watch. Pisa: ETS, 202–207.

Moran, M. 2018. Global Philanthropy. In Weiss, T.G., Wilkinson, R. (Eds.), *International Organization and Global Governance*. Abingdon: Routledge, 408–422.

Møgedal, S., 2004. Global funds: scaling up through linking efforts. *Health Policy and Planning*, 19(1), 52–55.

Muraskin, W., 2000. Paper presented to the Workshop on Public-Private Partnerships in Public health, Dedham, MA, 7–8 April.

Nantulya, V.M., 2004. The Global Fund to Fight AIDS, Tuberculosis and malaria: what makes it different. *Health Policy and Planning*, 19(1), 54.

Nishtar, S., 2004. Public-private 'partnerships' in health: a global call to action. *Health Research Policy and Systems*, 2(5), 1–7.

Pearson, L.B., 1969. *Partners in Development: Report of the Commission on International Development*. London: Commission on International Development.

Petras, J., Veltmeyer, H. 2001. *Globalization Unmasked. Imperialism in the Twenty-First Century*. London: Zed Books.

Poore, P., 2004. The Global Fund to fight AIDS, Tuberculosis and Malaria (GFATM). *Health Policy and Planning*, 19(1), 52–53.

Reich, M.R. 2000. Public-private partnerships for public health. *Nature Medicine*, 6(6), 617–620.

Richter, J., 2014. Time to turn the tide: WHO's engagement with non-state actors and the politics of stakeholder governance and con icts of interest. *BMJ*, 348(5), g3351–1.

Rist, G., 1996. *Le Dévelopment. Histoire d'une croyance occidental*. Paris: Presses de la Fondation Nationale de Sciences Politiques.

Ruckert, A., Labonte, R., 2014. Public-private partnerships (ppps) in global health: the good, the bad and the ugly. *Third World Q*, 35(9), 1598–1614.

SAGE, 2017. 2017 *Assessment Report of the Global Vaccine Action Plan Strategic Advisory Group of Experts on Immunization*. Geneva: World Health Organization.

Sandor, E., Scott, S., Benn, J. 2009. Innovative financing to fund development: progress and prospects. *DCD Issues Brief*, OECD, November.

Tesner, S., 2000. *The United Nations and Business: a Partnership Recovered*. New York: St. Martin Press.

UN, 2000. United Nations Millennium Declaration, UN document: Resolution A/RES/55/2, 18 September.

UN, 2015. *Transforming our world: the 2030 agenda for sustainable development*. New York: United Nations, 25 September. https://sustainabledevelopment.un.org/post2015/transformingourworld.

Utting, P., 2000. *UN-Business Partnerships: Whose Agenda Counts*. Seminar on Partnerships for Development or Privatization of the Multilateral System. Oslo: North-South Coalition, 8 December.

Utting, P., Zammit, A., 2006. *Beyond Pragmatism. Appraising UN-Business Partnerships*. United Nations Research Institute for Social Development, Programme Paper Number 1.

Waddell, S., 2011. *Global Action Networks. Creating our Future Together*. Basingstoke/Milan: Palgrave MacMillan/Bocconi University Press.

WHO, 2000. Guidelines on interaction with commercial enterprises to achieve health outcomes, EB107/20 (Annex), 30 November 2000. http://apps.who.int/iris/bitstream/10665/78660/1/ee20.pdf.

WHO, 2016. Framework of engagement with non-State actors. 69th World Health Assembly WHA69.10 Agenda item 11.3, 28 May.

Widdus, R., 2003. Public-private partnerships for health require thoughtful evaluation. *Bulletin of the World Health Organization*, 81(4), 235.

Witte, J.M., Reinicke, W., 2005. *Business Unusual: Facilitating United Nations Reform through Partnerships*. New York: United Nations Publications.

Yamey, G., 2001. Global vaccine initiative creates inequity, analysis concludes. News Roundup. *BMJ*, 322, 754.

Yamey, G., 2002. WHO in 2002. Why does the world still need WHO? *BMJ*, 325, 1294–1298.

Unless otherwise indicated, all websites were accessed on 9 August 2018.

10 Future challenges toward global governance for health

10.1 Introduction

As we tried to illustrate in the previous chapters, a growing number of international institutions and new transnational actors have contributed to changing health-related global governance. However, the complexity of the interactions among global actors and their role in influencing, establishing and implementing policies that may have an impact on populations' health and national systems has barely been mentioned.

The global health governance challenges that were identified at the beginning of the new century (Dodgson *et al.* 2002) remain ahead of us, possibly even exacerbated (see also Chapter 5). It is largely at the governance level, and thus at the level of the interaction between those actors, that the epochal challenge of building a new regulatory and ethical framework of reference will be faced. To modify the suicidal course imposed by the absolutely unsustainable development model of the globalized growth-society, with environmental, social, economic and cultural effects that have unprecedented impacts on health, a paradigmatic change is needed.

Current international institutions are becoming inadequate in facing the reality of a globalized world and its collective health needs.

The WHO's constitutional role of coordinating and directing authority is increasingly at stake. It would seem that the Organization no longer has the credibility and the support needed to fulfill that mandate. Meanwhile, the number of actors with very diverse interests, resources and skills challenging its role at the global level continues to grow. New private and hybrid players entrusted with unprecedented amounts of funding are actively shaping and reforming global health, eroding the centrality of international institutions such that the course of global governance in health may have been changed irreversibly (Helble *et al.* 2018).

The resources made available in the context of development assistance for health (DAH) have increased enormously (see Chapter 13). However, the allocation of these resources is still dominated by short-term and narrow thinking, exacerbated by the proliferation of "disease-specific" vertical approaches and global partnerships. At the same time, there is a growing awareness of the need to promote health and combat diseases, thus of prioritizing health in all policies and in all countries, in order to achieve "health for all, at all ages" (SDG3).

Except for the rather limited scope of the provisions of the International Health Regulations (IHR) and the application of the Framework Convention on Tobacco Control (FCTC), the WHO's action has remained limited by the exclusive "recommendation" character of its resolutions, without prescriptive powers, let alone sanctions, while a global health policy would require a more strategic and combined use of available instruments. These should include a wider and coordinated use of health-related internationally binding instruments, and the introduction of public health protection clauses in existing international agreements beyond the health sector (for example multilateral and regional trade agreements). In this sense, Health Impact Assessment (HIA) should be promoted as a prerequisite of any policy adopted internationally.[1]

Due to often contrasting priorities and interests of national, international and transnational actors, it is increasingly difficult to imagine a governance system that can guarantee on the one hand the necessary pluralism and representation and, on the other hand, the indispensable cohesion among the participants. Indeed, it appears rather utopian to believe in a "global society" made up of

> individuals and non-state entities all over the world that conceive of themselves as part of a single community and work nationally and transnationally to advance their common interests and values.
>
> (Fidler 1998 cited Dodgson *et al.* 2002)

While multiple governance mechanisms emerged to face single global health issues, a governance system alternative to the traditional bureaucratic model of post-war intergovernmental organizations is still absent.

Some of the issues related to the impact of consumerist neoliberal globalization on the population's health and current global policy and action responses will be explored in Chapter 11. Here we will try to briefly identify the governance challenges ahead and to deal with those issues in the perspective of global governance for health.

10.2 The "chaotic" nature of global health governance and its "narrative"

The post-World War II governance system was rooted in the UN as a center for harmonizing the actions of nations in the attainment of their common ends and was based on international law.

Starting in the 1980s and with the fall of the Berlin wall, neo-liberal paradigm shifts took place in international political and economic relations. Capital and market mechanisms progressively prevailed over state authority, creating governance gaps that have encouraged actors from business and civil society sectors to assume roles previously considered an exclusive prerogative of the state (Jang *et al.* 2016).

The proliferation of intergovernmental and transnational mechanisms is a striking trend, which led to the current complexity of global governance, characterized by being *multilayered*, with interactions at multiple levels, from global to sub-state; *multisector*, i.e. highly segmented in multiple different arenas; and *multi-actor*, due to the proliferation and increased power of very diverse transnational agents (Held 2018).

> Current global governance arrangements favour flexibility over rigidity, prefer voluntary measures to binding rules, choose partnerships over individual actions, and give rise to new initiatives and ideas.
>
> (Jang *et al.* 2016)

While the global political agenda is influenced by an increasing diversity of actors and voices, challenging the old multilateral post-war order, the original cooperative spirit envisaged by the architects of that arrangement may also be challenged by sovereignty, which "remains a powerful obstacle to the development and execution of policies in areas sensitive to the interests of leading states" (Held 2018). Recent changes in the political scenario, such as the US withdrawing from the Paris climate change agreement and from nuclear negotiations, or the recently initiated trade and tariffs war, increase uncertainty about the future.

Global health governance (GHG) follows similar patterns. The "diversification" characterizing the new governance architecture (Helble 2018), its "polycentric"[2] (Tosun 2017) or rather "chaotic nature" (McInnes and Lee 2012) represent a serious obstacle to effective collective action. GHG

> is characterized by different layers and clusters of rule making and rule implementation authority, operating in many separate domains by disease area, activity area, function or membership.
>
> (McInnes and Lee 2012)

The absence of a convergence in actors' expectations around agreed sets of explicit or implicit principles, norms, rules and decision-making procedures that characterize governance (see Chapter 5) leads McInnes and Lee (2012) to argue that "it can hardly be said that GHG exists at all". This is even more true for what we have defined as global governance *for* health, i.e. making populations' health a priority in all policies (see Chapter 5).

McInnes and Lee (2012) identify a number of different reasons for "certain forms of GHG", such as security (national interest), economism (financial necessity), an evidence-based approach (biomedicine) and social determinants of health, with the first three being identified as the dominant frames.

The "outbreak narrative" following the emergence of HIV/AIDS, and in general the emergence or re-emergence of acute and severe infectious diseases outbreaks, has prompted security concerns since the early 1990s. "Securitization"[3] of global health increased with HIV/AIDS being recognized as an issue of international security (Security Council 2000) and with a similar framing of a number of epidemics in the early 2000s, such as SARS and Avian influenza. The fact that the revised International Health Regulations (IHR) of 2005, a binding international instrument, was finally agreed two years after the SARS epidemic "was not coincidental" and many authors would definitively refer to the IHRs as a governance tool of global health security (McInnes and Lee 2012). The WHO later widened the concept of global health security to include any acute public health events that endanger the collective health of populations living across international boundaries, including epidemic-prone diseases, food-borne diseases, breaches in bio-safety (bio-terrorism), toxic-chemical accidents, radio-nuclear accidents and environmental disasters (WHO 2007); however, the predominant focus remained on infectious diseases.

The neo-liberal-based economism championed the limitation of state-provided health care, stressing the efficiency of the market in distributing health resources and delivering health care "viewing patients as consumers exercising rational choice to maximize benefits" and "arguing that unleashing the rationalism of competitive market forces" would produce the greatest benefits, as long as politics did not "interfere with the market" (McInnes and Lee 2012). By the end of the 1990s, a more Keynesian economism challenged the neoliberal view to a certain extent. The Jeffrey Sachs-led WHO

Commission on Macroeconomics and Health, which proved to be highly influential, argued in favor of public health investments (McInnes and Lee 2012). However, the focus was on an "essential package" of public health interventions (with GPPPs as mechanisms to support the package or some of its components, mainly centered on infectious diseases), maintaining health as a good investment, not a right in itself.

The evidence-based biomedical frame views health as a technical problem to which factual evidence leading to the identification of "magic bullets" (a drug, a vaccine, a technology, etc.) provides the response. This approach also tends to depoliticize health, emphasizing individual behaviors and responsibility, and de-emphasizing social determinants and their role in driving people's health-related choices. Again, politics are perceived as interfering in rational decision-making. Biomedical, quantitative and economic evidence has also provided the rationale for the creation of global health initiatives and their allocation of resources. Indeed, the way global health estimates are produced, the institutions involved, and their funding reflect some of the contemporary challenges in global health governance (see Chapter 3). Also the biomedical frame historically centered action on infectious diseases and favored vertical approaches (McInnes and Lee 2012). Now, there is a wide consensus that vertical spending on specific diseases has distorted the global DAH agenda and weakened health systems. Despite an increased focus on health systems and a wider scope if compared with health-related Millennium Development Goals (MDGs), Harman (2018) considers that Sustainable Development Goal 3 (SDG3) is a result of that approach and

> is in many respects a shopping list of global health's needs, mixing the MDG agenda, universal health coverage, and global health laws around pandemic preparedness and tobacco control with new pertinent issues such as road traffic accidents and drug abuse included.
>
> (Harman 2018)

Indeed, if one examines the nine targets and three "actions" against which the achievement of SDG3 will be measured, there is a sense of "shopping list". However, such a view leaves out the substantial novelty introduced with the Agenda 2030: the universality and indivisibility of its 17 SDGs. Thus "Ensure healthy lives and promote wellbeing for all at all ages" needs to be understood and pursued in its comprehensiveness and interconnection with all other SDGs (see Chapter 2). The SDGs brought into the global health agenda the urgent need for strategies to address noncommunicable diseases. If that international commitment is to be taken seriously, the main challenge will be to consistently frame global governance using the determinants of health perspective, promoting health as a priority in all policies and dealing more effectively with broader factors beyond the health sector, i.e. global governance *for* health.

10.3 Leadership *for* health

The Commission on Social Determinants of Health (CSDH 2008) recommended that WHO should be the leading advocate for health in the wider global governance arena. Despite known limitations of the WHO (see Chapter 6) a "credible alternative to the WHO does not exist" but "little consensus exists on how it ought to be reformed" (Harman 2018).

An inclusive and efficient governance of the complex problems facing global health requires the harmonization of different stakeholders. The WHO needs to adapt to the changing global health governance mechanisms and coordinate the efforts of multiple and very diverse actors to avoid duplication and efficiency losses in vertical interventions (Helble *et al.* 2018).

Clearly the Organization would not only need to regain its leadership and steering role in the current complex global health scenario, but should be able to push it beyond the health sector, being more proactive and timely in representing health interests in other fora, such as in trade or environmental negotiations, at regional and global levels, where businesses have privileged access to policy-makers and dominate the formulation of negotiating positions exerting heavy influence on the trade agenda (Lee *et al.* 2009). "WHO must become much more agile and astute in dealing with global forces and global flows that impact on health and respond with strategies that address global public goods and bads" (Kickbusch and Reddy 2015). A strategic link must be sought with other transnational agendas and the ability should be developed to position health priorities in the appropriate political spaces. It is paramount for WHO to clarify the interpretation of its mandate, which remains one of "coordinating and directing authority" but may need to reach out and set the challenge even "beyond the institutional mandate" (Harman 2018). Such a re-invented role obviously cannot be left to the sole leadership and diplomatic skills of WHO's Director-General but will require the commitment of heads of government from all the regions of the WHO, and decisive action by the member states at the highest level to "match WHO's constitutional authority with the political support and the financial resources to act" (Kickbusch and Reddy 2015). In this respect, the role of emerging countries may be determinant, due both to the increasing "soft power" of their diplomatic strategies and to their enhanced negotiation power deriving from the growing share of the contributions to the UN system in general and to WHO in particular (Gautier *et al.* 2014). At the same time the WHO could take advantage of strong alliances with civil society organizations that defend the public interest and identify global health as a common good (Missoni 2013, 2015).

10.4 Facing the challenge: which instruments?

An important challenge is related to the instruments that should be pursued to ensure appropriate policy outcomes. The adoption of a legally binding global health treaty, a framework convention on global health grounded in the right to health, with WHO at the center of the convention regime, has been proposed by a global coalition of civil society and academics – the Joint Action and Learning Initiative on National and Global Responsibilities for Health (JALI) (Gostin *et al.* 2015). Nevertheless, evidence remains unclear about the effectiveness of global health treaties to have an impact on people, places, products or policies compared with other instruments, such as political declarations, codes of practice or resolutions.

> The precise mechanism through which states make commitments to each other seems less important than the content of the commitment, the regime complexes it joins, financial allocations, dispute resolution procedures, processes for promoting accountability, and the support of states and other stakeholders to see commitments fully implemented. Arguments about "hard law" versus "soft law" and "binding"

versus "non-binding" seem less important than do strategic conversations about incentivizing elites, institutionalizing compliance mechanisms, and activating interest groups.

(Hoffman and Rattingen 2015)

Whatever the strategically most appropriate instrument, success will be highly dependent on wider alliances among institutions and sectors of civil society actively engaged with the promotion of the right to health and the Common Good at both the global and community levels (Missoni 2013, 2015).

One of the factors characterizing globalization is interconnectedness, and with the proliferation of and access to information and communication technologies "individuals' capabilities in information gathering, analysis and political projection" dramatically increased, and according to Jang *et al.* (2016) the corresponding trend of individual empowerment "is logically supposed to pave a wider road towards cooperative global governance, because peace is generally preferred over war by individual humans". Although this view may seem rather optimistic, as social networks have notably also channeled and amplified power interests and even prompted armed conflicts, there is no doubt that mobilizing communities throughout the world for a collaborative response for health and well-being will lead to both challenges as well as opportunities.

Ensuring a strong direct link between global responsibilities and leadership and people's ability to mobilize for their health needs and rights is paramount when facing the major challenge of the instability of the current global governance scenario.

Notes

1 Health Impact Assessment (HIA) is a means of assessing the health impacts of policies, plans and projects in diverse economic sectors using quantitative, qualitative and participatory techniques. See: www.who.int/hia/en/.
2 The simultaneous existence of a range of policy actions by multiple actors at different scales corresponds to the definition of polycentric governance.
3 Securitization refers to the discursive process by which an issue is socially constructed as a security threat through the speech and representation of relevant political actors. The central issue for securitization studies is not how much of a security threat a particular issue poses. Rather, it aims to understand who defines the threat to security and whose interests are being served by securitization (Global Health Watch 2017: 327).

References

Dodgson, R., Lee, K., Drager, N., 2002. Global Health Governance. A conceptual review. *Discussion Paper n. 1, Centre on Global Change & Health*. London and Geneva: London School of Hygiene & Tropical Medicine – Dept of Health & Development, World Health Organization.

Gautier, L., *et al.*, 2014. Reforming the World Health Organization: what influence do the BRICS wield? *Contemporary Politics*, 20(2), 163–181.

Global HealthWatch, 2017. *Global Health Watch 5. An Alternative World Health Report*. London: Zed Books.

Gostin, L. O., Sridhar, D., Hougendobler, D., 2015. The normative authority of the World Health Organization. *Public Health*, 129(7), 854–863.

Harman, S. 2018. Global health governance. In Weiss, G.T., Wilkinson, R. (Eds.), *International Organizations and Global Governance*. Abingdon: Routledge, 719–731.

Helble, M., Zulfiqar, A., Lego, J., 2018. A comparison of global governance across sectors: global health, trade, and multilateral development finance. *ADBI Working Paper Series*, Asian Development Bank Institute.

Held, D., 2018. The diffusion of authority. In Weiss, G.T., Wilkinson, R. (Eds.), *International Organizations and Global Governance*. Abingdon: Routledge, 63–66.

Hoffman, S. J., Rattingen, J.A., 2015. Assessing the expected impact of global health treaties: evidence from 90 quantitative evaluations. *Government, Law, and Public Health Practice*, 105(1), 26–40.

Jang, J., McSparren, J., Rashchupkina, Y. 2016. Global governance: present and future. *Palgrave Communications*, 2, 15045.

Kickbusch, I., Reddy, K.S., 2015. Global health governance – the next political revolution. *Public Health*, 129(7), 838–842.

Lee, K., Sridhar, D., Patel, M. 2009. Bridging the divide: global governance of trade and health. *The Lancet*, 373(9661), 416–422.

McInnes, C., Lee, K., 2012. *Global Health and International Relations*. Cambridge: Polity.

Missoni, E., 2013. Understanding the impact of global trade liberalization on health systems pursuing universal health coverage. *Value in Health*, 16(1), S14–S18.

Missoni, E., 2015. Degrowth and health: local action should be linked to global policies and governance for health. *Sustainability Science*. doi:10.1007/s11625-015-0300-1.

Security Council, 2000. Resolution 1308 (2000) Adopted by the Security Council at its 4172nd meeting, on 17 July 2000. United Nations, S/RES/1308 (2000).

Tosun, J., 2017. Polycentrism in global health governance scholarship. Comment on "our challenges that global health networks face". *Internaional Journal of Health Policy and Management*, 7(1), 78–80.

WHO, 2007. *The World Health Report 2007. A safer future: global public health security in the 21st century*. Geneva: World Health Organization.

Unless otherwise indicated, all websites were accessed on 9 August 2018.

SECTION 3
Global policies and issues

11 Neoliberal globalization, global policies and health

11.1 Introduction

This chapter explores the impact of consumerist neoliberal globalization on population health and global policy responses.

Structural ties exist between neoliberalism and contemporary globalization. In Chapter 2 we discussed how multiple factors interacted, thereby accelerating the globalization process, and highlighted economic transformations as being the most obvious contemporary features of that process.

Neoliberalism, "a way of governing capitalism that emphasizes liberalizing markets and making market forces the basis of economic coordination, social distribution, and personal motivation" (Sparke 2016: 224), has conditioned global governance through a set of norms that reconfigure politics in the shape of the market and covert the state into an entrepreneurial actor that governs through proliferating public-private partnerships responding to the interests of business and investors. Through multiple pathways of "conditionalization" of macro political-economic governance, down to the basic conditions in which people strive to live their everyday lives, neoliberalism has become embodied by health inequities and premature mortality and morbidity (Sparke 2016).

Among the positive, though highly contentious, claims made for neoliberal globalization, there is an emphasis on health as a result of liberalized markets and economic growth.

> This argument holds that trade and investment liberalization improves growth, which generates wealth that reduces poverty. Poverty reduction, in turn, improves health (poverty being the single greatest risk condition for disease), creating more productive and skilled workers, which spur the economy to even greater growth and more trickle-down health. It is by interrogating the links in this 'virtuous circle,' however, that globalization's health risks begin to emerge.
>
> (Labonté 2015)

Indeed, many development economists question "the assumption that liberalization is inevitably a 'global public good' for the economic growth it is presumed to engender" (Labonté 2015). In addition, economic growth in itself is arguably a factor of health promotion (see Chapter 2).

As the former Director-General of the World Health Organization (WHO) clearly stated, economic growth pursued "with single-minded purpose, as the be-all, end-all, cure-for-all" is not valid as "the assumption that market forces could solve most problems has not proved true" (Chan 2009).

Indeed, it is well-known that the neoliberal market-led global growth creates massive problems of inequality, volatility and precarity.

Labonté (2015) identifies three ways in which trade liberalization and global market integration poses specific health risks: spread of disease, loss of government policy space and capacity, and increased labor market insecurity.

Massive challenges of climate change, pollution and food and water insecurity are all strictly linked to market liberalization and the efforts to accommodate business interests globally. So are constraints placed on health systems and privatization imposed by international financial institutions, including structural adjustments and neoliberal austerity (Sparke 2016). Unconstrained and poorly regulated global market forces have had a heavy impact on labor and working conditions, severely affected the nutrition transition, expanded the production and consumption of health-damaging commodities, and led to the commodification of every aspect of human life and vital social determinants of health (CSDH 2008). Displaced and "superfluous" human beings occupy niches within occult economies, providing bodies, body parts, blood and biological material for consumption within medical and sexual domains (Berlinguer and Garrafa 1996; Rieder 2016).

Neoliberal globalization is also at the roots of "biomedicalization", and the emphasis put on techno-scientific advances in search of solutions to health problems, neglecting their social roots and leading to the creation of patients as consumers. "Pharmaceuticalization" maintains that drugs and vaccines are a necessary component of best practices in the treatment of diseases and disorders, thus influencing "experimentality and commercial, regulatory, and scientific priorities". Discussions of human rights are refocused on individual bodies and their biologies, and "geneticization" emphasizes the genetic basis of disease "obscuring the role of social and environmental health risks" (Rieder 2016).

In general, the structural asymmetries of the global institutional architecture are at the basis of and maintain the inequities in the processes and outcomes related to international trade activities, and of international relations in general.

In international trade negotiations, for example, the asymmetry between participating countries always penalizes poorer countries with weaker institutions and negotiating capacities. Trade agreements are mostly concluded without an appropriate evaluation of the social and health impact, including the increase of inequities in health. The same happens in most fora of economic debate. In fact, health advocates and policy-makers have most of the time been left out of trade negotiations. Trade negotiators tend to be accountable to economic and trade ministries, which are in turn accountable to economic and business interests. Neither tends to appreciate the health consequences of trade and trade policies. New generations of regional and bilateral agreements tend to undermine or adversely impact public health protection provided by multilateral agreements such TRIPS (CSDH 2008; Jarman 2017). However, especially in the field of international trade agreements, one cannot disregard that since the election of Mr. Trump to the presidency, the United States of America has seemed to distance itself from traditional American neoliberal policies. With China emerging as the second largest economy (in GNI terms), we can credibly believe that economic globalization will take new avenues with characteristics that are difficult to foresee.

If on the one hand it is particularly important to analyze the impact on health of economic and trade policies and practices, on the other hand it is vital to identify the policies and regulations that the WHO and other global actors have adopted, and can adopt and implement, to protect health and limit the impact of unconstrained global commerce, mainly along three lines:

> systematic resource *redistribution* between countries and within regions and countries to enable poorer countries to meet human needs, effective supranational *regulation* to ensure that there is a social purpose in the global economy, and enforceable social *rights* that enable citizens and residents to seek legal redress.
> (Labonté 2015)

To exemplify the relationship between neoliberal globalization and health, and the related existing policy response, in the following paragraphs we discuss a non-comprehensive list of issues with a clear link to globalization: the changes in the ecosystem, epidemics and the spread of infectious diseases, the global transformation of the food system, the tobacco epidemic, human migration, the macroeconomic processes and global financial crisis, intellectual property rights and access to drugs, and the challenge of eHealth.

11.2 Changes in the ecosystem[1]

The human being has always been highly dependent on ecosystems and the benefits they provide such as products and services (e.g. availability of fresh water, food and fuel sources) which are required for good health and productive livelihoods. People depend directly on ecosystems in their daily lives, including for the production of food, medicines, timber, fuel and fiber, but ecosystems also provide less tangible benefits, such as spiritual enrichment and areas for recreation and leisure. These and other important benefits are essential to our society, our economic development and our health and well-being.

However, since the 1950s, anthropogenic pressures, demographic changes and changes in production and consumption patterns associated with the globalization of the Western societal model have increasingly contributed to dramatic and potentially catastrophic changes in the ecosystem, as well as loss of biodiversity. This veritable ongoing attack by our species on nature is an aspect of human violence that cannot continue forever. Humanity needs to appraise its stocks and prospects, both socially and environmentally; indeed, the threats civilization faces are far higher than most experts and governments acknowledge (Butler 2017).

According to the World Health Organization (WHO), 23% of global deaths (and 26% of deaths among children under five) are due to modifiable environmental factors. Globally, environmental health risks cause an estimated 12.6 million deaths a year (Prüss-Ustün *et al.* 2016).

The WHO estimates that 3.7 million persons died prematurely in 2012 due to the effects of ambient air pollution, with the Western Pacific and South East Asian regions bearing most of the burden (WHO 2012). According to the WHO Global Urban Ambient Air Pollution Database (update 2018),[2] more than 80% of people living in urban areas where air pollution is monitored are exposed to air quality levels which are below the WHO standards. While all regions of the world are affected, populations in low-income countries are the most at risk: 97% of cities with more than 100,000 inhabitants in low- and middle-income countries do not meet WHO air quality guidelines. In high-income countries, that percentage decreases to 49%. As urban air quality declines, there is an increase in inhabitants' risk of stroke, heart disease, lung cancer and chronic and acute respiratory diseases, including asthma.

The relevance of water in daily life is always neglected or underestimated: safe water is important for public health whether it is used for drinking, domestic use, food production or recreational purposes. The huge increase in demand for water in agriculture, intensive livestock farming, modern industry and energy generation, together with overpopulation, urbanization and climate changes, exacerbates pressures on water quality and availability.

According to the WHO/UNICEF Joint Monitoring Program, in 2015, 71% of the global population, around 5.2 billion people, used a safely managed drinking-water service, i.e. one with uncontaminated water that is available when needed (WHO and UNICEF 2017).

Over 2 billion people had no access to safely managed water services in 2015, including 1.3 billion people with only basic services (access to an improved water source located within a round trip of 30 minutes), 263 million people with limited services (access to an improved water source requiring more than 30 minutes to collect water), 423 million people taking water from unprotected wells and springs, and 159 million people collecting untreated surface water from lakes, ponds, rivers and streams (WHO and UNICEF 2017).

The presence of pollutants in drinkable water may be related to natural or anthropic contamination, lack of adequate water sanitation systems, use of unsafe water distribution systems and low levels of hand-washing in many countries.

One important example of anthropic contamination is the inappropriate use of antimicrobials in health care, in swine and poultry production and in fish farming. Antimicrobials spread in water, soil and in the environment, facilitating growth and dissemination of antimicrobial-resistant bacteria, thus having a serious impact on public health.

Moreover, fertilizers, pesticides and herbicides from unsustainable agricultural practices and their dumping in water influence almost all living organisms, producing loss of biodiversity and a negative impact on human health; pesticides are known to be related to multiple health disorders due to their effects on the reproductive system, their teratogenic and carcinogenic effects, as well as their neurotoxicity and immunosuppressive action. It is becoming evident that exposure to most prevalent environmental pollutants may play a role in the long-term response of molecular processes such as epigenetics, with dramatic transgenerational effects (Skinner *et al.* 2010).

The presence of pathogenic microorganisms in freshwater can lead to transmission of water-borne diseases, many of which cause diarrheal disease, the third leading cause of death among children under five. Globally, almost 1000 children under five die every day from diarrheal diseases due to poor sanitation, poor hygiene, or unsafe drinking water.[3] Global climate change is expected to affect water-borne enteric diseases. There is a positive association between ambient temperature and diarrheal diseases, and an increase in diarrheal disease following heavy rainfall and flooding events (Levy *et al.* 2016). The spread of neglected infectious diseases like schistosomiasis, trachoma and intestinal worms, which affect more than 1.5 billion people every year, is linked to poor water, sanitation and hygiene.[4] An emerging issue regarding water quality is the worldwide presence of microplastics in the water regularly being ingested by people worldwide (83% of water samples collected worldwide and up to 94% in the USA contained microplastics), though very little is known about the effects of microplastic consumption on human health (*The Lancet* 2017).

Forests also play a fundamental role in relation to human health. On the one hand, 1.6 billion people totally depend on forests for their survival and 70% of them are indigenous people. On the other hand, 80% of all species live in forests and forests are essential in water-cycle regulation, playing a key role in CO_2 capture by absorbing the gas from the atmosphere and storing it in the form of carbon. Forests also protect coastal areas from erosion and help to reduce tsunami and big wave effects; they maintain soil quality, ensuring rich biodiversity, and are recognized as spiritual and holy places for burial and initiation. Thus, deforestation is an important threat to human health, biodiversity and the ecosystem in general (Aragão 2012).

Taking down trees to increase food production or transforming land for shepherding can directly alter the capacity of carbon sinks and thus further increase the risks of climate change. Deforestation and subsequent use of lands for agriculture or pasture, especially in tropical regions, are contributing strongly to global warming (Mahowald *et al.* 2017).

Climate change is one of the greatest challenges of our century, with widely recognized interconnected effects on human health and overall changes in the ecosystem. Global warming is unequivocal, with proven increase in global average air and ocean temperatures, widespread melting of snow and ice, rising global average sea level and slowing down of the ocean circulation that transports warm water to the North Atlantic (Pachauri and Reisinger 2007). There is wide scientific consensus on the fact that global warming is the direct result of anthropogenic activities, mainly related to the rapid rise of greenhouse gas emissions (Cook *et al.* 2016).

The 2001 Report of the Intergovernmental Panel on Climate Change (IPCC) noted that greenhouse gas emissions from human activities were growing at a pace between 0.5% and 1% per year (IPCC 2001). The average rate of change of global average surface temperature since 1901 has been 0.7–0.9°C century^{-1}. However, this rate of change has nearly doubled in the period since 1975 (1.5–1.8°C century^{-1}) (Blunden *et al.* 2018), and this temperature rise trend average will be about 4 degrees by 2100 (Costello 2009). Many of the changes observed since 1950 are without precedent in the history of the Earth. The atmosphere and the ocean are experiencing an increase in temperature, rain and snowfall has decreased, and sea levels are rising (IPCC 2014). These changes have already affected physical and biological systems in many parts of world, also causing a dramatic impact on biodiversity: reduction of freshwater levels in lakes and rivers, redistribution of fish towards the poles, loss of marine biodiversity, disappearance of tree species and the rise of vector-borne and water-borne diseases. These are all examples of the complex interaction between ecological factors and climate change (WHO and CBD 2015). There is increasing awareness that climate change represents the biggest threat for global health. According to the Lancet Commission on Climate Change and Health, the human symptoms of climate change are unequivocal, potentially irreversible and unacceptable (Watts 2017).

In 2000, about 160,000 deaths and 5.5 million DALYs, i.e. the number of years lost due to disability or premature death, were related to climate change (McMichael *et al.* 2004). These lost life years were mainly due to malnutrition, infectious diseases (especially malaria and diarrhea), heat waves and floods. A WHO study published ten years later estimated that around 250,000 the deaths per year will be due to climate change between 2030 and 2050. This is a conservative estimate as it is based only on the most widespread conditions, such as malnutrition and infectious diseases. Interestingly, according to the same study, in 2030 sub-Saharan Africa will be the most affected area, but by 2050 the greatest burden will be borne by South Asia (WHO 2014).

The effects of climate change may be classified into three groups: direct, indirect and indirect impacts mediated through societal systems (IPCC 2001). In the first case, there is a direct impact on DALYs (McMichael *et al.* 2003). This is the case with heat stress, a serious public health problem especially for the most vulnerable people living in urban areas, as in the case of the 2003 heatwaves in Europe (Mitchell *et al.* 2016). The World Meteorological Organization (WMO) defined heatwaves as extreme weather events with marked warming of the air, or the invasion of very warm air, over a large area; it usually lasts from a few days to a few weeks (WMO 2016). This first group also includes the effects of floods or cyclones, which are always more frequent and violent. In 2012, worldwide, 231 disasters caused 5469 deaths, affected 87 million people, and caused US$ 44.6 billion in economic damage.[5] Flood events in 2011 affected 112 million people, causing 3410 deaths (IPCC 2014).

The second group (indirect effects) includes all the health effects mediated by different types of complex, multi-step, diffuse or deferred causal paths and phenomena such as in the case of the spread of certain infectious diseases such as malaria and cholera (McMicheal and Lindgren 2011). For example, in Bangladesh, cyclones or heavy rainfall-mediated changes in turbidity and salinity gradients can significantly influence the abundance and distribution of estuarine cholera vibrios. Extended salt intrusion and higher turbidities in tropical estuaries by stronger and more frequent storms and deforestation-derived erosion favor vibrio growth, with increasing risks for aquatic resources and human health in that zone (Lara *et al.* 2009).

Increased salinity of drinking water sources affects not only the spread of cholera. It is estimated that about 844 million people still lack basic drinking water. This problem is exacerbated by rising sea levels due to climate change, and other contributing factors, like changes in fresh water flow from rivers and increased shrimp farming along the coastal areas. Another implication of rising salinity is the higher risk of (pre)eclampsia in pregnant women living in coastal areas (Khan *et al.* 2014). In some countries, desalination plants are used to partly remove salt and other minerals from water sources, but this is unlikely to be a sustainable option for low-income countries affected by high salinity (Vineis 2011).

As mentioned, another significant example is related to changes in the spread of vector-borne diseases. The biological basis that explains the persistence of malaria in the tropics is that the reproductive rate of the anopheles mosquito is much higher in the hot and damp lowlands of the tropics as compared to more temperate regions. This has historically made malaria eradication much more difficult in the tropical regions compared with temperate climates where malaria spread is less robust (Carminade *et al.* 2014). The most significant climate change effects on malaria are confined to some regions (highlands in Africa and some areas in South America and Southeastern Asia); in other regions climate change is likely to have no effect on malaria owing to other important socioeconomic factors (Carminade *et al.* 2014). Other vector-borne-diseases like dengue and chikungunya can also be affected by climate change.

Impacts mediated through societal systems include undernutrition and food insecurity from drastically altered agricultural production, mental disorders due to forced displacement, extreme weather events and social isolation, migration within and outside countries, and gender differences exacerbated by severe meteorological events. For example, disasters on average kill more women than men, and kill women at a younger age than men (WHO 2014).

Nowadays human mobility has reached an unprecedented level caused by a multiplicity of factors like poverty, conflicts and labor needs but also environmental determinants such as natural disasters and climate change. The environmental changes are seldom direct drivers of migration; instead they are secondary elements linked to socioeconomic factors that push people to move. In 2008 the increased number of sudden and extreme events, affecting most of all vulnerable communities, forced 22.5 million people to move within their countries or across borders. People living in coastal areas where the sea-level rise is the biggest hazard or living where droughts are always more frequent and the ecosystem is degraded try to adapt to these situations, but many of them are aware that they should move to another place to survive (Ionesco *et al.* 2017). According to the International Organization for Migration (IOM), it is impossible to estimate the correct number of environmental migrants, but future forecasts vary from 25 million to 1 billion environmental migrants by 2050.

Moreover, climate change will lead to increased risks not only for communicable diseases but also for noncommunicable diseases such as cardiovascular diseases, cancer and respiratory diseases (Table 11.1).

Table 11.1 The direct and indirect pathways from climate change to NCDs

Climate change impacts	Pathway from climate change to NCDs	NCD outcome	Direction of health risk
Direct			
More frequent and increased intensity of heat	Heat stress	CVD, respiratory disease	Increased risk
Increased temperatures and less rainfall	Higher ground-level ozone and other air pollutants	CVD, respiratory disease (e.g., bronchitis, asthma)	Increased risk
Changes in stratospheric ozone and in precipitation and cloud coverage	Increased exposure to solar UVR	Autoimmune diseases (multiple sclerosis)	Reduced risk
Higher winter temperatures in temperate latitudes		CVD, respiratory disease	Reduced risk
Extreme weather event (fires, floods, storms)	Structural damage	Injuries	Reduced risk
Indirect			
Drought, flooding	Impaired agriculture, reduced food yields, and nutrition insecurity	Poor general health	Increased risk
Extreme weather event (fires, flooding, storms)	Trauma	Mental health (posttraumatic stress disorder)	Increased risk

Abbreviations: CVD, cardiovascular disease; NCDs, noncommunicable diseases; UVR, ultraviolet radiation.

Source: adapted from Friel *et al.* (2011).

Climate change also poses important global equity issues. Comparing the cumulative emissions of carbon dioxide for the period 1950–2000 with WHO estimates for malaria, malnutrition, diarrhea and floods, it is clear that populations which have experienced the most significant increase in the burden of diseases attributable to the rise in temperature over the last 30 years are, ironically, the least responsible for greenhouse gas emissions (Patz 2007). In fact, WHO estimates show that 99% of the disease burden due to climate change is in developing countries (Patz 2007). This phenomenon is related to vulnerability, which IPCC defines as the propensity or predisposition to be adversely affected by climate change (IPCC 2007). Being exposed to a risk factor, sensitivity to that risk and capacity to adapt to it make specific populations vulnerable to the health consequences of climate change. There is a risk that vulnerability will be a crucial element in the process that further worsens the degree of health inequality at the global level.

Regarding environmental health-related policies, the WHO plays a fundamental role in providing guidelines and policy recommendations.

For example, it sets recommended limits for health-harmful concentrations of key air pollutants. In 2005 WHO issued the last update for air quality guidelines for particulate matter, ozone, nitrogen dioxide and sulfur dioxide (WHO 2005). As air pollution is the largest single environmental risk for health, killing 7 million people per year, in May 2015 the World Health Assembly (WHA) urged Member States to take action in order to comply with WHO guidelines, including furthering policy dialogue, establishing partnerships and strengthening multi-sectorial cooperation at national, regional and international levels, and prompted the WHO Director-General to strengthen WHO capacities in the field of air pollution and health through the development and regular updating of WHO air quality guidelines (WHO 2015).

The revision process of the air quality guidelines for outdoor air pollution was started only in 2016. In the past the guidelines mainly focused on providing guidance in the form of pollutant exposure specific recommendations, usually as "not to be exceeded" concentration levels of air pollutants. The next update of the guidelines should formulate recommendations concerning specific measures or interventions shown to decrease the levels of air pollutants and improve health. The focus will still be on the main air pollutants: particulate matter, ozone, nitrogen dioxide, sulfur dioxide and carbon monoxide (WHO EURO 2016a).

In environmental health, however, the "health in all policies approach" is strategic. The "indivisible" Sustainable Development Goals (SDGs) included in the UN "Agenda 2030" clearly show the need to link action to achieve SDG good health and well-being to other SDGs, such as SDG6 clean water sanitation, SDG7 affordable and clean energy, SDG9 industry, innovation and infrastructure, SDG11 sustainable communities, SDG13 combat climate change and impact, SDG12 responsible consumerism and production and SDG14 and SDG15 life below water and on land.

In the UN system WHO collaborates with the United Nations Environmental Programme (UNEP), among other organizations. As a follow-up to a Ministerial Declaration on Health, Environment and Climate Change calling for the creation of a global "Health, Environment and Climate Change" Coalition at the United Nations Framework Convention on Climate Change (UNFCCC) COP 22 in Marrakesh, Morocco in 2016, in January 2018 WHO and UNEP agreed to set up a more systematic framework for joint research, development of tools and guidance, capacity building, monitoring of Sustainable Development Goals, and global and regional partnerships.

Priority areas for collaboration were identified as air quality, climate-related health risks, water, and waste and chemicals management, particularly in the area of pesticides, fertilizers and the use of antimicrobials.[6]

In May 2018 the collaboration was extended to the World Meteorological Organization (WMO) with the launch of a global coalition on health, environment and climate change, with the purpose, among others, of organizing the Global Conference on Air Pollution and Health, to take place in Geneva in autumn 2018.[7]

The most remarkable event regarding environmental policies at the global level, however, has been the Paris Agreement. The Agreement was established within the United Nations Framework Convention on Climate Change (UNFCCC), dealing with greenhouse-gas-emissions mitigation, adaptation, and finance. It was signed on 12 December 2015, and entered into force on 4 November 2016 (UN 2015). The Paris Agreement was the first global response to climate change: after less than one year it had been ratified by 153 of 197 parties to the United Nations Framework on Climate Change (UNFCCC), covering 84.7% of greenhouse gas emissions (Watts 2017). This is an extraordinary result if we compare it with the Kyoto Protocol, which entered into force eight years after its signing (after the ratification by at least 55 parties responsible for 55% of global emissions). The Paris Agreement aims to curb greenhouse gas emissions to keep global warming well below 2°C compared to pre-industrial levels, commits countries to adaptation, including plans aimed to protect human health from climate change (preamble), and recognizes the value of voluntary mitigation actions and their co-benefits for health (decisions). Health co-benefits of climate change mitigations represent a protective mechanism intended not only to decrease greenhouse gases and global warming, but also to improve human health: active transport such as walking, running and cycling protects people from noncommunicable diseases and helps to reduce pollutants and emissions. This win-win strategy should be extended not only to transport, but also to energy, food and agriculture (Hosking *et al.* 2011).

In her "Ten Years in public health, 2007–2017" report, former WHO Director-General Dr Margaret Chan stated that "the Paris Agreement is not just a treaty for saving the planet from severe, pervasive, and irreversible damage. It is also a significant public health treaty, with a huge potential to save lives worldwide".

The IPCC reports, too, have put increased emphasis on the connection between climate change and health: the first IPCC report in 1990 only mentioned a few papers on the topic; later reports all included a specific chapter on health implications of climate change (Verner *et al.* 2016).

Undoubtedly, environmental issues and climate change are among the biggest challenges to global governance for health in the twenty-first century. In addition, the global environmental agenda may suffer setbacks due to sudden changes in the support from big players, as for example the United States' withdrawal from the 2015 Paris climate agreement announced in June 2017 by President Donald Trump,[8] which has left many scientists frustrated and dismayed.

11.3 Epidemics and the global spread of infectious diseases

As early as the 1840s, Rudolph Virchow claimed the proper response to the typhus epidemic in Prussia would be political, not medical. Indeed, Virchow believed that politics and social systems have profoundly positive or negative effects on public health and that all epidemics are *social* in origin (Walter and Scott 2017). The increasingly quick spread

198 *Global policies and issues*

of diseases determined by the acceleration of the globalization process requires a more complex and transnational analysis of the determinants and responses to the spread of infectious diseases and epidemics.[9]

Infectious diseases are mostly associated with poverty and inequality, and so are most of their epidemics. Although heat and humidity play a role, especially in the distribution of vector-borne diseases, the concept of "tropical diseases" conceptualized at the end of the nineteenth century to support colonial powers and colonial expansion (Doyal 1981) is absolutely inappropriate as those pathologies and their distributions are not bound up with latitude, but mostly associated with socioeconomic conditions (Missoni *et al.* 1988). Diseases such as malaria, cholera and intestinal parasitosis were present in nineteenth-century Europe, where they disappeared thanks to improvements in standards of living conditions and hygiene.

The failure to control the spread of infectious diseases in low-income countries is largely a consequence of structural drivers such as the colonial and capitalist expansion in past centuries and more recently the establishment of the hegemonic neoliberal societal model, leading to rising inequality and weakening of national health systems. The intensified global circulation of people (see section 11.6 in this chapter) and goods, which is among the characterizing features of globalization, has reduced the barriers to the spread of infectious agents, including through previously unknown routes of transmission (see for example the case of bovine spongiform encephalopathy described below).

Infectious diseases follow four main routes of transmission: fecal-related, air-borne, direct contact and vector-borne. Whatever the mechanism, both environmental and socioeconomic determinants influence transmission, incidence and fatality rate.

For example, in the past cholera epidemics often spread along the fecal-related route. With improved sanitation and hygiene, cholera outbreaks became rarer in advanced industrialized countries in the twentieth century, though they are still a threat in less-developed countries (especially when conflicts or natural disasters complicate already precarious health and sanitary conditions).

Influenza represents perhaps the most well-known example of an epidemic-prone airborne infectious disease. The "Spanish flu" pandemic of 1918 infected 500 million people across the world resulting in the deaths of 3–5% of the world's population. It was one of the deadliest disasters in human history (Taubenberger and Morens 2006). Evidence showed that both the incidence of influenza and its death rate were different across social classes and socioeconomic status, then as well as now (Mamelund 2006). Life and working conditions (i.e. human-animal contact, overcrowded dwellings, poor hygiene) have been associated with the recent epidemic spreads of variants of the influenza virus such as "avian flu" H5N1 (2003) and "swine flu" H1N1 (2009). Social and racial/ethnic disparities in exposure, susceptibility and access to timely and effective treatment have been documented even in high-income countries like the United States. Disparities can also be observed in pandemic preparedness plans, lacking systematic attention to differential social risks (Blumenshine *et al.* 2008).

Examples of epidemic-prone infections that spread through direct contact include Ebola and sexually transmitted diseases such as HIV/AIDS, which occur in every country in the world. However, there is a positive correlation between HIV prevalence and poverty. Poverty seems to increase susceptibility to HIV/AIDS and facilitate its spread (Fenton 2004). The distribution of HIV does not follow national borders, but rather spreads along the economic trails of migrant labor and sexual commerce (Farmer 1996; Fox 2012). In addition, nowadays HIV/AIDS has become a chronic condition for millions of people, especially in higher-income countries where treatment is accessible, posing new challenges to health systems.

The 2014–2016 Ebola epidemic claimed thousands of lives in Sierra Leone, Liberia and Guinea, three of the poorest countries of the world. Poverty and social exclusion have been clearly linked to the Ebola crisis and its severity, exacerbated by reforms designed to attract international investment. Populations faced increased risk of exposure, while lacking functional surveillance and with health systems weakened by decades of macroeconomic adjustment policies and donor-driven investments in vertical programs, unable to promptly respond to the epidemic to avoid spread across borders (Huff and Winnebah 2015; Kentikelenis et al. 2015) (see also Chapter 12, Box 12.1).

A recent example of a vector-borne disease epidemic is the Zika virus (ZIKV). In 2016 the WHO declared the Zika epidemic a "public health emergency of international concern" (PHEIC), due to its possible association with microcephaly and Guillain-Barré syndrome. The ZIKV infection shares its transmission route and vector, i.e. *Aedes* spp. mosquitoes, with dengue and yellow fever, and could have the characteristics to become the next pandemic (Baumgaertner 2016).

In May 2016 the IFRC called for immediate action to control a deadly yellow fever outbreak in Angola, which had already spread to the Democratic Republic of the Congo, Kenya and China, and could continue to spread internationally. Three main lessons had emerged from the West African Ebola crisis which should have been applied to the yellow fever outbreak: invest in local health systems and community surveillance; engage local communities in developing and driving the response; and provide early response targeted to local circumstances. The Ebola crisis also highlighted the consequences of the short-term and reductionist approach of global health donors. In all countries hit by Ebola, development assistance for health was largely focused on disease-specific initiatives with little investment in strengthening the health systems.

Nevertheless, according to IFRC, months later the lessons from Ebola were not being applied in the response to Angola's yellow fever outbreak. While an urgent and coordinated response was considered, WHO declined to deem the outbreak a PHEIC (As Sy 2016). Angola's yellow fever outbreak ended in July 2016; nevertheless structural health system weakness (inadequate disease surveillance systems, limited access to care, lack of financial and human resources) remains the real challenge to timely and adequate response. Although an effective vaccine exists, it appears to be in limited supply (only four factories produce yellow fever vaccines globally and production relies on an old low-tech process). Fifteen of the 34 countries that already include the vaccine in their routine immunization programmes reported stock-outs that affected national coverage between 2013 and 2015. The yellow fever virus may potentially spread in Asia where 2 billion people with no immunity to the virus live in densely populated areas (Anderson 2018).

Overlapping high population densities of mosquitoes and humans sustain infection focal points (e.g. for *Aedes* spp.-transmitted diseases such as dengue, yellow fever, chikungunya, Zika and others), which are often associated with poor peri-urban areas with uninsulated homes, inadequate hygienic and sanitary conditions, the piling up of non-biodegradable waste and lack of an adequate public health infrastructure (Castro et al. 2010).

Ecosystem changes (see section in this chapter) are modifying the geographical limits (latitude and altitude) and the seasonality of infectious diseases, especially those which are vector-borne (e.g. malaria or dengue) or food-borne (e.g. salmonellosis). However, climatic changes are likely to disproportionately affect the poorest populations and developing countries, exacerbating inequality (Patz 2007; Bathiany *et al.* 2018).

The privatization and trade of water has reduced water security and increased the incidence of water-related diseases and related epidemics (Huynen *et al.* 2005). In many parts of Africa, ecological perturbations linked to export-oriented mineral and timber extraction involving expansive land grabs have resulted in increased risk of disease among rural communities. International investments contributed to exceptional economic growth which did not reach the majority of the population, while often contributing to the spread of zoonotic diseases to peri-urban areas (Huff and Winnebah 2015).

The overuse of antibiotics in both the health and agricultural sectors has driven antibiotic resistance to levels where now previously controllable infections could result in catastrophic epidemics. Rising antimicrobial resistance is deeply linked to how health systems function and interact with the public and with the pharmaceutical industry. Trade-related mechanisms also play a significant role: the Agreement on Trade-Related Intellectual Property Rights (TRIPS) has created a global system of patent protection that may increase pharmaceutical prices and reduce access to drugs and vaccines (Smith and Correa 2009). The high cost of essential medicines may contribute to the trade of substandard and counterfeit drugs, especially in low-income countries, to enormous social, economic and political challenges to health security, and to undermined capabilities to curb infectious diseases (Labonté 2010). At the same time, lack of access to appropriate and timely treatment compounds the problem by increasing the risk of multi-drug resistance for diseases such as tuberculosis. In the agroindustry, antibiotics are widely used in meat and fish production as a growth promoter; beyond Europe their use on animals is unregulated, to the advantage of transnational industries. In 2015, the sixty-eighth World Health Assembly endorsed a global action plan to tackle antimicrobial resistance, and in 2016 the UN adopted a political declaration committing to raise awareness about the issue and to better monitor the use of antibiotics in the health and farming sectors (UNGA 2016).

Finally, prevention and response to epidemics heavily rely on well-functioning health systems, as individual health security largely depends on access to safe and effective health services, products and technologies. Notwithstanding the global commitment to universal access to care, in many countries health systems have been weakened over the years by financial cuts and increasingly fragmented funding of selective approaches to disease control.

The response to epidemics cannot be reduced to a technical problem to be dealt with only through medical rescue processes and public health interventions. Upstream sociopolitical processes that determine the modalities of response also need to be addressed; these are intimately related to global health governance.

Besides its non-binding resolutions, WHO can revert to normative and regulatory instruments, seldom used, to defend the right to health and to influence the response to epidemics and their socioeconomic determinants (see Chapter 6).

In 2005, following the 2003 outbreak of severe acute respiratory syndrome (SARS), which served as a strong reminder that disease does not require a passport to cross borders, the International Health Regulations (IHR) were broadened in scope. The IHR – which together with the Framework Convention on Tobacco Control (FCTC) is one of only two examples of the WHO exercising its regulatory capacity – seek to prevent and provide a public health response to the international spread of diseases "in ways that are commensurate with and restricted to public health risks, and which avoid unnecessary interference with international traffic and trade" (IHR 2008). The latter was a concern during the bovine spongiform encephalopathy (BSE) epidemics in Britain in the 1980s, where the attempt by a government veterinarian to publish a paper describing one of the first cases of BSE was suppressed because "of possible effects on exports and the political implications" (Pennington 2005).

Over the last decade, epidemics of international concern such as SARS (2003), Ebola (2014) and Zika (2016) have put the spotlight on the implementation of the IHR and raised the focus on responses to health emergencies as "global health security". Significant new global resources are being proposed and mobilized for emergency responses, such as new reporting systems, new global financing facilities and independent assessments by global actors. Yet "securitization" seems to reduce global public health efforts to emergency responses and infectious disease control, without addressing local, national and cross-border measures which would strengthen the capacity of health systems to provide universal access to care. In addition, the global health security approach pays little attention to the promotion of public health through public policies beyond the immediate competence of the health sector – i.e. policies aimed at controlling or reducing the impact of socioeconomic determinants.

Too often epidemics also elicit international public interest and mobilization only when they spread beyond developing countries. The WHO declared the Ebola outbreak a Public Health Emergency of International Concern only in 2014, after two American aid workers infected in Liberia were evacuated to the United States. This was five months after the first cases were reported to the WHO, after almost 1800 people were infected and almost 1000 had died. By this point the outbreak was no longer a humanitarian crisis affecting a few poor countries in Africa, but an international security threat to developed countries. A month later an emergency meeting of the UN Security Council was held, and the UN's first-ever emergency health mission was established, the United Nations Mission for Ebola Emergency Response (UNMEER), because "the unprecedented extent of the Ebola outbreak in Africa constitutes a threat to international peace and security". Even colonial legacies became prominent in the organization of Ebola response, with military assistance being delivered along old colonial lines (Benton and Dionne 2015).

The emphasis on technology is another common aspect of global response to epidemics that takes attention away from the underlying causes of the outbreak – such as weak healthcare systems and poor life conditions. The current system of drug and vaccine development is market-friendly and favors chronic diseases that primarily affect people in the developed world, rather than neglected and infectious diseases likely to cause epidemics. It is only in the presence of *transnational* epidemics that emphasis is placed on the search for a vaccine or a drug, often perceived as a "magic bullet". It was not until the "transnational" Ebola epidemic that investments were mobilized in search of a last-minute vaccine; only then famous personalities such as Bill Gates, Jeremy Farrar (Wellcome Trust) and Seth Berkley (GAVI The Vaccine Alliance) called for funding additional research into drugs, vaccines and diagnostic tests, as well as creating a system for accelerating the approval of these interventions during a crisis (Kaner and Schaack 2016). Similarly, as soon as the Zika epidemic hit the news of developed countries, emphasis was put on the need to develop a vaccine rather than on the relation of the disease and its vector to poor urban peripheries and the need to improve sanitation and waste control.

202 *Global policies and issues*

Structural health system weaknesses (i.e. inadequate disease surveillance systems, limited access to care, lack of financial and human resources) remain a real challenge to timely and adequate response.

Evidently, the global fight against twenty-first-century epidemics of infectious diseases cannot be narrowed to emergency responses; it also needs to address their social, economic, political and environmental determinants. Medical rescue processes and public health interventions in response to epidemics are last-resort measures.

Health sector response to preventing and controlling epidemics should be based on long-term health system strengthening, a process that begins locally, within countries focusing on comprehensive primary health care, universally accessible services, social protection and public health approaches capable of identifying, preventing and managing risk *before* an epidemic.

Nevertheless, many determinants of epidemics lie outside the health sector and the traditional domain of health authorities. They are heavily related to processes of production and consumption, to societal structure and to social, economic and political processes, interests and influences. Thus, prevention of epidemics must link epidemiological knowledge to political processes that involve challenges to current economic and social institutions and, to be faced, require proper alliances and global well-directed and coordinated strategies (Missoni 2017).

11.4 The transformation of the global food system

Globalization has had a major impact on the global food system. Changes are closely associated with urbanization, market liberalization and foreign investments. Competition for markets shares, rather than an increase in production to satisfy nutritional needs, has led to significant changes all along the food chain from production and processing to retail and marketing. The transformation in the global food system

> Include[s] massive use of agrochemicals and hybrid plants and [...] genetically modified plants; changes in food processing designed to produce uniform quality, size and shape, particularly suited for brand name products; and changes in distribution and marketing systems supported by computer systems for ordering, delivery and improved corporate control over markets.
>
> (Kennedy *et al.* 2004)

These food system features were already well established in developed countries, and rapidly moved into developing country markets in the last two decades, impacting agriculture systems, pushing small farmers out of business and contributing to urbanization.

Urban residents were the first to experience dramatic lifestyle and dietary changes driven by, among other factors, demands on time, increased exposure to advertising, availability of new foods and emergence of new food retail outlets. Eventually people living in less urbanized areas progressively experienced them as well (Kennedy *et al.* 2004).

Foreign investment has ubiquitously introduced fast food restaurants and supermarkets, influencing consumer food choices through the offer of greater variety, quality, convenience and competitive prices in high-value-added foods, in addition to perceived higher social desirability (Mendez and Popkin 2004).

Supermarket offers are dominated by packaged and processed foods that expose consumers to "exotic" food items, those with a long shelf-life, and many varieties of snack foods containing any kind and quantity of additives, such as sodium, sugar and sweeteners, fat, preservatives, food coloring, and others. These are added to food in the industrial process to increase the palatability of the product, create dependency and increase its consumption.

The rapid adoption and increased consumption of new foods is further pushed through subtle marketing and aggressive advertising strategies, in which the transnational food industry (Big Food) invests enormous amounts of resources.

For example, to boost consumption bulk-sized packages are offered at discounted prices. In the United States, the size of a fast food burger and beverages has increased considerably over the last decades (Young and Nestle 2002; Nielsen and Popkin 2003). In addition to fast food, supermarkets and large food chains also encourage wholesale shopping and oversized convenience food.

"The advertising budget of the largest food companies can exceed national expenditures on health promotion and health education by massive proportions" (Kennedy *et al.* 2004). At the global level, for each US dollar invested by the WHO for the promotion of healthy eating habits, the agri-food industry spends 500 to promote its processed products (IACFO 2003).

Thus, over the course of the twentieth century and starting in industrialized countries, while on the one hand the individual daily energy requirements have been progressively decreasing (work activities with lower energy consumption; development of means of transport; increasing sedentary activities in leisure time), on the other hand the daily caloric intake has increased and populations have moved from traditional diets high in fiber and micronutrients to diets based on highly processed food, high in sugar, fats and salt, low in fiber and less nutrient-dense – with these dietary changes accompanied by changes in eating behaviors (Popkin *et al.* 2012). These global changes in lifestyle, food culture and dietary consumption patterns had a dramatic impact on populations' nutritional status and health.

11.4.1 The impact on nutritional status and health

Worldwide, obesity among children increased from less than 1% (equivalent to 5 million girls and 6 million boys) in 1975 to nearly 6% in girls (50 million) and nearly 8% in boys (74 million) in 2016, with an additional 213 million children and adolescents of both sexes considered overweight in 2016. Meanwhile, in 2016, 75 million girls and 117 million boys worldwide were moderately or severely underweight (Abarca Gomez *et al.* 2017). Thus, the number of children and adolescents aged 5–19 years in the world who are moderately or severely underweight remains higher than those who are obese. Yet the transition from underweight to overweight and obesity can be rapid, as it was seen in east Asia and Latin America and the Caribbean. Although hunger seems again on the rise (FAO *et al.* 2018), if current trends continue, more children and adolescents will be obese than moderately or severely underweight by 2022 (Abarca Gomez *et al.* 2017)

In 2016, more than 1.9 billion adults 18 years and older (39% of adults) were overweight. Of these, over 650 million were obese (13% of adults). Most of the world's population lives in countries where overweight and obesity kills more people than underweight; this occurs in every region except parts of sub-Saharan Africa and Asia. Every year, 1500 children under five years of age die every day as a result of hunger.[10]

But the world's increasing obese and overweight population suffers from related chronic diseases that are also the leading cause of death worldwide and entail enormous economic and social costs. This dramatic shift in "the way the entire globe eats, drinks and moves have clashed with our biology to create major shifts in body composition", a phenomenon which is now global and that was described in 1994 as the "nutrition transition" (Popkin et al. 2012).

Not only is obesity increasing worldwide, but also in the last three decades not a single country recorded obesity reduction (Ng et al. 2014).

In low-income countries, obesity mainly affects rich, urban-dwelling, middle-aged adults (mostly women), while in high-income countries it affects both sexes and all ages but disproportionately affects disadvantaged groups (Swinburn et al. 2011). Inequality is therefore itself a risk factor. The prevalence of malnutrition and obesity is directly proportional to the internal inequality of countries, regardless of their national income (Wilkinson and Pickett 2010).

High body mass index is strongly associated with increased morbidity of a wide range of chronic diseases including cardiovascular disease (mainly heart disease and stroke), the leading cause of death, diabetes, musculoskeletal disorders (especially osteoarthritis) and some cancers (including endometrial, breast, ovarian, prostate, liver, gallbladder, kidney and colon). Childhood obesity is associated with a higher chance of obesity, premature death and disability in adulthood. But in addition to increased future risks, obese children experience breathing difficulties, increased risk of fractures, hypertension, early markers of cardiovascular disease, insulin resistance and psychological effects.[11]

It has also been extensively shown that susceptibility to obesity and chronic diseases is influenced by environmental exposures from the time of conception. Indeed, fetal nutritional insufficiency triggers a set of biological changes that enhance survival in a "resource-poor" environment. In a postnatal environment with plentiful food, these developmental adaptations will favor obesity and development of disease (Popkin et al. 2012).

11.4.2 Food security, food safety and food sovereignty

Paradoxically, despite the obesity pandemic, after steadily declining for over a decade, global hunger appears to be on the rise again and threatens to derail the international commitment to end hunger and all forms of malnutrition by 2030. Despite more than enough food production in the world to feed everyone, there has been an increase in the proportion of the world's population that is undernourished, and the absolute number of undernourished people on the planet has also increased to 821 million in 2017, up from 804 million in 2016. According to the latest FAO report, the main driver behind this increase is the greater number of conflicts, whose impacts are often exacerbated by climate-related shocks (FAO et al. 2018) and one of the greatest challenges the world faces is how to ensure *food security*[12] for a growing global population (projected to rise to around 10 billion by 2050), to guarantee they have enough food to meet their nutritional needs.

> Food security exists when all people, at all times, have physical and economic access to sufficient, safe and nutritious food that meets their dietary needs and food preferences for an active and healthy life.
>
> (Definition agreed at FAO, 2018)[13]

It should be noted that the definition refers not only to the availability of food but also to the quality of the diet, linking it to a healthy and active lifestyle. Malnutrition, in fact, does not only exist in the presence of a general condition of hunger, but also manifests itself with deficiencies of single nutritional components, with serious health consequences. For example, iodine deficiency causes brain damage and mental retardation, iron deficiency causes anemia, and vitamin A deficiency is the leading preventable cause of childhood blindness.

Food security is a complex condition requiring a comprehensive approach to all forms of malnutrition, the productivity and incomes of small-scale food producers, resilience of food production systems and the sustainable use of biodiversity and genetic resources.

International trade of agricultural and food products substantially increased over the last decades. Between 1995 and 2016 export of agricultural products tripled in real terms from US$ 361 billion to US$ 1073 billion.[14] Nevertheless, vast areas of the planet are exposed to serious shortages of food; evidently, food distribution is an important issue.

The balance between national production, distribution and access to international markets is a critical aspect of food security at the country level. Many developing countries do not produce a sufficient quantity of staple foods and must import them to satisfy their needs. To this end, availability of foreign exchange is essential to buy imports, and the needed financial resources are generally the result of exports of raw materials, which are also largely linked to agricultural production. Thus, national food security is affected primarily by a country's ability to earn enough foreign exchange to import the food it needs. However, trade liberalization may reduce self-sufficiency in basic food production and increase reliance on imports.

Thus, agricultural exports remain a cornerstone of the economies of many developing countries and it is "no surprise that developing countries have been very active, for instance, in the on-going WTO negotiations on agriculture" (WTO/WHO 2002).

Trade barriers raised by industrialized countries (as in the case of the EU and the US, which act mainly through incentives for domestic agricultural production) are an obstacle to poor countries' exports. Trade liberalization policies in this area could have positive effects on global food security. Trade, in itself, is neither a threat nor a panacea, it presents at the same time opportunities and risks (Table 11.2) that need to be assessed to ensure that countries' food security and development needs are considered in a coherent and systematic way (FAO 2015).

The other major issue in the relationship between trade and food is *food safety*, i.e. ensuring that food does not harm health. Food production, processing and consumption may endanger health through contaminants that include, but are not limited to, pesticides and other agrochemicals, environmental/industrial contaminants, processing/storage-derived contaminants, contact-material-derived contaminants, biotoxins, antimicrobials, biological contaminants (such as bacteria and viruses), natural or artificial allergens and illegal food adulterants. In addition, new technologies such as genetic modification and nanotechnologies pose growing concerns in terms of food safety.

National policies are often put in place to ensure the safety of foods, though they are implemented with a variety of approaches and protection standards. However, this national priority may compete with international trade and multilateral regulations aiming to ensure that no barriers are raised against the free circulation of goods.

Table 11.2 Food security: risks and opportunities linked to global trade liberalization

	Potentially positive effects	*Potentially negative effects*
Availability	Trade boosts imports and increases both the quantity and variety of food available. Dynamic effects on domestic production: greater competition from abroad may trigger improvements in productivity through greater investment, R&D, technology spillover.	For net food-exporting countries, higher prices in international markets can divert part of production previously available for domestic consumption to exports, potentially reducing domestic availability of staple foods. For net food-importing countries, domestic producers unable to compete with imports are likely to curtail production, reducing domestic supplies and foregoing important multiplier effects of agricultural activities in rural economies.
Access	For net food-importing countries, food prices typically decrease when border protection is reduced. In the competitive sectors, incomes are likely to increase as the result of greater market access for exports. Input prices are likely to decrease. The macroeconomic benefits of trade openness, such as export growth and the inflow of foreign direct investment, support growth and employment, which in turn boosts incomes.	For net food-exporting countries, the domestic prices of exportable products may increase. Employment and incomes in sensitive, import-competing sectors may decline.
Utilization	A greater variety of available foods may promote more balanced diets and accommodate different preferences and tastes. Food safety and quality may improve if exporters have more advanced national control systems in place or if international standards are applied more rigorously.	Greater reliance on imported foods has been associated with increased consumption of cheaper and more readily available high-calorie/low-nutritional-value foods. Prioritization of commodity exports can divert land and resources from traditional indigenous foods that are often superior from a nutrition point of view.
Stability	Imports reduce the seasonal effect on food availability and consumer prices. Imports mitigate local production risks. Global markets are less prone to policy- or weather-related shocks.	For net food-importing countries, relying primarily on global markets for food supplies and open trade policies reduces the policy space to deal with shocks. Net food-importing countries may be vulnerable to changes in trade policy by exporters, such as export bans. Sectors at earlier stages of development may become more susceptible to price shocks and/or import surges.

Source: adapted from FAO 2015.

For example, the WTO Sanitary and Phytosanitary Agreement (SPS) (described in Chapter 6) aims at preventing public health protection measures from being used as a pretext for raising trade barriers. The WTO allows for restrictive trade measures only if consolidated scientific evidence exists about the health hazards related to specific goods, and standards have been adopted internationally (as in the Codex Alimentarius[15] and IRA[16]). In their absence, it is up to the WTO member to provide that evidence. The case of meat from animals reared using hormones provides a good example. A WTO panel ruled in 1997 against a European Union (EU) ban on artificial hormone-treated beef.

> Since 1988, the EU has banned the sale of beef from cattle treated with artificial hormones and has applied the ban in a nondiscriminatory fashion to both domestic and imported beef products. Exposure to the artificial hormones themselves have been linked to cancer and the premature pubescence in girls, although the risk to humans of artificial hormone residues in the meat they consume has yet to be conclusively measured (…). The U.S. beef and biotechnology industries have long opposed this EU policy. In January 1996, the US challenged the ban the WTO. In 1998, a WTO panel ruled that the beef hormone ban was an illegal measure under SPS rules (…) and the EU was ordered to begin imports of U.S. artificial hormone-treated beef (…). After the EU refused to comply with the WTO panel ruling (…) the WTO approved a U.S. request to impose retaliatory sanctions against European-made products. In its beef hormone ruling, the WTO effectively declared that food safety regulations enacted in advance of scientific certainty were not allowed.
>
> (Wallach and Sforza 1999)

Although standards such as the Codex Alimentarius are based on databases which include a vast array of agents and issues (including animal feed, antimicrobials, biotechnology, contaminants, pesticides and others), the choice to rely exclusively on scientific evidence and international standards cannot exclude with certainty risks to human health from unexplored or insufficiently studied potentially harmful agents. In addition, the Codex Alimentarius itself also has accountability limits, being exposed to the pressure exerted by the economic world; its decision-making process is no longer based on consensus but on voting (Ni 2013). Although nominally intergovernmental the Codex Alimentarius appears to be industry-dominated. "Industry representatives vastly outnumber consumer or general public-interest non-governmental organization (NGO) representatives, both in plenary sessions and in committee meetings." In addition "a 1997 study found that only 11 of the NGOs recognized by Codex were not industry-funded" (Büthe and Harris 2011: 225). Also developing country members are under-represented, as they often lack the institutions, expertise and resources to influence the standard-setting process. This results in a relative marginalization of developing countries in Codex, and their membership is at risk of only existing to legitimize advanced countries' global rule-making (Büthe and Harris 2011).

Indeed, the current level of scientific knowledge does not always allow one to distinguish between what is harmful and what is not. In specific circumstances where scientific evidence has been insufficient but preliminary, and where objective scientific evaluation has provided an indication of potentially dangerous effects on the environment, human, animal or plant health, the "precautionary principle" has been adopted in some legislation, like in the EU, where it is entrenched in a number of laws. Although the precautionary principle may have been invoked in ways that aim to boost or protect opportunities for local producers, thus discriminating against foreign producers, the core motivation is indeed to protect the environment and health (McNeill *et al.* 2017).

As an alternative model to the industrial food systems, *food sovereignty* was introduced in 1996 by La Via Campesina (LVC), possibly the most important transnational social movement in the world. Food sovereignty is presented as an alternative model based on the democratization of food systems, and aims to include small-scale farmers and sustainable production. Food sovereignty is based on six founding principles with a focus on agrarian rights and food production:

- autonomy of peoples and communities to define their food and agricultural systems;
- pluralism and the democratic control of localized food systems to achieve food security with sustainable production;
- women's rights, i.e. – addressing the inequalities that persist in the community, group and family unit, rather than hiding different agrarian classes in the notion of a homogeneous community;
- localization, without precluding long-distance trade; it emphasizes local food systems and short-distance trade;
- complexity of societies requiring enough flexibility in delivering social justice and food, allowing food sovereignty to be implemented in different settings;
- adaptability, as food sovereignty is a process, rather than an outcome, allowing for a wide-range of interpretations, now inclining towards the inclusion of whole food systems.

A "second generation" of thinking and action in terms of food sovereignty

> is broadening the original focus on 'agrarian sovereignty' to incorporate consumers, cities, and urban food security through a broader food systems approach. As the critique of conventional market-based approaches to development becomes more mainstream due to the convergence of economic, social and environmental crises, it is likely that food sovereignty will emerge as a 'connecting concept', capable of uniting various streams of theory and practice, from systems thinking to post-growth economics and social innovation.
>
> (Dekeyser *et al.* 2018)

11.4.3 The global framework of policies and response

The response to food-system-related health issues can be traced along the lines of different levels of global policy-making.

The 2030 Agenda for Sustainable Development (see Chapters 2 and 4) incorporates food-related health challenges in Sustainable Development Goal (SDG) 2 "End hunger, achieve food security and improved nutrition and promote sustainable agriculture" and SDG3 "Ensure healthy lives and promote well-being for all at all ages", specifically target 3.4 "By 2030, reduce by one third premature mortality from noncommunicable diseases through prevention and treatment and promote mental health and well-being" (UN 2015a).

Neoliberal globalization 209

At the global level, nutrition priorities and policies have been discussed intersectorally by three main bodies: The World Health Assembly, the Committee for Food Security (CFS)[17] and the United Nations General Assembly (UNGA). The WHO has dealt with broader nutrition policy issues since the First International Conference on Nutrition in 1992, when it endorsed a Plan of Action on Nutrition which incorporated nutrition objectives in national development programs (Branca and Ellis 2017). In response to obesity and related diseases, the WHO has been implementing its Action Plan on "Global Strategies on Diet, Physical Activity and Health" since 2004 (WHO 2004). The Plan sets out a series of recommendations which may be adopted by national governments to ensure that the obesity epidemic is adequately tackled. The recommendations include encouraging individuals to eat healthy foods (fruit and vegetables) and to gradually decrease the intake of saturated animal fats (instead giving preference to unsaturated vegetable fats) as well as salt and sugars. As a follow-up to the Plan, WHO has also developed a set of recommendations on marketing foods and beverages to children (Branca and Ellis 2017).

In the following years the focus shifted to the direct link between the food system, nutrition and NCDs, involving the highest level of the UN system as the UN General Assembly adopted the Political Declaration of the High-level Meeting on the Prevention and Control of Noncommunicable diseases, which expressed

> deep concern at the ongoing negative impacts of the financial and economic crisis, volatile energy and food prices and ongoing concerns over food security, as well as the increasing challenges posed by climate change and the loss of biodiversity, and their effect on the control and prevention of non-communicable diseases.
>
> (UN 2012)

Among other interventions, the UNGA committed to reduce risk factors through the implementation of

> cost-effective interventions to reduce salt, sugar and saturated fats and eliminate industrially produced trans-fats in foods, including through discouraging the production and marketing of foods that contribute to unhealthy diet, while taking into account existing legislation and policies

while also encouraging

> policies that support the production and manufacture of, and facilitate access to, foods that contribute to healthy diet, and provide greater opportunities for utilization of healthy local agricultural products and foods, thus contributing to efforts to cope with the challenges and take advantage of the opportunities posed by globalization and to achieve food security.
>
> (UNGA 2012)

With the Second International Conference on Nutrition (ICN2), in 2014, further progress was made in achieving intersectoral integration, and the WHA also called for the implementation of policies across the health sector, the food system, education and the environment. With the Rome Declaration, which considered the "broken" food system, world leaders committed "to fix the global food system" and to ensure that everyone has access to safe, healthy and affordable diets. To this end, the Declaration suggested options such as building sustainable food systems and intervening in international trade and investment (Branca and Ellis 2017).

Building on the commitments made in the ICN2 and in the framework of the 2030 Agenda for Sustainable Development, world leaders at the UNGA proclaimed the UN Decade of Action on Nutrition from 2016 to 2025, providing an umbrella for all relevant stakeholders to consolidate and align action across different sectors.

The UN Conference on Climate Change (COP21) in 2015 also addressed nutrition, framing vulnerabilities in food production systems as one of the negative consequences of climate change (Branca and Ellis 2017).

11.5 The tobacco epidemic

Though cigarette consumption was popularized in the nineteenth century, only in the 1950s was the scientific community able to demonstrate its adverse health effects thanks to the results of a seminal study conducted by Doll and Hill (1954).

As James B. Duke and his American Tobacco Company shaped the modern tobacco industry, the manufactured cigarette became the dominant form of tobacco consumption in the twentieth century, surpassing other forms of use (NCCDPHP: National Center for Chronic Disease Prevention and Health Promotion (US) Office on Smoking and Health 2014). At the beginning of the twentieth century, lung cancer was only a reportable disease, but now it has become the commonest cause of death from cancer in both men and women in the developed world, and before long it will reach that level in the developing world as well (Spiro and Silvestri 2005).

Following the demonstration of the relationship between smoking and lung cancer by Doll and Hill (1954), the first control measures and public awareness campaigns were initiated. The campaigns led to a progressive reduction in smoking in developed countries since the 1990s, demonstrating that strong scientific evidence on the relationship between risk factors and disease helps to counteract health-damaging phenomena such as smoking.

Despite these efforts, in the late 1990s the Global Burden of Disease study estimated that tobacco was the cause of 6% of deaths worldwide (Murray and Lopez 1996). More recently, the WHO has estimated that 7 million deaths are caused each year by tobacco consumption and exposure to tobacco smoke (equivalent to one death every five seconds); this is more than the combined deaths due to HIV, tuberculosis and malaria, the three diseases whose control is the focus of SDG3 (WHO 2017). These figures are expected to increase to more than 8 million a year by 2030[18] as a result of both population growth and the fact that, in some large populations, generations of few heavy smokers are being replaced by generations in which heavy smoking is widespread. If current trends persist, smoking will kill around one billion people in this century, mostly in low- and middle-income countries. About half of these deaths will occur before the age of 70 years (Jha and Peto 2014). Smoking, therefore, is one of the main components of the global burden of disease, along with alcohol consumption, hypertension and high blood cholesterol levels (Ezzati *et al.* 2005).

In recent decades, a reduction in tobacco use in industrialized countries has been accompanied by a sharp increase in the rest of the world, linked to the aggressive marketing strategies (advertising, sponsorship, brand promotion) that transnational companies implemented in these countries. Since the 1960s, in response to the fall in sales in Western industrialized countries, the main transnational companies moved their target to the growing economies of Latin America, and in the 1980s to the newly industrialized countries of Asia (Taiwan, South Korea and Thailand). In the 1990s, they moved towards Eastern Europe, China and Africa, increasingly targeting young people and women (Bettcher et al. 2000). In these countries, advertising messages often combined cigarettes with Western, especially North American, images of freedom and prosperity (Collin and Lee 2003). Over the years, tobacco transnational companies have developed sophisticated strategies to make their products increasingly attractive. The work done by Philip Morris for the Marlboro brand is extremely symbolic. The advertising campaign focused on the image of the Marlboro Man was launched in 1954 and represents one of the longest-lasting advertising campaign ever. Over 40 years Philip Morris has invested more than one billion dollars in that image, creating one of the world's most famous brands (Klein 2002).

In terms of the penetration of world markets, the tobacco transnational industry also benefited from the trade agreements established during the Uruguay Round negotiations which led to the creation of the World Trade Organization (WTO); these included for the first time the liberalization of unmanufactured tobacco products (Bettcher et al. 2000).

The reduction of trade barriers has had a large impact on low-income countries; although smaller, the impact on middle-income countries is also relevant (Taylor and Bettcher 2000). Consumption has increased because of greater demand. Besides increased advertising by the tobacco industry, among factors that stimulated demand reduction in tobacco prices has played an important role, being linked to trade liberalization and the related competition regime introduced in countries where the tobacco market was previously monopolistic. Trade liberalization is therefore presumably a further challenge in the control of tobacco consumption.

In the context of WTO trade agreements, tobacco control policies could be challenged at various levels, such as in the Technical Barriers to Trade (TBT) Agreement in relation to product requirements such as packaging and labeling, in the Agreement on Agriculture in relation to state support for tobacco production, in the General Agreement on Trade in Services (GATS) agreement in relation to cigarette advertising restrictions, and in the TRIPS agreement in relation to trademark protection and the disclosure of product-related information that producers consider confidential (WTO/WHO 2002).

In addition, two articles present in the General Agreement on Tariffs and Trade (GATT), which was in force before the establishment of the WTO, may interfere with tobacco control policies: Article XI on the general elimination of quantitative restrictions, which may restrict limitations on imports of cigarettes from abroad; and Article III on national treatment for internal taxation and regulation, which can affect cigarette taxation.

Since the early 1990s several proposals have emerged for the elaboration of international responses to the global tobacco epidemic. In May 1995, at the 48th World Health Assembly (WHA), the idea of an international binding agreement to combat smoking habits was launched. The following year, the WHA committed the WHO Director-General to work on the development of an International Tobacco Control Treaty. It was only in 2003, after several years of work, that the WHA unanimously adopted the WHO Framework Convention on Tobacco Control (FCTC), which is the first international convention designed to reduce worldwide smoking-related deaths and diseases (WHO 2003). The FCTC entered into force in 2005, once the required number of ratifications was achieved. The FCTC requires countries to impose restrictions on cigarette advertising, sponsorship and promotional campaigns, to establish new packaging and labeling for cigarette packets, to establish indoor air quality controls, and to strengthen legislation to combat tobacco smuggling (WHO 2003). Even before the conclusion of the negotiations on the FCTC, concerns about the possible incompatibility with WTO agreements were examined in a joint WTO/WHO study. According to that document

> None of the provisions of the FCTC seem to be inherently WTO-inconsistent; and many of the restrictions called for by some of its provisions may well be determined to be "necessary" for health protection under WTO rules. However, the relationship between WTO rules and the FCTC will depend on the direction taken by future negotiations on the FCTC, and the manner in which its rules are applied by governments.
>
> (WTO/WHO 2002: 14–15)

In the following decade, 177 countries have ratified and started to implement the FCTC's provisions. The success has been mitigated by new challenges. As mentioned above, tobacco use has decreased in countries that are members of the Organization for Economic Cooperation and Development (OECD), but increased in low- and middle-income countries, in part as a result of illicit trade and the spread of low-cost products from China and other unregulated state monopolies (Yach 2014). In addition, the tobacco industry systematically hinders existing tobacco control legislation and aggressively counteracts control policies. Tobacco companies have often resorted to national litigation and international dispute settlements to discourage countries from implementing effective policies against tobacco use, though not always with success. In 2015, for example, Australia obtained a major victory over Philip Morris, which was suing the government for its decision to ban brands on packets of cigarettes (i.e. to require plain packaging) in order to reduce the commercial attractiveness of the product, especially among young people. In the wake of that success, the French National Assembly also approved an anti-tobacco plan, which since May 2016 has required neutral cigarette packaging, all identical, which can include the name of the manufacturer but without a logo. Other countries are studying the possibility of following the same path, despite threats from big tobacco companies (Maciocco 2015).

The sixth WHO report on the global tobacco epidemic testifies to the remarkable progress many countries have made to reduce tobacco use. In 2007 WHO first introduced the six MPOWER measures[19] to help countries implementing the FCTC. In 2007, only 42 countries were protected by at least one measure at best-practice level. After ten years, 121 countries have adopted at least one of these measures. Tobacco taxation is still the least implemented measure in terms of population coverage (since 2014 global coverage has remained steady at 10%), yet it is considered the most impactful and cost-effective of all the MPOWER measures (WHO 2017).

In addition, some authors remark that no progress will be made until interferences from the tobacco industry as referred to in Article 5.3[20] of the FCTC are prohibited (Gilmore et al. 2015). Tobacco companies often use international trade agreements as instruments to limit smoking control measures at the national level. Other authors argue that bilateral and regional free trade agreements, such as the Trans-Pacific Partnership (TPP) between the United States and 11 other countries in the Asia region, could provide the tobacco industry with new legal instruments to challenge measures taken by states to protect public health (Mitchell and Sheargold 2015). Of course, this is a trend that concerns not only tobacco use. At a time when multilateral agreements are at a stalemate, countries are trying to establish new agreements that, on a smaller territorial scale, will make it possible to increase trade.

11.6 Human migration

Migration is a global phenomenon, with around 3% of the world's population living temporarily or permanently outside their country of origin. International migration is a complex phenomenon that touches on a multiplicity of economic, social and security aspects affecting daily lives in an increasingly interconnected world (IOM 2018).

The International Organization for Migration (IOM) defines a migrant as "any person who is moving or has moved across an international border or within a State away from his/her habitual place of residence, regardless of the person's legal status; whether the movement is voluntary or involuntary; what the causes for the movement are; or what the length of the stay is".[21]

A refugee is "a person who, owing to well-founded fear of persecution for reasons of race, religion, nationality, membership of a particular social group or political opinions, is outside the country of his nationality and is unable or, owing to such fear, is unwilling to avail himself of the protection of that country".[22]

The term "asylum-seeker" refers to a person asking for international protection under international refugee law, but whose claim has not yet been finally decided on by the country in which he or she has submitted it. Not every asylum-seeker will ultimately be recognized as a refugee, but every refugee is initially an asylum-seeker (WHO EURO 2016)

According to WHO there are an estimated 1 billion migrants in the world today, of whom around one-quarter are international migrants and three-quarters are internal migrants. Globally, there are an estimated 65 million people who have been forcibly displaced from their homes, of whom 86% are hosted in low-income countries.[23]

Globally, there were an estimated 258 million international migrants in 2017. Of these, nearly 57% lived in developed regions, while developing regions hosted 43% of the world's migrants. Of the 146 million international migrants living in the developed regions in 2017, 89 million, or 61%, originated from a developing country, while 57 million, or 39%, were born in developed regions. Meanwhile, 97 million, or 87%, of the 112 million international migrants residing in the developing regions in 2017 originated from other parts of the developing regions, while 14 million, or 13%, were born in the developed regions (UN 2017). International migration increased in the last 27 years but has remained relatively stable as a proportion of the world's population since 1990 (IOM 2018) (Figure 11.1).

The proportion of migrants who are refugees, however, is increasing. According to the UN Refugee Agency (UNHCR), 37.5 million people were forcibly displaced by war in 2005. Of the total 65 million forcibly displaced from their homes in 2015, 22.5 million are refugees, half of whom are under 18.[24] The median age of international migrants worldwide was 39 years in 2015 (IOM 2015).

Climate change, urbanization and expanded trade are likewise driving increased population mobility within and between countries (IOM 2011).

It should be noted that the heterogeneity of the literature on the international migration determinants is very high (Maastricht University and GMDAC 2016). Three main

214 *Global policies and issues*

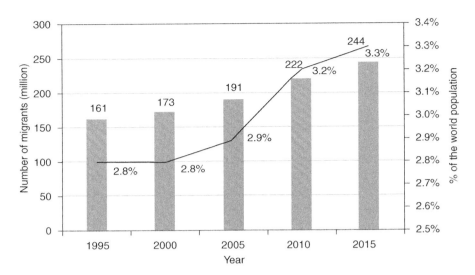

Figure 11.1 Migrant population between 1995 and 2015.
Source: adapted from IOM 2018.

points seem to emerge quite strongly: first, economic and political factors generally seem to prevail over demographic and environmental factors in explaining international mobility; secondly, specifically in the irregular and forced migration domains, recent studies emphasize the important role played by migrant formal and informal networks in facilitating migration; and third, migrants are a highly heterogeneous group, and migration decisions are never static (Maastricht University and GMDAC 2016).

The challenges for public health and health systems relate to migrants' individual health problems, whether they affect the resident population, and how to adequately respond to their needs, including access to health care.[25] In spite of the common perception of an association between migration and the importation of infectious diseases, there is no systematic association. Communicable diseases are associated primarily with poverty. Migrants often come from communities affected by war, conflict or economic crisis and undertake long, exhausting journeys that increase their risk of disease.[26]

Migrants are too heterogeneous as a group to make sweeping generalizations about their health. It is important to examine country of origin, country of destination and the circumstances of migration (Marmot 2016). A more process-oriented and integrated framework is needed; health aspects of migration should be considered in terms of the migratory process itself (Gushulak 2017).

Zimmerman *et al.* (2011) propose the following framework for understanding the migratory process in terms of five phases of migration: Pre-Departure Phase (which comprises the time before individuals leave from their place of origin), Travel Phase (which encompasses the period when individuals are between their place of origin and a destination or an interception location), Destination Phase (when individuals settle either temporarily or long-term in their intended location), Interception Phase (which is characterized by situations of temporary detention or interim residence) and Return Phase (when individuals go back to their place of origin) (Figure 11.2).

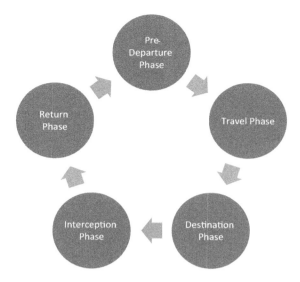

Figure 11.2 Migration phases framework.
Source: adapted from Zimmerman *et al*. 2011.

A careful analysis of the health needs of immigrant communities represents the fundamental precondition for identifying appropriate health and social policies. This involves a commitment to quantitative and qualitative research, possibly with the involvement of the same migrant communities. When not properly supported by appropriate inter-sectoral policies, immigrants will be exposed to hostile circumstances that leave them vulnerable to negative experiences which, in turn, influence their life chances (Marceca 2016). Unfortunately, especially in Europe, increasingly complex measures used to deter refugees have placed an emphasis on protection *from* the refugee above protection *of* the refugee (Smith 2016). As a result, UNITED for Intercultural Action has attributed 33,305 refugee deaths to the policing and border control measures in place across Europe, and most probably thousands more are never found.[27]

A general issue for health systems of countries that are destinations for migrants is how to deal with the intercultural dimension, or the encounter between different cultures. The challenge is how to guarantee care to patients who have different expectations according to their culture, which also includes traditional medicines. WHO provides very general guidance in this regard. On the one hand WHO defines traditional medicine as "the sum total of the knowledge, skills, and practices based on the theories, beliefs, and experiences indigenous to different cultures, whether explicable or not, used in the maintenance of health as well as in the prevention, diagnosis, improvement or treatment of physical and mental illness" (WHO 2000). On the other hand, in 2003, with Resolution 56.31 the WHA encouraged Member States to formulate and implement national policies and regulations in the field of non-conventional medicine, focusing on staff training (WHO 2003a).

Furthermore, what still hasn't been widely discussed is the enormous burden of mental-health disorders in migrants and refugees. For example, a large cohort study published in March 2016 looked at 1.3 million people who had arrived in Sweden before

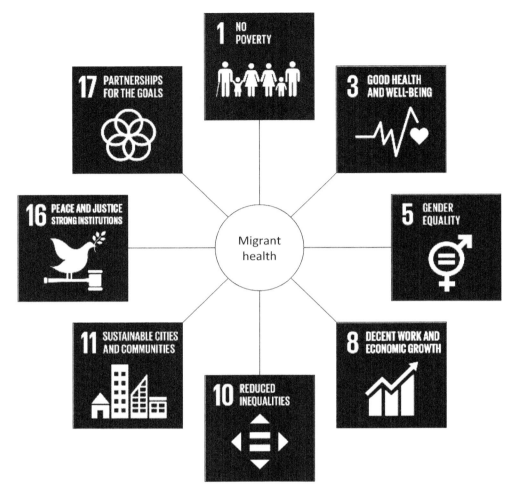

Figure 11.3 Migrant health and SDGs.

2011. Refugees had a threefold higher incidence of schizophrenia and other psychotic disorders than native-born Swedes, and a 66% higher incidence than migrants who were not refugees.[28] Mental health is a dimension that cuts across all phases of the migration process. It could be the first aspect to be taken into account in protecting migrants' health because it is closely linked to their well-being.

Finally, the health of migrant women deserves a special mention. Pregnant women and adolescent migrants are affected by inadequate access to medical care; the central role of women as caregivers means that poor health has a heavy impact on families and communities.[29] Compared with women in host countries, migrant women often have poorer maternal health and this is often related to risk factors that already precede and contextualize migrant maternal health (family planning, health-seeking behavior and asylum procedures) (Keygnaert *et al*. 2016). Women are doubly disadvantaged because they are discriminated as women and as migrants. Female migrants are also highly vulnerable to acts of sexual abuse, rape and violence (Adanu and Johnson 2009). A group at particular risk, especially in some cultural areas, is women and girls who have undergone or are at risk of undergoing female genital mutilation (FGM). It is estimated that more than 200 million girls and women have undergone FGM in the countries where the practice is concentrated. FGM has been documented in 30 countries across Africa, the Middle East and Asia. Growing migration has increased the number of girls and women living outside their country of origin who have undergone FGM or who may be at risk in Europe, Australia and North America.[30]

Migration and development are interdependent processes. The 2030 Agenda for Sustainable Development recognizes the positive contribution of migrants towards sustainable development. Migrants are recognized as populations in vulnerable situations that must be empowered (UN 2015a). The health and well-being of migrants and refugees is essential to the achievement of the SDGs,[31] and the health of migrants can be traced in at least eight of the 17 SDGs.

Migrant-specific health vulnerabilities can be addressed through the achievement of these goals and targets (IOM 2016).

Migration features high on the UN agenda (Kumar *et al.* 2018). In 2016, the IOM became part of the UN system (UN 2016), and the UN General Assembly issued the New York Declaration for Refugees and Migrants, which expresses the political will of world leaders to save lives, protect rights and share responsibility on a global scale (UN 2016a).

In 2017, the World Health Assembly issued the Resolution WHA70.15 urging Member States, in accordance with their national context, priorities and legal frameworks, to consider promoting the framework of priorities and guiding principles (Table 11.3), as appropriate, at global, regional and country levels (WHO 2017a).

Furthermore, the Committee on Economic, Social and Cultural Rights (CESCR), which is the UN treaty body monitoring the implementation of the International Covenant on Economic, Social and Cultural Rights (ICESCR), has articulated that nationality must not be used as a ground for discrimination in relation to health care and other rights in the Covenant. Article 12 of the ICESCR provides the most comprehensive articulation, recognizing "the right of everyone to the enjoyment of the highest attainable standard of physical and mental health" (IOM, WHO, UNHCHR 2013).

11.7 Macroeconomic processes and global financial crises

The macroeconomic changes linked to globalization, characterized by deregulation policies and liberalization of financial markets, have an impact on health. Although the mechanisms influencing the relationship between economic development, globalization and health are hard to measure, there are several ways these dynamics affect population health.

First, the expansion of commercial approaches to a growing number of human life domains, the increased privatization of vast economic sectors coupled with a reduced role played by national states have had an impact on universal accessibility to essential public goods and services such as water, energy, education and social and health services. Second, the globalized economy, with the increasing power held by transnational food corporations, along with the Westernization of lifestyles, has promoted the consumption of unhealthy products such as tobacco, alcohol or foods rich in fat, salt and sugar. Third, the economic and social inequalities, fostered by neoliberal globalization

218 *Global policies and issues*

Table 11.3 Guiding principles and priorities to promote the health of refugees and migrants

Guiding principles	Priorities
The right to the enjoyment of the highest attainable standard of physical and mental health	Advocate mainstreaming refugee and migrant health in the global, regional and country agendas and contingency planning
Equality and non-discrimination	Promote refugee- and migrant-sensitive health policies, legal and social protection and program interventions
Equitable access to health services	Enhance capacity to address the social determinants of health
People-centered, refugee- and migrant- and gender-sensitive health systems	Strengthen health monitoring and health information systems
Non-restrictive health practices based on health conditions	Accelerate progress towards achieving the Sustainable Development Goals including universal health coverage
Whole-of-government and whole-of-society approaches	Reduce mortality and morbidity among refugees and migrants through short- and long-term public health interventions
Participation and social inclusion of refugees and migrants	Protect and improve the health and well-being of women, children and adolescents living in refugee and migrant settings
Partnership and cooperation	Promote continuity and quality of care
	Develop, reinforce and implement occupational health safety measures
	Promote gender equality and empower refugee and migrant women and girls
	Support measures to improve communication and counter xenophobia
	Strengthen partnerships, intersectoral, intercountry and interagency coordination and collaboration mechanisms

Source: adapted from WHO 2017b.

processes, have been associated with worse health outcomes (CSDH 2008). There is in fact convincing evidence that the countries with the greatest economic inequalities have worse population health indicators than those where income is more evenly distributed in the population (Wilkinson and Pickett 2010).

In the 80s and 90s of the last century, policies of structural adjustment imposed by international financing institutions on developing countries after the debt crisis contributed to a reduction in access to essential health services. As a consequence, the structural adjustment policies had consequences on the health of the population in these countries (see Chapter 4).

History repeats itself. The current economic crisis is the most serious global economic crisis since end of the Second World War. It began in the summer of 2007 when the increasing insolvency of mortgage loans granted in the United States determined a substantial depreciation of several financial assets. The consequences were dramatic and included a drastic fall in financial product values, a trust crisis which in turn led to a limitation of credit given by banks to companies and individuals, as well as huge losses suffered by banks. In the United States and in Europe some financial institutions failed. The losses due to the collapse of the equity markets and the fall in property prices have been estimated to be in the tens of thousands of billions.

After 2008, the financial crisis also became an economic crisis, first in the United States, then in other industrialized economies, and eventually in the whole world. The slowdown in economic development then became a recession. In 2009, for the first time since World War II, there was a reduction of world product, with an even greater fall of industrial production and world trade volumes (Spaventa 2009). The consequences of what happened between 2007 and 2009 are still challenging the economies of various countries, especially in Europe. Nevertheless, people living in low income countries and with wide disparities between rich and poor are likely to suffer more than those in other countries (Levy and Sidel 2009).

In general, the economic crises led to higher unemployment rates that in turn have had a health impact, with short-term increases in suicides. Further challenges to population health conditions include increases in malnutrition, substance abuse, depression, and other mental health problems, mortality, child health problems, violence, environmental and occupational health problems, social injustice and violation of human rights, and decreased availability, accessibility and affordability of quality medical and dental care.

These negative health effects seem be mitigated when investments in policies to revitalize labor markets are substantial (Stuckler *et al.* 2009).

The recent financial and economic crisis has had a significant impact on health in several countries. The most frequently cited example is the experience of Greece. In 2008, Greece entered a deep financial crisis. In 2012, the total number of deaths was 116,670, the highest number since 1949. However, analysis of mortality data shows that in 2012, after four years of austerity policies, the age-adjusted mortality rate was actually lower than in 2008. In 2011–2012, this trend was reversed and there was an increase in the age-adjusted mortality rate, driven by the increase in deaths among people over 55 (about 2200 excess deaths); this was probably the first short-term consequence of austerity policies on mortality in Greece. This trend was probably linked to barriers to health care for patients suffering from chronic diseases due to the drastic health funding cuts (Vlachadis *et al.* 2012). Indeed, after 2008, in accordance with the prescriptions of the so-called "Troika", i.e. the European Commission, European Central Bank and International Monetary Fund, and under the pressure of the global financial market, the Greek government had to implement several packages of tough austerity measures and budget reforms, including cutting public health expenditure, in an effort to reduce the country's fiscal deficits and public debt.

Health expenditure in Greece decreased sharply from 2008 and in 2012 it was 25% lower compared to 2008. The public expenditure cuts affected all levels of the health system from public health and preventions programs to the hospital sector. The consequences of these austerity measures were on both adult and child health. In addition, the percentage of children at risk of poverty increased dramatically (28.2% in 2007 and 30.4% in 2011), and infant mortality rates for children born in the public sector increased by 21% between 2008 and 2011. Neonatal mortality is related to lack of access to timely and effective care in pregnancy and in the first month of life, while post-neonatal deaths indicate a general worsening of socioeconomic conditions (Kentikelenis *et al.* 2014). In parallel, outbreaks of infectious pathogens were also observed (Bonovas and Nikolopoulos 2012). Adhering to strict austerity policies may risk a worsening of infectious disease outcomes, as is the case in countries undergoing severe economic crisis. For example, during the 1990s in former Soviet Union countries, the incidence, prevalence and mortality of tuberculosis, as well as of other infectious

220 *Global policies and issues*

diseases, rose markedly and improper treatment led to the emergence of drug-resistant strains (Suhrcke *et al.* 2011).

Yet, the health impact of the recent crisis and austerity policies is not limited only to Greece. A study conducted in 2011 on 128 developing countries confirmed that austerity policies were rapidly expanding. In 70 developing countries the reduction in overall health expenditure was, on average, almost 3% of GDP in 2010. In addition, 91 developing countries expected to reduce health expenditures in 2012 (Ortiz *et al.* 2011). Private health expenditure was also affected, as documented by the decline in sales of prescription drugs, especially in countries with high reliance on out-of-pocket spending (Suhrcke *et al.* 2011).

Other European countries hit by the crisis such as Spain and Portugal also adopted strict fiscal austerity; their economies continued to recede and their health-care systems were increasingly restrained. Iceland, on the other hand, rejected the IMF's prescribed austerity measures through a popular vote and instead invested in social protection, with the Icelandic people drawing on strong reserves of social capital; there, the financial crisis seems to have had few or no discernible effects on health. "The interaction of fiscal austerity with economic shocks and weak social protection is what ultimately seems to escalate health and social crises in Europe" (Karanikolos *et al.* 2013)

In a completely different context, a similar lesson can be learned from analysis of the experience of Cuba in the 1990s during the so-called Special Period following the fall of the communist bloc. In those years, Cuba experienced almost a decade of negative economic growth due to declining production and consumption rates and had to adapt to shrinking resources and to local and labor-intensive production modes. Despite the disastrous conditions in which it had to develop, in contrast to other crises of comparable scale, that period brought about lifestyle changes with tangible health benefits, including reduced sedentariness and healthier nutrition. This was made possible thanks to a strong prioritization of health and social cohesion, and the government control over central aspects of socioeconomic life, though it allowed for some private initiative and problem-solving (Borowy 2013).

While healthcare spending is important, it is only one of the factors linking the economic crisis and health. In 2008, the WHO Commission on Social Determinants of Health illustrated how the set of conditions in which people are born, grow, live and work affects their opportunities to have a healthy life, and it showed that social injustice remains today a cause of death on a large scale (CSDH 2008).

Thus, also in crisis, cross-sectoral approaches that address the unequal distribution of power and resources in each country and between countries play a role in mitigating the impact of the social determinants of health (Richards 2012).

In others words, it is necessary to act beyond healthcare systems, promoting health as an objective in all policies.

11.8 Trade, intellectual property rights and access to drugs

Increased trade and trade liberalization are defining features of globalization, directly and indirectly affecting health and health systems. The protection of population health has always been challenged by trade interests and the free circulation of goods and services.

The Agreement on Trade-Related Intellectual Property Rights (TRIPS) represented an important step for harmonizing national legislation concerning international trade, with important consequences for global health.

While several experts have pointed to possible negative consequences of TRIPS, many others have highlighted the potential positive impacts for global health. In fact, many people considered the inclusion of medicines under TRIPS a major advance, since the extension of patent protection worldwide could stimulate investments in research and development for new medicines and medical technologies. Furthermore, protecting intellectual property rights could foster the transfer of technology to low-income countries, improving the availability of medicines and vaccines in these countries, especially in countries that would be able to adjust their legislation to attract foreign investments (Bale 1999). Indeed, the ideological basis of patent protection is to guarantee a return on investment to reward innovation. In theory, these rewards would then stimulate reinvestments in research and development that in turn would lead to further innovation, creating a virtuous circle: innovation – protection – innovation.

However, this argument does not consider the fact that the effects of such mechanisms are related to the types of research and development that is funded. Patent protection works only for medicines and medical technologies that can be sold at prices high enough to ensure a return on investment. Apart from HIV/AIDS, many of the diseases affecting the poor (malaria, African trypanosomiasis, also known as "sleeping sickness", and other "neglected" infectious diseases) are present only in low-income countries and affect mainly the most disadvantaged population groups that cannot afford to pay for medicines. As a result, big multinational pharmaceutical companies have no interest in investing in developing medicines for these diseases.

Between 1975 and 1999, only 13 out of the 1393 medicines developed were for treatment of the so-called "neglected tropical diseases", which under this definition included malaria but excluded HIV/AIDS and tuberculosis (Trouillier 2002). In the following decade, only 16 new products were developed for those diseases, of which 11 were for malaria. The percentage of approved products for infectious diseases (including HIV/AIDS and tuberculosis) sponsored by the private industry fell from 83% to 46% in the same period, while the share sponsored by product development partnerships, such as IAVI (International AIDS Vaccine Initiative), increased from 15% to 46%. Furthermore, in the same period 97 relevant products were registered as under development, out of which 68 were for HIV/AIDS, tuberculosis and malaria. There has therefore been some progress, especially for malaria, but very limited or none for many other diseases such as dengue fever, ulcer of Buruli, trachoma, rheumatic fever or typhus (Cohen *et al.* 2010).

Driven mainly by global initiatives, the number of patients who received antiretroviral therapies went from half a million to 10 million in 10 years (Pascual 2014). These figures are particularly important if we consider that in recent years the number of new medicines developed decreased despite the growth in research and development investment (WHO 2012). The research and development investments to develop medicines for diseases prevalent mainly (e.g. HIV/AIDS) or only (e.g. malaria) in low-income countries remain limited. In 2010, about 3.2 billion dollars (only 2% of total research and development expenditure) was invested for these diseases. Access to health services and technologies is a serious challenge particularly for the 767 million people (10.7% of the world population) who live on less than 1.90 dollars a day, of whom 50.7% live on the African continent.[32]

The second argument in support of TRIPS, technology transfer, is based on Article 7 of the agreement itself:

> The protection and enforcement of intellectual property rights should contribute to the promotion of technological innovation and to the transfer and dissemination of technology, to the mutual advantage of producers and users of technological knowledge and in a manner conducive to social and economic welfare, and to a balance of rights and obligations.
>
> (WTO 1994)

Some people argue that "the universal harmonization of patent protection" will bring benefits for low-income countries, due to the "development of new drugs by local pharmaceutical companies, the increase of foreign direct investments, and improvement in population health ensured by the increased availability of high quality medical technologies" (Mirza 1999: 92).

According to this argument, the implementation of TRIPS could provide incentives for pharmaceutical companies based in low-income countries to invest in research and development. In addition, transnational pharmaceutical companies would have an incentive to invest in those countries, attracted by the cheap labor. The mechanism could work if, in developing countries, the necessary conditions existed, starting with research and development capacity. However, pharmaceutical companies in developing countries are mainly active in the field of reproduction of existing technologies rather than in innovation. At best they can produce copies of already patented drugs at low cost. In these countries, in fact, there is a lack of infrastructure and capital needed to invest in research and development (Correa 2001). Under these circumstances it is highly unlikely that they can benefit from the conditions established in TRIPS.

It is illustrative that the history of patent protection in the Western world was characterized by three distinct phases: absence of patents, patents on processes, and patents on processes and products. "Through the WTO agreements, developed countries have succeeded to prohibit developing countries this type of industrial strategy" (Brauman 2002: 149–150), imposing the transition from the absence of patents, to patents on almost everything. This in turn presents a further risk to developing countries.

> It is likely that in many low-income countries the local pharmaceutical industry will face the competition of multinationals companies, without positive effects in terms of technology transfer, jobs and drug prices. The disappearance and weakening of the national pharmaceutical industry will represent, for many countries, the foreseeable consequence of the abolition of protectionist measures.
>
> (Brauman 2002: 149–150)

While recognizing these risks, some experts believe that the introduction of patents can produce positive effects even in low-income countries, but only if preceded by a series of policies designed to offset their potential negative effects. These measures would include tax benefits for pharmaceutical industries which authorize the use of their own technologies in low-income countries, measures to foster access to scientific databases, and the implementation of policies to contain medicines prices (CIPR 2002).

For low-income countries, the greatest concern related to the application of TRIPS is the risk of higher medicines prices. Of course, the price of medicines does not depend only on the patents. Many factors determine medicines prices: demand and supply factors; prescription and consumption models; production costs; the degree of competition within the market; taxes and exchange rates; wholesale and retail price increases;

the degree of elasticity to the price of the various drugs; and above all the payment policies of national health systems, social health insurance agencies and private health insurances schemes (WTO / WHO 2002).

However, several expert opinions argue that greater patent protection leads to an increase in medicine prices and represents a further obstacle for access to essential drugs. The report published by the British Commission on Intellectual Property Rights (CIPR)[33] states that

> International comparisons show that copies of drugs patented elsewhere are much cheaper in markets which do not offer patent protection. (…) This literature demonstrates that the introduction of patent regimes into such developing countries has, or is predicted to have, the effect of raising prices. The estimates range widely depending on the drugs and countries being considered – from 12% to over 200%, but even the lower estimates imply very substantial costs for consumers. The range of estimates is indicative of the degree of uncertainty about the dynamic effect of introducing patents, and suggests that the outcome will be very much determined by market structure and demand, in particular the degree of competition.
> (CIPR 2002)

A similar commission established by the WHO by the mandate of the 56th World Health Assembly, the Commission on Intellectual Property Rights, Innovation and Public Health (CIPH), argued that patent protection reduces the research and development capacity of low-income countries for developing medicines they actually need, and generates very high costs to ensure access to products already available on market. "Where pharmaceutical patents are in force, in impoverished countries, medicines are out of reach of those who need them" (Dentico 2013).

The major concerns relate to access to the so-called essential drugs. These are medicines that meet the needs of the majority of the population and must therefore always be available in sufficient quantities under the appropriate pharmaceutical form. Inclusion criteria for the List of Essential Medicines (published by the World Health Organization) are efficacy and proven safety, clear therapeutic properties and reasonable cost or price (Hoen 1999). This last criterion automatically excludes numerous life-saving medicines, recently developed and of proven efficacy but marketed at a high price.

With patent protection under the TRIPS agreement, the number of life-saving drugs that would not meet the price criterion is likely to increase, even for drugs with a patent that is expiring. It is in fact possible to extend the patent lifetime of old medicines (which may already be part of the Essential Medicines List), even if only by means of the so-called "evergreening approaches". Evergreening is achieved by seeking extra patents on variations of the original drug – new forms of release, new dosages, new combinations or variations, or new forms. Big Pharma refers to this as "lifecycle management". Even if the patent is dubious, the company can earn more from the higher prices than it pays in legal fees to keep the dubious patent alive (Correa 2001).

In some cases the market conditions allow arbitrary increases of prices for medicines with expired patents, even without resorting to "evergreening". The most recent example is the 5000% increase in the price of Daraprim, a medicine used in the United States primarily to treat toxoplasmosis in AIDS patients, imposed by a reckless entrepreneur who also acquired exclusive marketing rights on the drug in order to deter other pharmaceutical companies from producing the generic form of the drug, pyrimethamine, whose patent expired in the 1970s. The drug's limited patient population, the absence of competing manufacturers, and a lack of therapeutic alternatives created an effective monopoly and allowed the entrepreneur to set a high price for Daraprim. Similar mechanisms allowed prices of other off-patent drugs to grow, including drugs used in the treatment of diverse conditions ranging from heart failure to multi-drug-resistant tuberculosis (Tallapragada 2016).

A long debate surrounded the reinterpretation of certain clauses in the TRIPS agreement, which finally made it possible for countries to grant access to patent-protected drugs in order to protect population health. With the "Doha Declaration on the TRIPS Agreement and Public Health" of 14 November 2001, the WTO, while reaffirming the commitments established in the TRIPS agreement, intervened with important clarifications and some changes on the right of States to protect public health. Specifically, the Doha Declaration affirms that "the TRIPS Agreement does not and should not prevent Members from taking measures to protect public health" (WTO 2001).

In this regard, the Doha Declaration enshrines the principles that WHO has publicly advocated and advanced over the years, namely the reaffirmation of the right of WTO Members to make full use of the safeguard provisions of the TRIPS agreement in order to protect public health and enhance access to medicines for poor countries.

The discussion about the number of diseases to which safeguard clauses could be applied initially caused the negotiation to stall. The United States wanted to limit its application exclusively to HIV/AIDS, tuberculosis and malaria. WHO, although not involved in the debate, instead emphasized the inadequacy of the global list of disease priorities, due to the need to consider each country's epidemiological conditions and priorities.

The Doha Declaration (WTO 2001) and the subsequent "Decision on the Interpretation of Paragraph 6" (WTO 2003) affirmed the rights of member countries to independently determine which situations represent a public health emergency, to grant compulsory licenses for the production of patent-protected drugs, to determine the criteria on which to grant such licenses, and, for countries without adequate production capacity, to import drugs produced in third countries under compulsory licensing.

The flexibilities provided for in the TRIPS agreement, i.e. compulsory licenses and parallel imports, were thus reaffirmed. Currently, these flexibilities facilitate availability of medicines at affordable prices in low-income countries. For example, in 26 member countries which are among those with the lowest income in the world, thanks to the adoption of a legislation that is based on the provisions contained in the Doha Declaration the import of generic drugs is allowed regardless of the status of the related patents (Owoeye 2014). Some measures adopted by the WTO are set out in Table 11.4.

It is useful to remember that the Doha Declaration has not only a political value, but also a legal one. The interpretations it provides are binding for the decision-making bodies of the WTO (Correa 2002). Although the Doha Declaration confirmed the right of middle- and low-income countries to use the exceptions foreseen by TRIPS, there is still reluctance in implementing those flexibilities due to concerns about the reactions of trade partners. In a globalized world, maintaining the reputation of reliable business partners committed to protecting intellectual property rights has so far been prioritized over access to medicines (Kerry and Lee 2007).

In some cases, the threat of applying the compulsory license can be used as a negotiation tool. For example, Brazil has successfully used this approach to achieve substantial reductions in the prices of patented pharmaceutical products, thereby extending access

Table 11.4 World Trade Organization (WTO) measures taken in response to the TRIPS agreement

Provision	Objective
Least-Developed Country Members – Obligations Under Article 70.9 of the TRIPS Agreement with Respect to Pharmaceutical Products[a]	Allows least developed countries to refuse to maintain the standards imposed by TRIPS in respect of pharmaceutical products until 1 January 2016 with an option for possible extension
Implementation of Paragraph 6 of the Doha Declaration on the TRIPS Agreement and Public Health[b]	Enables countries to produce and export medicines pursuant to a compulsory licence to countries that cannot produce them locally
Amendment of the TRIPS agreement[c]	It incorporates provisions of the Implementation Decision as an amendment to the TRIPS Agreement; enters into force once accepted by two-thirds of all WTO members
Extension of the Transition Period Under Article 66.1 for Least Developed Country Members[d]	Extends the time for least developed countries to implement the minimum standard of intellectual property protection required by the TRIPS Agreement to 1 July 2021

a World Trade Organization. Least-developed country members – obligations under article 70.9 of the TRIPS Agreement with respect to pharmaceutical products, decision of 8 July 2002(1) (WT/L/478). Geneva: WTO; 2013. Available from: www.wto.org/english/tratop_e/trips_e/art70_9_e.htm.
b World Trade Organization [Internet]. Implementation of paragraph 6 of the Doha Declaration on the TRIPS Agreement and Public Health: General Council Decision of 30 August 2003 (WT/L/540). Geneva: WTO; 2013. Available from: www.wto.org/english/tratop_e/trips_e/implem_para6_e.htm.
c World Trade Organization [Internet]. Amendment of the TRIPS Agreement: General Council decision of 6 December 2005 (WT/L/641). Geneva: WTO; 2013. Available from: www.wto.org/english/tratop_e/trips_e/wtl641_e.htm.
d World Trade Organization [Internet]. Extension of the transition period under Article 66.1 for least developed country members: decision of the Council for TRIPS of 11 June 2013 (IP/C/64). Geneva: WTO; 2013. Available from: www.wto.org/english/tratop_e/trips_e/ta_docs_e/7_1_ipc64_e.pdf.

Source: Owoeye 2014.

to larger portions of the population. Unfortunately, not many low-income countries can afford to take similar positions. In many cases they cannot afford to initiate public health assistance programs without international support. Furthermore, they lack not only the administrative infrastructure and legal capacity to use and manage mandatory licenses, but also the technological and productive capacity, as well as adequate national legislation.

Most developing countries will continue to import pharmaceutical products. Africa, which has the highest burden of disease worldwide, will continue to depend on imported pharmaceuticals (Stirner and Thangaraj 2013). At the same time, measures to protect patents that benefit mainly transnational companies who hold them (especially US, European and Japanese companies) inhibit the production of generic drugs whose availability has always contributed to lowering costs and ensuring a constant and sufficient supply of medicines for the poorest countries.

With the progressive adoption of intellectual property protection policies by emerging economies (such as Brazil, China, India and Mexico) which are traditionally large producers of generic medicines, it is expected that the availability on the global market of generic low-price formulations of new patented drugs will gradually decline, and the availability of generics will be increasingly limited to old off-patent drugs. Access

226 *Global policies and issues*

to the latest patented drugs will become more difficult (Birn *et al.* 2009; Stirner and Thangaraj 2013).

On the other hand, pharmaceutical companies do not like the trend of some emerging countries to use compulsory licenses, competition law and stricter patent standards to enable the production of generics in therapeutic areas with patented drugs previously intended to serve almost exclusively the markets of high-income countries (Williams *et al.* 2015).

As already mentioned above (see Chapter 6), after the 2003 stalling of negotiations aimed at promoting trade liberalization through multilateral channels (WTO), the major industrialized countries intensified negotiations to establish bilateral or regional free trade agreements outside the WTO, the so-called "TRIPS-plus" agreements. These agreements have imposed on weaker partners even more penalizing conditions regarding the protection of public health. The TRIPS-plus have narrowed the options for the use of compulsory licenses and parallel import. In some cases, like in the North American Free Trade Agreement (NAFTA) between the United States, Canada and Mexico, they have included in the dispute settlement mechanism the possibility for investors (i.e. large transnational companies) to sue governments (in the WTO agreements dispute settlement only concerns governments) that implement policies that may go against their interests[34] (Birn *et al.* 2009). For example, in 2013, the Federal Court of Canada revoked the patents of two drugs of the American company Eli Lilly which did not meet the Canadian patent law standards. The pharmaceutical company claimed compensation of $481 million from the Canadian government on the basis of the provisions in NAFTA (Cattaneo 2014), though the tribunal eventually rejected Eli Lilly's allegations.

The TRIPS-plus agreements were negotiated bilaterally, for example between the USA and Jordan, or Chile and Australia. They extended the duration of protection of the patents, a measure also included in the Free Trade Agreement of the Americas (FTAA) negotiated between the countries of the American continent. This extension, among other things, removed the possibility of resorting to compulsory licenses until after the patent expires, unless under conditions of "national emergency" (Kerry and Lee 2007). In the case of free trade agreements between partners with similar levels of economic development, as in the case of the Transatlantic Trade and Investment Partnership (TTIP) which is being negotiated between the USA and the European Union, there are concerns about the effects on the drug prices, the lowering of standards and the possibility for transnational drug companies to claim compensation for measures that governments have taken to reduce pharmaceutical spending, considered as interference with the free market (Cattaneo 2014).

Regarding intellectual property, the WHO's above-mentioned CIPIH report (see Box 11.1)

BOX 11.1 CIPIH report: main recommendations

"The independent Commission on Intellectual Property Rights, Innovation and Public Health (CIPIH) was set up by WHO Member States at the World Health Assembly (WHA) in May 2003 to investigate how to improve access to health products for diseases that mainly affect developing countries, given current international and national rules on patent rights. The commission's final report, Public health, innovation and intellectual property rights, was published on 3 April 2006.

WHO Member States will debate the issues it raises at the WHA from 22 to 27 May 2006, and decide whether to adopt a resolution on the subject. Resolution EB117. R13 on intellectual property rights has been submitted to the WHA for consideration already. Among more than 50 recommendations of the CIPIH report were the following:

Governments should:

- avoid provisions in bilateral trade agreements that could reduce access to medicines in developing countries
- increase funding for research projects run by public-private partnerships and by developing countries, and make that funding more sustainable
- develop advance purchase schemes to contribute to the development of vaccines, medicines and diagnostics
- incorporate digital libraries of traditional medical knowledge into their patent offices' data to ensure that data contained in them are considered when patent applications are processed
- make available reliable information on the patents they have granted
- amend their laws to allow compulsory licensing for export consistent with the TRIPS Agreement
- eliminate tariffs and taxes on healthcare products.

Governments of developing countries should:

- promote health research that is in line with public health needs
- promote the use of research exemption as part of their patent law
- invest appropriately in health delivery infrastructure
- improve financing of the purchase of medicines and vaccines
- make use of compulsory licensing provisions, where this will promote innovation or access to medicines.

WHO and other international agencies should:

- develop a global plan of action to secure more sustainable funding to develop new products and make those products more accessible
- encourage the creation of patent pools where this would facilitate product development
- monitor the impact of intellectual property rights from a public health perspective.

Companies should:

- adopt transparent and consistent pricing policies
- reduce prices for developing countries
- avoid filing patents or enforcing them in low-income developing countries in ways that would inhibit access to their products."

Source: WHO website www.who.int/bulletin/volumes/84/5/CIPIH_report/en/.

proposed 60 recommendations addressed to all governments, to international organizations and to the WHO itself. An Inter-Governmental Working Group (IGWG) was created in 2006 to ensure that CIPIH recommendations were translated into government policies.

228 *Global policies and issues*

The IGWG process is the first multilateral attempt to open a debate on complementary approaches, or even alternative approaches, to the classic interpretation of the TRIPS agreement. During the intergovernmental debate, important issues are discussed such as public funding of clinical trials, the formulation of new incentives (patent pools, innovation awards, open source management of medical research) and the proposal to develop a new international agreement on research and development of new medicines as an alternative to TRIPS (Dentico 2013).

The output of these negotiations was the "Global Strategy and Plan of Action on Public Health, Innovation and Intellectual Property" (GSPA), approved by the World Health Assembly in 2008 (see Box 11.2). The main goal identified by the Global Strategy was a substantial reform of the research and development system of pharmaceutical products, aimed at developing new medicines for diseases that affect most of the world's population living in developing countries.

BOX 11.2 The Global Strategy and Plan of Action on Public Health, Innovation and Intellectual Property

"Today, 4.8 billion people live in developing countries and 2.7 billion of them (43%) live on less than US$ 2 a day. Communicable diseases account for half of the diseases in these countries. Recognizing that poverty, among other issues, affects access to health products and that new products to fight diseases affecting developing countries are needed, governments, the pharmaceutical industry, foundations, NGOs and others have undertaken initiatives in recent years to address these challenges. But more needs to be done. To foster innovation and improve access for people in developing countries, the World Health Assembly adopted in May 2008 resolution WHA61.21, and resolution WHA62.16, on a global strategy and plan of action on public health, innovation and intellectual property.

The global strategy

The strategy proposes that WHO should play a strategic and central role in the relationship between public health and innovation and intellectual property within its mandate. Member States endorsed by consensus a strategy designed to promote new thinking in innovation and access to medicines, which would encourage needs-driven research rather than purely market-driven research to target diseases which disproportionately affect people in developing countries.

Elements of the strategy

The eight elements of the global strategy are designed to promote innovation, build capacity, improve access and mobilize resources. These include:

- prioritizing research and development needs
- promoting research and development
- building and improving innovative capacity
- transfer of technology
- application and management of intellectual property to contribute to innovation and promote public health

- improving delivery and access
- promoting sustainable financing mechanisms
- establishing and monitoring reporting systems."

Source: WHO website www.who.int/phi/implementation/phi_globstat_action/en/.

The new Global Strategy represents a major advance with respect to the Doha Declaration, introducing more flexibility and opening new paths for sharing knowledge for the benefit of all. The United Nations Human Rights Council (UNHRC) has also recognized the possible regulatory role of GSPA with regard to pharmaceutical policies, both globally and nationally (Dentico 2013).

Given on the one hand the deadlock of WTO multilateral negotiations, and on the other hand the progression of TRIPS-plus agreements, it is difficult to imagine that the new proposal can actually develop into an instrument with binding commitments.

11.9 eHealth and the global "health 4.0" challenge

Interconnectedness is a defining feature of globalization, and the development and worldwide diffusion of information and communication technologies (ICT) are at its roots. Use of the internet, computers, smartphones and other electronic devices has dramatically increased over recent decades. Mobile-broadband subscriptions have grown more than 20% annually in recent years reaching 4.3 billion globally by end 2017. Younger generations are the most involved and are paving the way. In 104 countries, more than 80% (830 million) of the youth population aged 15–24 is online. However, the digital gap is consistent: nearly nine out of ten young individuals not using the internet live in Africa or Asia and the Pacific (ITU 2017).

The use of the internet has provided on one hand clear benefits to individual and institutional users, and on the other hand new risks to health and new governance and policy challenges.

eHealth is the term that WHO has adopted to refer to the use of ICT for health.[35] Other terms such as internet health, telehealth, or mHealth are also used to refer to specific uses or approaches in the use of ICT for health.

11.9.1 Internet-related health risks

Globally, the exponential use of the internet and electronic devices over recent decades has been associated with documented cases of excessive use and negative health consequences, reaching in some countries the magnitude of a significant public health concern.

Consequences on health of excessive use of the internet have mostly been studied and discussed under the lens of behavioral addictions. These are usually characterized by an "irresistible urge, impulse or drive to repeatedly engage in an activity (non-substance use) and an inability to reduce or cease this behavior (loss of control) despite serious negative consequences to the person's physical, mental, social and/or financial well-being" (WHO 2015a). These internet-mediated addictions include among others gambling, viewing pornography, video gaming, internet-based single-player and multi-player gaming, and excessive use of social media and smartphone applications (apps).

230 *Global policies and issues*

The highest prevalence of internet use disorders, as well as cell phone addiction and social network site addiction, is among adolescents and young adults. This is not surprising given the recent development of this technology. "In Korea internet addiction has been identified as the largest health problem experienced among kids" (WHO 2015a).

Besides addiction, the use of the internet and increasingly of mobile devices may be associated with a variety of physical, psychosocial and socio-behavioral consequences, which in most cases still need further study due to the recent emergence of the phenomenon.

Devices such as the smartphone have become almost a "prosthesis" of the body for millions of human beings worldwide and their physical effects are already debated as a global public health concern. Visual symptoms are associated with prolonged exposure to smartphones' blue-light screens; musculoskeletal problems are related to fixed posture in the use of the device (e.g. "text neck") (Cuéllar and Lanman 2017); hearing problems and permanent hearing damage are associated with the extended exposure to harmful levels of sound generated by the devices used with headphones (WHO 2015a). Human exposures to electromagnetic fields including those produced from the use of mobile phones have been classified as "possibly carcinogenic to humans" by the WHO (IARC 2013).

Excessive use of the internet and electronic devices is frequently associated with psychosocial pathologies such social withdrawal, sleep deprivation and low self-esteem, and may lead to clinically significant distress and/or impaired functioning. These disorders have the potential to become chronic, relapsing and resistant to treatment (WHO 2015a).

Modern technologies and the internet enable increasingly widespread cyber-bullying, which is associated with serious psychosocial consequences. Other socio-behavioral consequences may include social withdrawal, sometimes dangerous unreal social interactions online and increased risky sexual behavior. They can lead to aggressive behaviors, family problems, marital breakdown and reduced work and academic performance. Due to their distracting power while performing other tasks, smartphones have been increasingly associated with injuries and traffic accidents (WHO 2015a). "Drivers using mobile phones are approximately 4 times more likely to be involved in a crash than drivers not using a mobile phone".[36]

The internet is also the most important vehicle for a cross-border supply of health services to individual consumers.[37]

"Health" is one of the most searched-for topics online, and the internet is also a worldwide marketplace for health information and products. In addition to access to valuable services, however, the internet also channels new types of exploitation and fraud, including the sale and use of health data of individuals and the illegal promotion and sale of medicines (including counterfeits, adulterated or unapproved drugs) and other products, posing severe risks to both individual and collective health (e.g. antimicrobic resistance promoted by below-standard drugs) and undermining legitimate trade and the correct functioning of health systems (WHO 1998; WHO 2016).

11.9.2 eHealth potential and challenges

In 2005 the World Health Assembly defined eHealth as:

the cost-effective and secure use of information communication technologies (ICT) in support of health and health-related fields, including health-care services, health surveillance, health literature, and health education, knowledge and research.

(WHO 2005a)

That same year, WHO launched the Global Observatory for eHealth (GOe), to support countries in developing and managing national eHealth strategies.

Since then "the potential impact" of the advances in information and communication technologies on healthcare delivery, public health, research and health-related activities for the benefit of both low- and high-income countries has expanded considerably, together with new challenges. To date, 58% of countries have established an eHealth national strategy.[38]

Different aspects of eHealth have been considered and pose different governance challenges.

The internet has radically transformed telehealth, i.e. the interaction between a healthcare provider and a patient when the two are separated by distance, which relied until the mid-1990s mostly on slow and expensive telephone and satellite connections and radiocommunications in remote poorer areas of the world. Today, telehealth can be synchronous (e.g. real-time consultation via video conference) or asynchronous (when input and feedback are separated in time), with the latter being easier to organize and requiring less-costly infrastructure. Remote patient monitoring is an increasingly important application of telehealth in high-income countries, where patients, often at home, transmit information about their condition from sensors and monitoring equipment to external monitoring centers.

With the advent of mobile communications using smart mobile devices supporting fast broadband data transmission, mHealth, i.e. the use of mobile devices for medical and public health practice, has been a main attraction among research and business communities. mHealth is at the cutting edge of healthcare innovation. Mobile phones are nowadays almost ubiquitous, even in most remote parts and in very low-resource settings, and often provide more affordable services than many other forms of technology or health service infrastructure. mHealth systems have a strong impact on typical healthcare monitoring and alerting systems, clinical and administrative data collection, record maintenance, healthcare delivery programs, medical information awareness, and detection and prevention systems, as well as on drug-counterfeiting and theft (Silva *et al.* 2015). mHealth, through its capacity to individualize access to health information and services, promises to revolutionize health systems and to eventually become a key component of universal health coverage (UHC), and also to make the health market even more pervasive, helping to build what is already envisaged as Health 4.0 (Comptesse 2017).

Use of social media such as Facebook, WhatsApp, Twitter, YouTube and others has also experienced a huge expansion; however, "only 29% of the world's 3.4 billion people living in rural areas benefit from the 3G-coverage that is needed to enable a rich social media experience" (WHO 2016). Nevertheless, social media is changing the dynamics of interactions among and between healthcare consumers, health professionals and healthcare organizations, allowing them to share information, debate issues and promote new ideas. The number of health-related apps increases daily (according to estimates there are already more than 300,000) and may roughly be divided into three categories: treatment-related apps, prediction and prevention-related apps, and lifestyle-related apps (UNESCO 2017).

While social media may contribute to improving access to health information and care, it can also provide a phenomenal channel for additional exposure to legal and illegal marketing looking for "health" consumers.

The rapid expansion of social media comes with important challenges to privacy, confidentiality and security linked to the enormous production of aggregate social media information, requiring "a strategic vision that contemplates the need to include people, processes and policies to ensure their adoption" (WHO 2016).

Indeed, the market already works on Big Data, data mining, cloud computing and complex algorithms that are changing the way information is captured and processed. Health 4.0 includes individually tailored care and predictive medicine, with patients as active players influencing the type of care they will receive. "Apps" such as calorie trackers, memory builders, step counters and vital function monitors feed personalized data into Big Data systems that will provide responses, with individual behaviors determining diagnoses and proposed care (Comptesse 2017). However, such a scenario may not contribute to health system sustainability; rather, if left unattended, it will leave even more people behind, further undermining the control of structural health determinants.

> In worst-case scenarios, however, big data would be an expensive distraction driven by high-income countries, focused on disease specific outcomes and unintelligible to those who most need data access. Breaches of data security could threaten personal safety, and the global health community could oversee the spending of huge amounts of money on big data, with potentially little to show for the investment.
> (WHO 2016)

Among the features of a national eHealth strategy, WHO includes electronic health record (EHR) systems. Indeed, such a dynamic repository of the population's health data may provide important benefits if it is implemented by the national health authority and makes patient medical histories available to authorized health professionals in healthcare institutions, linking related services such as pharmacies, laboratories, specialists and emergency and medical imaging facilities. An EHR system may become an important component of the provision of UHC, contributing to the quality, accuracy and timeliness of patient information at the point of care. It may also play an important role in reducing costs, supporting patient mobility and increasing reliability of information. In combination with other health and social information systems, it could highlight areas of concern in health services delivery, public health and social determinants (WHO 2016). However, the quality and effectiveness of such a system will highly depend on the overall organization and governance of national and supranational health systems. Indeed, "the policy framework needs further and urgent examination, both by government organizations in general and health organizations in particular" (WHO 2016).

From a public health perspective, a less contradictory component of eHealth is eLearning, i.e. the use of ICT for education. The global healthcare workers crisis calls for innovative solutions in health workforce development, and eLearning provides a valuable approach in addressing educational needs of health professionals, especially in remote and low-resource settings. Combining multiple technologies and tools, and through multiple and diverse approaches, eLearning allows for a broadened audience, promotes collaboration and better use of existing educational resources, and allows health workers at all levels to update their knowledge and skills in a flexible, efficient and personalized manner. However, the development and implementation of eLearning in health faces important challenges. It requires significant human and financial resources, given that evidence about cost-effectiveness is still scarce and evaluation standards are still lacking (WHO 2016). In addition, socioeconomic and cultural distance between the provider and the learner, especially in the context of transnational eLearning programs, is linked to a number of interculturality issues (Lapsang 2007).

11.9.3 eHealth policy and governance

At the global level, eHealth standardization has been on the International Telecommunications Union (ITU)[39] agenda since 2003.[40]

In 2005, the World Health Assembly (WHA) passed its first resolution on eHealth (WHO 2005a). An eHealth unit was created to promote and strengthen the use of ICT in health development, from applications in the field to global governance.

Previously, in 1998, the WHO Executive Board (EB) tackled the potential impact on health of the advertising and promotion of medical products via the internet (WHO 1998).

The ITU felt the need to build on the collaboration with the WHO to create a global, open environment for the development and promotion of eHealth standards. In 2012, the 12th World Telecommunications Standardization Assembly (WTSA-12)[41] adopted a resolution regarding ITC applications and standards for improved access to eHealth. Among issues needing global attention in order to ensure the successful adoption of eHealth applications, responses that were considered were: the conformity with standards to increase interoperability among systems, the safeguarding of privacy and security and the reduction of the cost of devices through economies of scale.

Many technical aspects are examined in collaboration between International Institutions, mainly the ITU, and private stakeholders such as the Personal Connected Health Alliance (PCHA), which is an international not-for-profit industry organization whose members are prominent ITC, health technology and pharmaceutical companies.[42] The PCHA promotes adoption of the Continua Design Guidelines, which are recognized by ITU as the international standard for safe, secure and reliable exchange of data to and from personal health devices.

However, the above-described trend toward Health 4.0 may require a deeper analysis on what is really at stake in terms of human rights, universal access to health services and further commodification of health needs. Indeed, at ITU and in its collaboration with WHO, discussions around eHealth deal with a variety of fields in addition to technical aspects, including legal, ethical, cultural and economic issues.[43]

Many of the regulations at the international level have been developed mainly due to trade in health services in the context of transnational data flows; one example is the United Nations Conference on Trade and Development (UNCTAD)'s Data protection regulations and international data flows (UNCTAD 2016).

The UNESCO International Bioethics Committee (IBC) has specifically analyzed the complex issues concerning Big Data in health. The IBC identified four measures which are crucial for protecting individual rights and fostering public good (though they recognized the unavoidable loss of control by individuals about the use of their data in times of Big Data): governance, education, capacity-building and benefit-sharing.

234 *Global policies and issues*

Regarding the first point, the following principles were identified for directing the governance of Big Data in health:

> Governance systems for Big Data should protect the fundamental rights of the persons from whom the data originates, including their freedom to make decisions, and aim at maintaining the trust of the public. Thus, guiding principles for governance have to include the respect of autonomy and the right to information, voluntariness, privacy and data protection, transparency, equality and lawfulness. Data governance should guarantee that citizen involvement, engagement, participation and sharing of data will not be subject to exploitation, manipulation and improper control.
>
> (UNESCO 2017)

Health-related internet domains have also been among the issues debated at a global level. In 2012, the Internet Corporation for Assigned Names and Numbers (ICANN) opened a new round of applications for generic top-level domain (gTLD) names. The entry of new, commercial players applying to create health-related names (e.g. "health", "doctor", "med") reopened the debate on the global safeguards and policies needed to protect consumers (Eysenbach 2014).

In 2013 the WHA recognized the need for health data standardization as part of eHealth systems and services, and the importance of proper governance and operation of health-related gTLD names, including "health" (WHO 2013). The resolution emphasized that health-related gTLDs in all languages, including "health", should be operated in a way that protects public health, including by preventing the further development of illicit markets for medicines, medical devices and unauthorized health products and services. According to the governing principles, regulating the .health domain was considered key in ensuring the internet can play its proper role in supporting global public health. Thus, the WHO urged ICANN's Governmental Advisory Committee (GAC) and Board to postpone the attribution of "health" until adequate baseline conditions for its operation were elaborated, and their implementation and observance could be ensured (WHO 2018). In addition, a number of authors voiced their predictions that effectively privatizing all future uses of the .health domain would have profound effects on health information access and quality for generations to come (Mackey *et al.* 2014).

Despite those recommendations, in 2015 the .health gTLD was awarded to the private company DotHealth.[44] The company submitted Public Interest Commitments (PICs)[45] declaring it would "establish .health as the most trusted top-level domain for population health management, health education and healthcare innovation worldwide" (dotHealth 2013).

Citing the risks of poor or biased information and of misleading health and well-being advice on the internet, experts insisted on some degree of content oversight and control. That position was opposed by the advocates of an unrestricted and open internet, who countered that once compromised that principle could be definitively lost (Solomonides and Mackey 2015).

Failing a global negotiation to prevent ICANN awarding the domain without requested guarantees, due to the global nature of the internet, national legislators will have difficulty in ensuring that the management and operation of .health and other health-related gTLDs will be consistent with public health goals.

Through the Global Observatory for eHealth (GOe) WHO has since 2010 been updating an online directory of eHealth-related national policies and strategies from Member States;[46] however, a comprehensive and strategic global policy is still missing.

At the national level, comprehensive legislation will need to address a long list of issues that many low-income countries will find difficult to introduce and sustain autonomously. The list of regulatory issues relevant for eHealth identified as key includes: access to and ownership of data, security and access to clinical information systems, privacy and confidentiality, informed consent for data use, access rights, integrity of data, patient safety, secure transmission of patient data, electronic and physical security, reliability of electronic portable medical devices used with eHealth, accuracy and reliability of online information for patients, sustainability of accuracy and integrity of electronic patient medical records, validity and reliability of clinical decision-support systems, quality of care using eHealth processes, availability of efficient and effective communication systems, and reliability and dependability of telemedicine and telemonitoring. It has been argued that regulatory priorities for eHealth development should focus on privacy, confidentiality, security and standards (WHO 2016).

Clearly, eHealth governance covering multiple areas mentioned above is a challenging issue of our times and needs input from global policy-makers.

> In a global environment, the current complex sets of national laws and regulations are not enough to prevent the sale of health-search information, the exposure of health and other personal data online, and concerns over cybersecurity of medical devices and hospital networks.
>
> (WHO 2018)

Notes

1 Benedetta Rossi contributed to this paragraph.
2 www.who.int/airpollution/data/cities/en/.
3 www.unwater.org/water-facts/water-sanitation-and-hygiene/.
4 www.dandc.eu/en/article/world-needs-work-together-beat-neglected-tropical-diseases-good.
5 www.unisdr.org/archive/30026.
6 www.who.int/en/news-room/detail/10-01-2018-un-environment-and-who-agree-to-major-collaboration-on-environmental-health-risks.
7 www.who.int/globalchange/coalition/en/.
8 However, the terms of the Paris agreement prevent any Partner from withdrawing from the pact for four years. Thus, also the final word on US participation would not come before November 4th, 2020.
9 An epidemic is defined as a sudden increase in the number of infections/cases well above the expected average for a given population.
10 www.who.int/news-room/fact-sheets/detail/obesity-and-overweight.
11 www.who.int/en/news-room/fact-sheets/detail/obesity-and-overweight.
12 Food security can be defined in terms of food availability, food access and food utilization. Food availability is achieved when sufficient quantities of food are consistently available to all individuals within a country. Food access is ensured when households and all individuals within them have adequate resources to obtain appropriate food for a nutritional diet. Food utilization is the proper biological use of food, requiring a diet providing sufficient energy and essential nutrients, potable water, and adequate sanitation.

13 FAO, 2018. Food Security and the Right to Food. Available from: www.fao.org/sustainable-development-goals/overview/fao-and-the-post-2015-development-agenda/food-security-and-the-right-to-food/en/.
14 https://knoema.com/cduhihd/world-exports-and-imports-of-agricultural-products.
15 The Joint FAO/WHO Codex Alimentarius Commission was set up in 1962 to establish food safety standards. It currently has 188 member countries and one member organization (the European Union), which with the help of independent technical experts selected by FAO and WHO revise and update the Codex, which is a collection of internationally adopted food standards and related texts presented in a uniform manner. These food standards and related texts aim at protecting consumers' health and ensuring fair practices in the food trade. See: www.fao.org/fao-who-codexalimentarius/home/pt/.
16 The World Organization for Animal Health (OIE) developed guidelines to assess risks associated with trade in animals and their products, known as Import Risk Analysis (IRA). Risk analysis is an approach to assess both the likelihood and consequences of undesirable events, known as hazards. It is used to support decision-making in the face of uncertainty. The assessment of risk necessarily involves prediction and uncertainty, which can result, on occasion, in controversy, particularly in the area of food safety, for example disputes over imports of hormone-treated beef to the EU (Peeler *et al.* 2013).
17 The Committee on World Food Security was established in 1974 in order to review food security policies. It is hosted by the Food and Agriculture Organization (FAO). It was reformed in 2009 to ensure that voices of other stakeholders were heard, and it aims at being the most inclusive international and intergovernmental platform for all stakeholders to work together in a coordinated way to ensure food security and nutrition for all. See: www.fao.org/cfs/home/about/en/.
18 www.cdc.gov/tobacco/global/index.htm.
19 These are the measures suggested by WHO: Monitor tobacco use and prevention policies; Protect people from tobacco smoke; Offer help to quit tobacco use; Warn about the dangers of tobacco; Enforce bans on tobacco advertising, promotion and sponsorship; Raise taxes on tobacco.
20 In setting and implementing their public health policies with respect to tobacco control, Parties shall act to protect these policies from commercial and other vested interests of the tobacco industry in accordance with national law (WHO 2003).
21 www.iom.int/who-is-a-migrant.
22 www.who.int/migrants/about/definitions/en/.
23 www.who.int/migrants/about/en/.
24 https://blogs.bmj.com/bmj/2018/01/02/richard-smith-migrant-health-political-hysteria-but-insufficient-attention-to-an-issue-that-will-increase-substantially/.
25 www.europarl.europa.eu/thinktank/en/document.html?reference=EPRS_BRI%282016%29573908.
26 www.euro.who.int/__data/assets/pdf_file/0005/293270/Migration-Health-Key-Issues-.pdf?ua=1&ua=1.
27 http://unitedagainstrefugeedeaths.eu/about-the-campaign/about-the-united-list-of-deaths/.
28 www.nature.com/news/the-mental-health-crisis-among-migrants-1.20767.
29 www.euro.who.int/__data/assets/pdf_file/0017/330092/6-Migrant-womens-health-issues-irregular-status.pdf?ua=1.
30 www.who.int/reproductivehealth/topics/fgm/prevalence/en/.
31 www.euro.who.int/__data/assets/pdf_file/0014/352130/10.7-SDG-Fact-sheet-Migration-and-Health_FINAL.pdf.
32 World Bank most recent estimates (2013). See: www.worldbank.org/en/publication/poverty-and-shared-prosperity.
33 The Commission was set up by the British government to look at how intellectual property rights might work better for poor people and developing countries. The first Commission

meeting was in London on 8–9 May 2001, and the final report was published on 12 September 2002. See: www.iprcommission.org/home.html.
34 The Investor-state dispute settlement (ISDS) or investment court system (ICS): a system through which investors can sue countries for alleged discriminatory practices. ISDS is an instrument of public international law and provisions are contained in a number of bilateral investment treaties.
35 www.who.int/ehealth/en/.
36 www.who.int/en/news-room/fact-sheets/detail/road-traffic-injuries.
37 Mode 1 under the General Agreement on Trade in Services, GATS. See Chapter 6, section 6.6.3.
38 www.who.int/ehealth/en/.
39 The International Telecommunication Union (ITU) is the United Nations specialized agency in the field of telecommunications, information and communication technologies (ICTs).
40 www.itu.int/en/ITU-T/e-Health/Pages/default.aspx.
41 The World Telecommunication Standardization Assembly (WTSA), which meets every four years, establishes the topics for study by the ITU-T study groups which, in turn, produce Recommendations on these topics. The ITU Telecommunication Standardization Sector (ITU-T) is a permanent organ of ITU, which is responsible for studying technical, operating and tariff questions and issuing Recommendations on them with a view to standardizing telecommunications on a worldwide basis.
42 The mission of PCHA is "advancing personal connected health solutions". PCHA is itself an "HIMSS innovation Company"; the Healthcare Information and Management Systems Society (HIMSS) in turn is a global, cause-based, not-for-profit organization focused on better health through information and technology. www.himss.org/.
43 www.itu.int/en/ITU-T/e-Health/Pages/default.aspx.
44 www.icann.org/resources/agreement/health-2015-02-11-en.
45 PICs are voluntary amendments that applicants can create, sign and undertake along with the general registry agreement in order to hold their registry operations to certain standards. https://icannwiki.org/Public_Interest_Commitments.
46 www.who.int/goe/policies/en/.

References

Abarca-Gómez, L., et al. 2017. Worldwide trends in body-mass index, underweight, overweight, and obesity from 1975 to 2016: a pooled analysis of 2416 population-based measurement studies in 128·9 million children, adolescents, and adults. *The Lancet*, 390(10113), 2627–2642.

Adanu, R.M., Johnson, T.R., 2009. Migration and women's health. *International Journal of Gynaecology and Obstetrics*, 106(2), 179–181.

Anderson, T. 2018. Stepping up local efforts to stop global spread of yellow fever. *Bulletin of the World Health Organization*, 96, 374–375.

Aragão, L., 2012. Environmental science: the rainforest's water pump. *Nature*, 489, 217–218.

As Sy, E. 2016. Yellow fever in Angola: Are we repeating the mistakes of Ebola? 1 July. Available from: www.ifrc.org/es/noticias/discursos-y-articulos-de-opinion/articulos-de-opinion/2016/yellow-fever-in-angola-are-we-repeating-the-mistakes-of-ebola-72340/.

Bale, H., 1999. Pharmaceutical access and innovation: challenges and issues, *Development*, 42(4), 84–86.

Bathiany, S., Dakos, V., Scheffer, M., Lenton, T.M., 2018. Climate models predict increasing temperature variability in poor countries. *Science Advances*, 4 (5), eaar5809.

Baumgaertner, E., 2016. Could yellow fever become the next pandemic? *Scientific American*, 15 August. Available from: www.scientificamerican.com/article/could-yellow-fever-become-the-next-pandemic/.

Benton, A., Dionne, K.Y., 2015. International political economy and the 2014 West African Ebola outbreak. *African Studies Review*, 58(01), 223–236.

Berlinguer, G., Garrafa, V., 1996. *La merce finale. Saggio sulla compravendita di parti del corpo umano*. Milan: Baldini & Castoldi.

Bettcher, D., Yach, D., Guindon, G.E., 2000. Global trade and health: key linkages and future challenges. *Bulletin of the World Health Organization*, 78(4), 521–534.

Birn, A.-E., Pillay, Y., Holtz, T.H., 2009. *Textbook of International Health. Global Health in a Dynamic World* (3rd edn.). Oxford: Oxford University Press.

Blumenshine, P., Reingold, A.L., Egerter, S., Mockenhaupt, R., et al., 2008. Pandemic influenza planning in the United States from a health disparities perspective. *Emerging Infectious Diseases*, 14(5), 709–715.

Blunden, J., Arndt, D.S., Hartfield, G. (Eds.), 2018. State of the climate in 2017. *Bulletin of the American Meteorological Society*, 99(8), Si–S332.

Bonovas, S., Nikolopoulos, G., 2012. High-burden epidemics in Greece in the era of economic crisis. Early signs of a public health tragedy. *Journal of Preventive Medicine and Hygiene*, 53(3), 169–171.

Borowy, I., 2013. Degrowth and public health in Cuba: lessons from the past? *Journal of Cleaner Production*, 38(C),17–26.

Branca, F., Ellis, C.H., 2017. Global and national public health nutrition approaches. In Buttris, J.L., Welch, A.A., Kearney, J.M., Lanham-New, S.A. (Eds.), *Public Health Nutrition*. Chichester: Wiley-Blackwell, 359–372.

Brauman, R. (Ed.), 2002. *Utopie sanitarie*. Milan: Feltrinelli, 149–150.

Büthe, T., Harris, N., 2011. Codex Alimentarius Commission. In Hale, T., Held, D. (Eds.) *Handbook of Transnational Governance*. Malden: Polity Press, 219–228.

Butler, C. D., 2017. Limits to growth, planetary boundaries, and planetary health. *Current Opinion in Environmental Sustainability*, 25, 59–65.

Caminade, C., et al., 2014. Impact of climate change on global malaria distribution. *Proceedings of the National Academy of Sciences*, 4, 111(9), 3286–3291.

Castro, A., Khawja, Y., Johnston, J., 2010. Social inequalities and dengue transmission in Latin America. In Herring, A., Swedlund, A. (Eds.), *Plagues and Epidemics: Infected Spaces Past and Present*. New York: Berg, 231–250.

Cattaneo, A., 2014. Trattati bilaterali di libero commercio e salute. *Sistema Salute*, 58(4), 431–439.

Chan, M., 2009. Steadfast in the midst of perils. Keynote address at the 12th World Congress on Public Health. Istanbul, Turkey 27 April. Available from: www.who.int/dg/speeches/2009/steadfast_midst_perils_20090428/en/.

CIPR, 2002. Integrating Intellectual Property Rights and Development Policy. Report of the Commission on Intellectual Property Rights, London. Available from: www.iprcommission.org/papers/pdfs/final_report/CIPRfullfinal.pdf.

Cohen, J., Dibner, M.S., Wilson, A., 2010. Development of and access to products for neglected diseases. *PLoS One*, 5, e10610. http://dx.doi.org/10.1371/journal.pone.0010610 pmid: 20485552.

Collin, J.E., Lee, K., 2003. *Globalisation & Transborder Health Risk in the UK*. London: The Nuffield Trust.

Comptesse, X., 2017. *Santé 4.0 Le tsunami du numérique*. Chêne-Bourg: Georg.

Cook, J., et al., 2016 Consensus on consensus: a synthesis of consensus estimates on human-caused global warming. *Environmental Research Letters*, 11, 048002.

Correa, C., 2001. Health and intellectual property right. *Bulletin of the World Health Organization*, 79(5), 381.

Correa, C., 2002. *Implications of the Doha declaration on the TRIPS agreement and public health*. WHO, Geneva. www.who.int/medicines/areas/policy/WHO_EDM_PAR_2002.3.pdf.

Costello, A., et al., 2009. Managing the effects of climate change. *The Lancet*, 373, 1693–1733.

CSDH, 2008. *Closing the gap in a generation Health equity through action on the social determinants of health*. Final Report of the Commission on Social Determinants of Health. Geneva: World Health Organization.

Cuéllar, J.M., Lanman, T.H., 2017. "Text neck": an epidemic of the modern era of cell phones? *The Spine Journal*, 17, 901–902.

Dekeyser, K., Korsten, L., Fioramonti, L., 2018. Food sovereignty: shifting debates on democratic food governance. *Food Security*, 10,. 223–233.

Dentico, N., 2013. Conciliare l'innovazione medica e accesso ai faramci essenziali: la Commissione su salute pubblica, innovazone e diritti di proprietà intellettuale. In Cattaneo, A., Dentico, N. (Eds.), *OMS e diritto alla salute: quale futuro*. Osservatorio Italiano sulla Salute Globale, 61–71.

Doll, R., Hill, A.B., 1954. The mortality of doctors in relation to their smoking habits. *British Medical Journal*, 1(4877), 1451–1455.

DotHealth, 2013. Public Interest Commitments. The .health Top Level Domain Registry, Application ID number 1-1684-6394, March 5. https://gtldresult.icann.org/applicationstatus/viewstatus (accessed August 2018).

Doyal, L., 1981. *The Political Economy of Health*. Boston, MA: South End Press.

Eysenbach, G., 2014. The new health-related top-level domains are coming: will cureforcancer.health go to the highest bidder? *Journal of Medical Internet Research*, 16(3), e73.

Ezzati, M., Henley, S.J., Thun, M.J., Lopez, A.D., 2005. Role of smoking in global and regional cardiovascular mortality. *Circulation*, 112(4), 489–497.

FAO, 2015. *The State of Food Insecurity in the World 2015*. Rome: Food and Agriculture Organization.

FAO, IFAD, UNICEF, WFP and WHO, 2018. *The State of Food Security and Nutrition in the World 2018. Building climate resilience for food security and nutrition*. Rome: FAO.

Farmer, P. 1996. Social inequalities and emerging infectious diseases. *Emerging Infectious Diseases*, 2(4), 259–269.

Fenton, L., 2004. Preventing HIV/AIDS through poverty reduction: the only sustainable solution? *The Lancet*, 364(9440), 1186–1187.

Fox, A.M., 2012. The HIV–poverty thesis re-examined: poverty, wealth or inequality as a social determinant of HIV infection in sub-Saharan Africa? *Journal of Biosocial Science*, 44(4), 459–480.

Friel, S., 2011. Climate change, noncommunicable diseases, and development: the relationships and common policy opportunities. *Annual Review of Public Health*, 32, 133–147.

Gilmore, A.B., *et al.*, 2015. Exposing and addressing tobacco industry conduct in low-income and middle-income countries. *The Lancet*, 385(9972), 1029–1043.

Gushulak, B., 2017. Health, health systems and global health, Thematic Discussion Paper, 2nd Global Consultation on Migrant Health: 21–23 February 2017 – Colombo, Sri Lanka. Available from: www.iom.int/sites/default/files/our_work/DMM/Migration-Health/Global%20Health%20paper%2C%20final%20Sept%202017.pdf.

Hoen, E., 1999. Acccess to essential drugs and globalization. *Development*, 42(4), 87–91.

Hosking, J., Mudu, P., Dora, C., 2011. *Health co-benefits of climate change mitigation – Transport sector. Health in the green economy*. Geneva: World health Organization. http://doi.org/10.2471/BLT.13.128413.

Huff, A.R., Winnebah, T. 2015. Ebola, politics and ecology: beyond the "outbreak narrative. *IDS Practice Paper in Brief*, 1–4.

Huynen, M.M., Martens, P., Hilderink, H.B., 2005. The health impacts of globalization: a conceptual framework. *Global Health*, 1(1), 14.

IACFO, 2003. *Broadcasting bad health. Why food marketing to children needs to be controlled*. Report by the International Association of Consumer Food Organizations for the World Health Organization consultation on a global strategy for diet and health, Cambridge.

IARC, 2013. *Non-ionizing radiation, part II: radiofrequency electromagnetic fields. IARC monographs on the evaluation of carcinogenic risks to humans*, vol. 102. Lyon: International Agency for Research on Cancer.

IHR, 2008. *International Health Regulations (2005)*. Geneva: World Health Organization.

IOM, 2011 *An analysis of migration health in Kenia.* Geneva: International Organization for Migration.
IOM, 2015. *International Migration Report 2015.* Geneva: International Organization for Migration.
IOM, 2016. *Migration health – Annual review 2016.* Geneva: International Organization for Migration.
IOM, 2018. *World Migration Report 2018.* Geneva: International Organization for Migration.
IOM, WHO, UNHCHR, 2013. *International Migration, Health and Human Rights.* Geneva: International Organization for Migration.
Ionesco, D., Mokhnacheva, D., Gemenne, F., 2017. *The Atlas of Environmental Migration.* Oxford: IOM / Routledge.
IPCC, 2001. *Climate change: IPCC third assessment report.* Geneva: Intergovernmental Panel on Climate Change.
IPCC, 2007. *Climate change: IPCC fourth assessment report.* Geneva: Intergovernmental Panel on Climate Change.
IPCC, 2014. *Climate change: IPCC fifth assessment report.* Geneva: Intergovernmental Panel on Climate Change.
ITU, 2017. *ICT Fact and Figures 2017.* Geneva: International Telecommunications Union.
Jarman, H., 2017. Trade policy governance: what health policymakers and advocates need to know. *Health Policy*, 121(11), 1105–1112.
Jha, P., Peto, R., 2014. Global effects of smoking, of quitting, and of taxing tobacco. *New England Journal of Medicine*, 370, 60–68.
Kaner, J., Schaack, S., 2016. Understanding Ebola: the 2014 epidemic. *Globalization and Health*, 12, 1–7.
Karanikolos, M., et al., 2013. Health in Europe 7. Financial crisis, austerity, and health in Europe. *The Lancet*, 381(9874), 1323–1331.
Kennedy, G., Nantel, G., Shetty, P., 2004. Globalization of food systems in developing countries:a synthesis of country case studies. In *Globalization of Food Systems in Developing Countries: Impact on Food Security and Nutrition.* FAO – Food and Nutrition Paper 83. Rome: Food and Agriculture Organization, 1–25.
Kentikelenis, A., et al., 2014. Greece's health crisis: from austerity to denialism. *The Lancet*, 383(9918), 748–753.
Kentikelenis, A., et al., 2015. The International Monetary Fund and the Ebola outbreak. *The Lancet Global Health*, 3(2), e69–e70.
Kerry, V.B., Lee, K., 2007. TRIPS, the Doha declaration and paragraph 6 decision: what are the remaining steps for protecting access to medicines? *Globalization and Health*, 3(3). http://doi.org/10.1186/1744-8603-3-3.
Keygnaert, I., et al., 2016. *What is the evidence on the reduction of inequalities in accessibility and quality of maternal health care delivery for migrants? A review of the existing evidence in the WHO European Region.* Copenhagen: WHO Regional Office for Europe (Health Evidence Network (HEN) synthesis report 45).
Khan, A.E., et al., 2014. Salinity in drinking water and the risk of (pre)eclampsia and gestational hypertension in coastal Bangladesh: a case-control study. *PLoS One*, 30; 9(9). doi:10.1371/journal.pone.0108715
Klein, N., 2002. *No Logo.* London: Picador.
Kumar, B.N., et al., 2018, Migrant health is global health. *Tidsskr Nor Legeforen.* Available from: https://tidsskriftet.no/en/2017/12/global-helse/migrant-health-global-health.
Labonté, R., 2010. *Global Health Policy: Exploring the Rationale for Health in Foreign Policy.* Ottawa: Globalization and Health Equity Institute, Population Health, University of Ottawa, 1–108.
Labonté, R., 2015. *Globalization and Health. International Encyclopedia of Social & Behavioral Sciences* (2nd edn.). Amsterdam: Elsevier, 198–205. http://doi.org/10.1016/B978-0-08-097086-8.14022-X.

Lapsang, A., 2007. Cross-cultural delivery of e-learning programmes: perspectives from Hong Kong. *IRRODL*, 8(3). www.irrodl.org/index.php/irrodl/article/view/426/937.
Lara, R.J., *et al.*, 2009. Influence of catastrophic climatic events and human waste on Vibrio distribution in the Karnaphuli estuary, Bangladesh. *Ecohealth*, 6, 279–286.
Levy, B.S., Sidel, V., 2009. The economic crisis and public health. *Social Medicine*, 4(2), 82–87.
Levy, K., *et al.*, 2016. Untangling the impacts of climate change on waterborne diseases: a systematic review of relationships between diarrheal diseases and temperature, rainfall, flooding, and drought. *Environmental Science & Technology*, 50(10), 4905–4922.
Maastricht University and the Global Migration Data Analysis Center (GMDAC), of the International Organization for Migration, 2016. Significant Pull/push factors for determining of asylum-related migration. A literature review. Available from: www.easo.europa.eu/sites/default/files/publications/the%20push%20and%20pull%20factors%20of%20asylum%20-%20related%20migration.pdf.
Maciocco, G., 2015. Conflitti d'interesse (ovvero business as usual). *Salute Internazionale*, 18 December. Available from: www.saluteinternazionale.info/2015/12/conflitti-di-interesse-business-as-usual/.
Mackey, T., Liang, B.A., Attaran, A., Kohler, J.C., 2014 Health domains for sale: The need for better global eHealth governance of health information online. *Annals of Global Health*, 80(3), 209–210.
Mahowald, N.M., *et al.*, 2017. Are the impacts of land use on warming underestimated in climate policy? *Environmental Research Letters*, 12, 094016.
Mamelund, S.E., 2006. A socially neutral disease? Individual social class, household wealth and mortality from Spanish influenza in two socially contrasting parishes in Kristiania 1918–19. *Social Science & Medicine*, 62(4), 923–940.
Marceca, M., 2016. Migration and health from a public health perspective. Available from: www.intechopen.com/books/people-s-movements-in-the-21st-century-risks-challenges-and-benefits/migration-and-health-from-a-public-health-perspective.
Marmot, M., 2016. Society and health of migrants. *European Journal of Epidemiology*, 31, 639–641.
McMichael, A.J., Lindgren, E., 2011. Climate change: present and future risks to health, and necessary responses. *Journal of Internal Medicine*, 270, 401–413.
McMichael, A.J., *et al.* (Eds.), 2003. *Climate Change and Human Health: Risks and Responses*. Geneva: World Health Organization.
McMichael, A.J., *et al.*, 2004. Climate change. In Ezzati, M, *et al.* (Eds.), *Comparative Quantification of Health Risks: Global and Regional Burden of Disease Due to Selected Major Risk Factors*. Geneva: World Health Organization.
McNeill, D., *et al.*, 2017. Trade and investment agreements: implications for health protection. *Journal of World Trade*, 51(1), 159–182.
Mendez, M.A., Popkin, B.M., 2004. Globalization, urbanization and nutritional change in the developing world. In FAO, *Globalization of food systems in developing countries: impact on food security and nutrition*. FAO – Food and Nutrition Paper 83. Rome: Food and Agriculture Organization, 55–80.
Mirza, Z., 1999. WTO/TRIPs, pharmaceuticals and health: impacts and strategies. *Development*, 42(4), 92–97.
Missoni, E. 2017. The political economy of epidemics. In Fantini, B. (Ed.), *Epidémies et sociétés, passé, present et futur*. Pisa: Edizioni ETS, 171–186.
Missoni, E., *et al.*, 1988. Remedies for Third World diseases. *The Lancet*, 332(8605), 282.
Mitchell D., *et al.*, 2016. Attributing human mortality during extreme heat waves to anthropogenic climate change. *Environmental Research Letters*, 11, 074006.
Mitchell, A., Sheargold, E., 2015. Protecting the autonomy of states to enact tobacco control measures under trade and investment agreements. *Tobacco Control*, e2, e147–153.
Murray, C.J.L., Lopez, A.D. (Eds.), 1996. *The Global Burden of Disease: A Comprehensive Assessment of Mortality and Disability from Diseases, Injuries, and Risk Factors in 1990 and*

Projected to 2020. Harvard School of Public Health on behalf of the World Health Organization and the World Bank.

NCCDPHP, 2014. *The Health Consequences of Smoking—50 Years of Progress: A Report of the Surgeon General. Atlanta (GA): Centers for Disease Control and Prevention (US); 2, Fifty Years of Change 1964–2014*. National Center for Chronic Disease Prevention and Health Promotion (US) Office on Smoking and Health. Available from: www.ncbi.nlm.nih.gov/books/NBK294310/.

Ng, M., Fleming, T., Robinson, M., et al., 2014. Global, regional, and national prevalence of overweight and obesity in children and adults during 1980–2013: a systematic analysis for the Global Burden of Disease Study 2013. *The Lancet*, 384(9945), 766–781.

Ni, KJ., 2013. Does science speak clearly and fairly in trade and food safety disputes? The search for an optimal response of WTO adjudication to problematic international standard-making. *Food and Drug Law Journal*, 68(1), 97–114, ii–iii.

Nielsen S.J., Popkin, B.M., 2003. Patterns and trends in food portion sizes, 1977–1998. *JAMA*, 289(4), 450–453.

Ortiz, J., et al., 2011. *Austerity Measures Threaten Children and Poor Households: Recent Evidence in Public Expenditures from 128 Developing Countries*. New York: United Nations Children's Fund (UNICEF).

Owoeye, O.A., 2014. Compulsory patent licensing and local drug manufacturing capacity in Africa. *Bulletin of the World Health Organization*, 92(3), 214–219.

Pachauri, R.K., Reisinger, A. (Eds.), 2007. *Contribution of Working Groups I, II and III to the Fourth Assessment Report of the Intergovernmental Panel on Climate Change*. Geneva: IPCC.

Pascual, F., 2014. Intellectual property rights, market competition and access to affordable antiretrovirals. Antiviral Therapy, 19, Suppl., 57–67.

Patz, J.A., et al., 2007. Climate change and global health: quantifying a growing ethical crisis. *EcoHealth*, 4, 397–405.

Peeler, E.J., Reese, R.A., Thrush, M.A., 2013. Animal disease import risk analysis – a review of current methods and practice. *Transboundary and Emerging Diseases*, 62, 480–490.

Pennington, H., 2005. Science, policy, and politics: the case of BSE. *The Lancet*, 366, 885–886.

Popkin, B.M., Adair, L.S., Ng, S.W., 2012. Now and then: the global nutrition transition: the pandemic of obesity in developing countries. *Nutrition Reviews,* 70(1), 3–21.

Prüss-Ustün, et al., 2016. *Preventing Disease through Healthy Environments. A Global Assessment of the Burden of Disease from Environmental Risks*. Geneva: World Health Organization.

Richards, T., 2012. The crusade for health equity. *BMJ*, 344, e4414.

Rieder, S., 2016. Interrogating the global health and development nexus: critical viewpoints of neoliberalization and health in transnational spaces. *World Development Perspectives*, 2(C), 55–61.

Silva, B.M.C., Rodrigues, J.J.P.C., la Torre Díez, de, I., López-Coronado, M., Saleem, K., 2015. Mobile-health: a review of current state in 2015. *Journal of Biomedical Informatics*, 56(C), 265–272.

Skinner, M.K., Manikkam, M., Guerrero-Bosagna, C., 2010. Epigenetic transgenerational actions of environmental factors in disease etiology. *Trends in Endocrinology & Metabolism*, 21(4), 214–222.

Smith, J. et al., 2016. Borders and migration: an issue of global health importance. *The Lancet*, 4(2), e85–e86.

Smith, R.D., Correa, C., Oh, C. 2009. Trade TRIPS and pharmaceuticals. *The Lancet*, 373, 684–691.

Solomonides, A., Mackey, T., 2015. Emerging ethical issues in digital health information: ICANN, health information, and the dot-health top-level domain. *Cambridge Quarterly of Healthcare Ethics*, 24(3), 311–322.

Sparke, M., 2016. Health and the embodiment of neoliberalism: pathologies of political economy from climate change and austerity to personal responsibility. In Springer, S., Birch, K., MacLeavy, J. (Eds.), *Handbook of Neoliberalism*. New York: Routledge, 223–237.

Spaventa, L., 2009. La grande crisi del nuovo secolo. www.treccani.it/enciclopedia/la-grande-crisi-del-nuovo-secolo_%28XXI-Secolo%29/.
Spiro, S.G., Silvestri,G.A., 2005. One hundred years of lung cancer. *American Journal of Respiratory and Critical Care Medicine*, 172(5), 523–529.
Stirner, B., Thangaraj, H., 2013. Learning from practice: compulsory licensing cases and access to medicines. *Pharmaceutical Patent Analyst*, 2(2), 195–213. doi:10.4155/ppa.12.91.
Stuckler D., et al., 2009. The public health effect of economic crises and alternative policy responses in Europe: an empirical analysis. *The Lancet*, 374(9686), 315–323.
Suhrcke, M., et al., 2011. The impact of economic crises on communicable disease transmission and control: a systematic review of the evidence. *PLoS ONE*, 6(6), e20724–12.
Swinburn, B.A, et al., 2011. The global obesity pandemic: shaped by global drivers and local environments. *The Lancet*, 378(9793), 804–814.
Tallapragada, N.P., 2016. Off-patent drugs at brand-name prices: a puzzle for policymakers. *Journal of Law and the Biosciences*, 3(1), 238–247.
Taubenberger, J.K., Morens, D.M.. 2006. 1918 Influenza: the mother of all pandemics. *Emerging Infectious Diseases*, 12(1), 15–22.
Taylor, A.L., Bettcher, D.W., 2000. WHO Framework Convention on Tobacco Control: a global "good" for public health. *Bulletin of the World Health Organisation*, 78 (7), 920–928.
The Lancet Planetary Health, 2017. Microplastics and human health—an urgent problem. *The Lancet Planetary Health*, 1(7), e254.
Trouiller, P., et al., 2002. Drug development for neglected diseases: a deficient market and a public-health policy failure. *The Lancet*, 359, 2188–2194.
UN, 2012. Political Declaration of the High-Level Meeting of the General Assembly on the Prevention and Control of Non-Communicable Diseases. Resolution adopted by the 66th General Assembly. A/RES/66/2.
UN, 2015. United Nations. Climate Change. The Paris Agreement. Available from: https://unfccc.int/process-and-meetings/the-paris-agreement/the-paris-agreement.
UN, 2015a. *Transforming our world: the 2030 agenda for sustainable development*. New York: United Nations, 25 September. Available from: https://sustainabledevelopment.un.org/post2015/transformingourworld.
UN, 2016. The United Nations General Assembly. Resolution adopted by the General Assembly on 25 July 2016. Agreement concerning the Relationship between the United Nations and the International Organization for Migration.
UN, 2016a. *New York Declaration for refugees and migrants*. United Nations.
UN, 2017. *International Migration Report 2017* (ST/ESA/SER.A/403). United Nations, Department of Economic and Social Affairs, Population Division.
UNCTAD, 2016. Data protection regulations and international data flows: Implications for trade and development. United Nations Conference on Trade and Development: Geneva. http://unctad.org/en/PublicationsLibrary/dtlstict2016d1_en.pdf .
UNESCO, 2017. Report of the IBC on Big Data and Health. SHS/YES/IBC-24/17/3 REV.2 Paris, 15 September. Unesdoc.unesco.org/images/0024/002487/248724e.pdf .
UNGA, 2012. *Political Declaration of the High-level Meeting of the General Assembly on the Prevention and Control of Non-communicable Diseases*. Resolution adopted by the General Assembly. A/RES/66/2.
UNGA, 2016. *Endorsed Political Declaration on AMR-1616108*, United Nations General Assembly, 21 September.
Verner, G., et al., 2016. Health in climate change research from 1990 to 2014: positive trend, but still underperforming. *Global Health Action*. 9:10.3402/gha.v9.30723.
Vineis, P., Chan, Q., Khan, A., 2011. Climate change impacts on water salinity and health. *Journal of Epidemiology and Global Health*, 1(1), 5–10.
Vlachadis, N., et al., 2012. Mortality and the economic crisis in Greece. *The Lancet*, 383, 691.
Wallach, L., Sforza, M., 1999. *The WTO. Five Years of Reasons to Resist Corporate Globalization*. New York: Seven Stories Press.

Walter, E., Scott, M., 2017. The life and work of Rudolf Virchow 1821–1902: "Cell theory, thrombosis and the sausage duel". *Journal of the Intensive Care Society*, 18(3), 234–235.

Watts, N., et al., 2017. The Lancet Countdown on health and climate change: from 25 years of inaction to a global transformation for public health. *The Lancet*, 391, 581–630.

WHO and CBD, 2015. *Connecting global priorities: biodiversity and human health.* Geneva: World Health Organization and Convention on Biological Diversity.

WHO and UNICEF, 2017. *Progress on drinking water, sanitation and hygiene: 2017 update and SDG baselines.* Geneva: World Health Organization (WHO) and the United Nations Children's Fund (UNICEF).

WHO EURO, 2016. *Toolkit for assessing health system capacity to manage large influxes of refugees, asylum-seekers and migrants.* Copenhagen: World Health Organization.

WHO EURO, 2016a. *WHO Expert Consultation: Available evidence for the future update of the WHO Global Air Quality Guidelines.* Copenhagen: World Health Organization Regional Office for Europe.

WHO, 1998. Cross-border advertising, promotion and sale of medical products through the internet. Executive Board 101st session, agenda item 9, EB101.R3. Geneva: World Health Organization. www.who.int/iris/handle/10665/79504.

WHO, 2000. *General Guidelines for Methodologies on Research and Evaluation of Traditional Medicine.* Geneva: World Health Organization.

WHO, 2003. *World Health Assembly Resolution 56.1 – WHO Framework Convention on Tobacco Control.* Geneva: World Health Organization. Available from: www.who.int/tobacco/framework/final_text/en/index1.html.

WHO, 2003a. World Health Assembly, 2003. *Resolution WHA 56.31.* 28 May.

WHO, 2004. *Global Strategy on Diet, Physical Activity and Health.* Geneva: World Health Organization.

WHO, 2005. *Air quality guidelines for particulate matter, ozone, nitrogen dioxide and sulfur dioxide.* Geneva: World Health Organization.

WHO, 2005a. *eHealth.* World Health Assembly Resolution WHA58.28. Fifty-Eighth World Health Assembly 16–25 May 2005. Geneva: World Health Organization.

WHO, 2012. *Research and Development to Meet Health Needs in Developing Countries: Strengthening Global Financing and Coordination Report of the Consultative Expert Working Group on Research and Development: Financing and Coordination.* Geneva: World Health Organization. www.who.int/phi/CEWG_Report_5_April_2012.pdf .

WHO, 2013. *eHealth standardization and interoperability.* World Health Assembly Resolution WHA66.24. Sixty-sixth World Health Assembly 27 May. Geneva: World Health Organization.

WHO, 2014. *Gender, Climate Change and Health.* Geneva: World Health Organization.

WHO, 2015. *Health and the Environment: Addressing the health impact of air pollution.* A68/A/CONF./2 Rev.1 26 May, 2015. Geneva: World Health Organization.

WHO, 2015a. *Public health implications of excessive use of the internet, computers, smartphones and similar electronic devices: meeting report. Tokyo, Japan, 27–29 August 2014.* Geneva: World Health Organization.

WHO, 2016. *Global diffusion of eHealth: making universal health coverage achievable. Report of the third global survey on eHealth.* Geneva: World Health Organization.

WHO, 2017. *WHO report on the global tobacco epidemic, 2017, Monitoring tobacco use and prevention policies.* Geneva: World Health Organization.

WHO, 2017a. World Health Assembly, 2017. Resolution WHA70.15, 31 May.

WHO, 2017b. World Health Assembly, 2017. Resolution WHA70.24, 29 May.

WHO, 2018. eHealth. The Health Internet. www.who.int/ehealth/programmes/governance/en/.

Wilkinson, R., Pickett, K., 2010. *The Spirit Level. Why Equality is Better for Everyone.* London: Penguin Books.

Williams, O.D., Ooms, G., Hill, P.S., 2015. Cautionary notes on a global tiered pricing framework for medicines. *American Journal of Public Health*, 105(7), 1290–1293.

WMO, 2016. Guidelines on the definition and monitoring of extreme weather and climate events. Available from: www.wmo.int/pages/prog/wcp/ccl/opace/opace2/documents/Draftversionofthe GuidelinesontheDefinitionandMonitoringofExtremeWeatherandClimateEvents.pdf.

WTO, 1994. Agreement on Trade-Related Aspects of Intellectual Property Rights. Annex 1C of the Marrakesh Agreement. Available from: www.wto.org/English/docs_e/legal_e/27-trips_01_e.htm.

WTO, 2001. Declaration on the TRIPS agreement and public health. Adopted on 14 November 2001, Doha WTO Ministerial 2001: TRIPS. WT/MIN(01)/DEC/220 November. Available from: www.wto.org/english/thewto_e/minist_e/min01_e/mindecl_trips_e.htm.

WTO, 2003. Implementation of paragraph 6 of the Doha Declaration on the TRIPS Agreement and public health. Decision of the General Council of 30 August 2003. WT/L/540 and Corr.1. Available from: www.wto.org/english/tratop_e/trips_e/implem_para6_e.htm.

WTO/WHO, 2002. *WTO agreements and public health. A joint study by the WHO and the WTO Secretariat*. World Trade Organization-World Health Organization, Geneva www.wto.org/english/res_e/booksp_e/who_wto_e.pdf .

Yach, D., 2014. The origins, development, effects, and future of the WHO Framework Convention on Tobacco Control: a personal perspective. *The Lancet*, 383(9930), 1771–1779.

Young, L.R., Nestle, M., 2002. The contribution of expanding portion sizes to the US obesity epidemic. *American Journal of Public Health*, 92(2), 246–249.

Zimmerman, C., Kiss, L., Hossain, M., 2011. Migration and health: a framework for 21st century policy-making. *PLoS Medicine*, 8(5), e1001034.

Unless otherwise indicated, all websites were accessed on 9 August 2018.

12 Health systems in the global health landscape

12.1 Introduction

The 2000 World Health Report, the first such report devoted to health system performance, defined health systems as "all those activities whose main purpose is to promote, restore and maintain health" (WHO 2000). This includes efforts to influence determinants of health as well as more direct health-improving activities. This conceptualization of health systems goes beyond the boundaries of the healthcare system, including broader areas such as disease prevention and health promotion through policies and interventions that are not strictly health-related, such as those aimed at improving the quality and safety of food products (e.g. organic farming), environmental safety (e.g. the elimination of lead from petrol) or road safety (e.g. the obligation to wear safety belts).

Health systems therefore include healthcare systems that provide individuals or populations with prevention and curative (or palliative) and rehabilitative services (WHO 2000). The core objectives of health systems, based on the approach proposed by the World Health Organization (WHO 2000, 2007, 2010), are:

1. Health: protecting and improving the health of the population they serve and reducing health inequalities.
2. Responsiveness and participation: responding to people's non-medical expectations and enabling participation in decisions that have an impact on their health and health systems.
3. Equity: protecting individuals from the risk of financial hardship due to the costs of health services through risk-pooling mechanisms, ensuring fairness for individual contributions and equity in access to services, i.e. access to and coverage for effective health interventions according to needs.
4. Efficiency: ensuring the best use of available resources to reach the aforementioned three objectives.

While policies in other sectors also influence the attainment of the first objective, the other three objectives are specific to the healthcare system. To reach their goals, healthcare systems rely on four functions, which are not all under the direct responsibility of the health sector (WHO 2000):

1. Leadership: responsibility and oversight of the system by health authorities and government institutions, and overall governance.

2. Generating resources, including:
   a. Human resources: the health workforce trained by schools, universities, and other training institutes.
   b. Financial resources: where citizens contribute as taxpayers or purchasers depending on the financing model of healthcare systems.
   c. Technology and infrastructure: medical technologies, medicines, vaccines, and medical devices, and other non-medical technologies.
3. Collecting, allocating and pooling financial resources: either by the state and/or by any financial intermediaries (insurance companies, mutual societies, etc.) that purchase the health services.
4. Delivery of health services: these are differentiated according to the level of care (primary, secondary or tertiary), the nature of providers (public, private), the degree of organization or the type of medicine practiced (conventional, unconventional).

The WHO Health Systems Framework summarizes health system components with six "building blocks" (Figure 12.1) (WHO 2007). Information systems are captured as one of the building blocks, and are of increasing importance in supporting the overall functioning of the system. The six building blocks do not alone constitute a system; the system is the result of the multiple interactions among the blocks and with the people at its center (WHO 2009) (Figure 12.2).

A wide variety of actors are involved in healthcare systems. The actors include all the "individuals or groups with an interest in the healthcare system, including patients and their families, nurses, physicians, laboratory technical staff, and other external entities as regulators, insurance companies, and healthcare organizations" (Wickramasinghe et al. 2008).

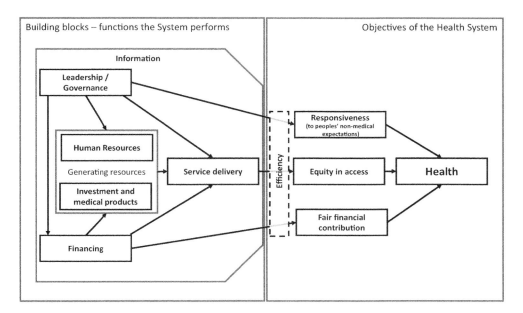

Figure 12.1 Health systems' building blocks and goals.

248 *Global policies and issues*

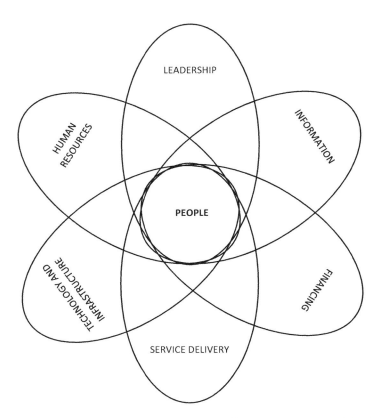

Figure 12.2 The dynamic architecture and interconnectedness of health system building blocks.

12.2 The Universal Health Coverage movement

As we described in Chapter 4, health system reforms were the central topic of the international debate during the 1980s. These reforms were heavily influenced by International Financial Institutions and the Structural Adjustment Programs they imposed on developing countries, which resulted in the reduction of public health expenditure, decentralization, privatization and introduction of user-fees with significant social costs.

Healthcare financing remains challenging in several countries. In fact, millions of people in the world are unable to seek care because they cannot afford the related costs, which may result in financial hardship and/or impoverishment. In several countries, including high-income countries, many people face financial hardship as a result of healthcare costs (Franklin 2017). For some people, out-of-pocket payments act as a deterrent to the use of health services or to continuity of care; for others to access the health services they need, they must cut their spending on food, clothing and housing. Postponing healthcare-seeking may have detrimental health consequences and can lead to higher costs: for example, when people let their health deteriorate and are then required to use expensive hospital emergency care as a last resort.

This has led the WHO to engage in the promotion of Universal Health Coverage (UHC) aimed at "ensuring that all people have access to needed health services (including prevention, promotion, treatment, rehabilitation and palliation) of sufficient quality to be effective while also ensuring that the use of these services does not expose the user the financial hardship".[1]

In 2005, the World Health Assembly (WHA) committed all member states of WHO to develop health financing systems conducive to UHC (WHO 2005), with the goal to contribute to the enjoyment of the highest attainable standard of health as stated in the WHO Constitution (1946). This commitment is also consistent with the concept of health for all and the Alma Ata Declaration of 1978 (Kieny and Evans 2013). Since then, several influential global health stakeholders such as the Rockefeller Foundation, bilateral donors such as USAID, and the governments of increasingly influential countries such as China and India have explicitly supported the emerging movement towards UHC.

In 2010 the WHO dedicated the World Health Report 2010 (WHR) to "Health systems financing: the path to universal coverage" (WHO 2010a). The publication of this report was a key step in establishing UHC as a priority for global health policy, eliciting the interest of several low- and middle-income countries (LMICs).

The following year, the WHA approved a new resolution which placed UHC in the broader context of health systems and not only as a health financing objective: "affordable universal coverage and access for all citizens" should respond to "equity and solidarity" criteria (WHO 2011).

The global commitment to UHC was reaffirmed in 2012 with a resolution of the United Nations General Assembly recognizing:

> that effective and financially sustainable implementation of universal health coverage is based on a resilient and responsive health system that provides comprehensive primary health-care services, with extensive geographical coverage, including in remote and rural areas, and with a special emphasis on access to populations most in need, and has an adequate skilled, well trained and motivated workforce, as well as capacities for broad public health measures, health protection and addressing determinants of health through policies across sectors, including promoting the health literacy of the population.
>
> (UN 2012)

In 2015, UHC was explicitly included in the Sustainable Development Goals (SDGs). SDG3 (Ensure healthy lives and promote wellbeing for all at all ages) includes a target (3.8) to "achieve universal health coverage, including financial risk protection, access to quality essential healthcare services, and access to safe, effective, quality, and affordable essential medicines and vaccines for all". A related target (3.7) adds the goal to: "by 2030, ensure universal access to sexual and reproductive health-care services, including for family planning, information and education, and the integration of reproductive health into national strategies and programmes."[2]

12.2.1 Policies towards Universal Health Coverage

The goal of UHC relates to the aspiration that all people will obtain the quality health services they need while not suffering financially as a result of seeking health care. Many countries have embraced the concept of UHC, which has become relevant to policy debates and reforms in LMICs (Tediosi *et al.* 2016). Around half of the countries in the world are in fact engaged in health reforms that aim to move towards UHC by either extending, deepening or otherwise improving coverage with needed health services and/or financial protection (Boerma *et al.* 2014).

Moving towards UHC would require countries to expand the availability of essential health services and to include more people in risk-pooling mechanisms, such as health insurance, in order to reduce out-of-pocket expenditure. For the poorest countries, the greatest challenge is not only reaching the people currently not benefiting from quality health services, but also guaranteeing that their financial situation is not worsened by having to pay for the services they receive (Boerma *et al.* 2014). Related challenges include: the large informal sector that makes collecting revenues difficult; the increasing burden of chronic noncommunicable diseases and injury that requires different service delivery models, a focus on prevention and expensive technologies for treatment; and the limited pooled resources sometimes fragmented in a multiplicity of public and private insurance schemes resulting in small risk pools that exclude the poorest segments of the population (Boerma *et al.* 2014; WHO 2010b).

In addition, in LMICs millions of people do not obtain the health services they need for several reasons: they are unavailable or of poor quality; people, particularly the poor, are unaware of their entitlements; people do not trust the health system; or there are financial and non-financial barriers to accessing health services that lead to exclusion (Obrist *et al.* 2007). At least half of the world's population cannot obtain essential health services, and each year large numbers of households are being pushed into poverty because they must pay for health care out of their own pockets.

In LMICs there are major challenges to understanding how to increase and sustain coverage, reach people in the informal sector, and ensure effective essential health services as well as financial risk protection for the poorest segments of the population and other groups who are excluded. In addition to the need for more funding, it is important to develop effective approaches to define appropriate service packages, to better identify and target the excluded poor, and to ensure that the rights of citizens who are less likely to be covered are properly addressed. It is also critical to understand who is excluded from needed services and from financial protection and why. Mechanisms to hold healthcare purchasers and service providers accountable to the patients need to be in place so that patients can get high-quality and affordable healthcare services.

Policies moving towards UHC should consider the three key dimensions embraced by the concept: expanding the number of people benefiting from social health protection systems such as health insurances or national health services, expanding the breadth of high-quality health services included in the benefit packages, and increasing the proportion of the total costs of the services that is pre-paid by the social health protection schemes with consequent reduction of the out-of-pocket payments. As stated by WHO:

> extending the coverage from pooled funds along the three dimensions calls for health financing reforms and actions leading to an increase of available funds for health, to an increase in the share of these funds collected through prepayment and the arrangements for pooling them, to efficiency gains and to upholding and increasing the quality of health services.[3]

Ensuring that all countries have sustainable pooled health resources is crucial to the goal of UHC (Global Burden of Disease Health Financing Collaborator Network 2018). This is particularly challenging in low-income countries (LICs).

Currently, 800 million people spend at least 10% of their household budgets on health expenses for themselves, a sick child or other family member (World Bank 2017). Every year more than 100 million people fall into poverty as a result of direct healthcare costs (Haider and Nibb 2017); 150 million people are forced to spend nearly half their incomes on medical expenses. This is because in many countries people have no access to social health protection, affordable health insurance or government-funded health services.[4]

Fragmentation of health systems tends to worsen the situation, reducing health system efficiency and seriously challenging equity. In countries where external aid plays a significant role, fragmentation and management difficulties are exacerbated by the presence of a growing number of international development cooperation actors (bilateral agencies, international institutions, NGOs, philanthropy and transnational companies, global public-private partnerships). These actors have their own objectives, strategies, intervention modalities, financing and execution times, and monitoring and evaluation needs, which weigh on the already weak partner countries' institutions and their weak administrative and management capacities, while also failing to respect the well-known core principles of aid effectiveness (ownership, alignment, harmonization, management by results and mutual accountability) (OECD/DAC 2005) (see Chapter 13).

Strengthening health systems is crucial to pursue the goal of UHC. Frenk (2015) even claimed that there is a need for "a third generation[5] of health-system reforms, which implies a comprehensive scope of policy interventions, including the introduction of explicit ethical frameworks, the enhanced attention to financial arrangements, and the transformation of major dimensions of the organization of health systems". Financial sustainability needs to be built into the system from the beginning "by exploring options to broaden revenue sources and prioritise the appropriate use of resources. Reforms in delivery systems should prioritise investment in non-hospital services, delivering stronger, high-quality primary and community care services, as well as public health programmes" (OECD 2016).

The journey towards UHC is affected by global forces and health determinants linked to the overall objectives of the Development Agenda, although some of the SDGs may not seem to be related to UHC. In turn, UHC in itself can make a major contribution to the achievement of several SDGs, including boosting a more inclusive economic growth in line with SDG8 (Promote sustained, inclusive and sustainable economic growth, full and productive employment and decent work for all) (Kieny *et al.* 2017).

12.3 Global challenges to health system sustainability

Health systems are facing several challenges everywhere. One of them is the sustainability of the health system in the contemporary increasingly complex context. The sustainability of health systems is often considered only in terms of financial constraints, which is a reductionist way to look at this issue. If fact, in order to be sustainable health systems should have three main features:

Affordability: First, health systems should be affordable for the population and for all the different entities that form them: healthcare providers, social health protections schemes, governments, manufacturers of biomedical technologies etc. In the last decades, health expenditure has almost always been growing at high rates in most countries. In several countries, the health expenditure growth has been far higher than the growth of the GDP, thereby increasing the share of the wealth created in each country which is spent on healthcare services. According to the latest report of the Institute of Health Metrics and Evaluation (IHME, 2018), in 2015 the global health expenditure was around $9.7 trillion, with over 50% of this spending occurring in six high-income countries. Health expenditure is correlated with national income, although there is dramatic variability in country-level spending even within income groups and geographical regions. Health expenditure growth was relatively constant even in the period between 1995 and 2015 when several countries were hit by the financial crisis. In these decades health expenditure grew at an annualized rate of 3.1%, and the largest growth occurred in upper-middle-income and lower-middle-income countries (5.4% and 4.2% respectively) (IHME 2018).

Yet, overall spending on health care in low-income and lower-middle-income countries is still tiny compared to upper-middle-income and high-income countries, even though in some countries it is reaching proportions of the GDP (6%) similar to those of upper-middle-income countries. At an aggregate level, out-of-pocket expenditure still represents the largest portion of healthcare spending in these countries, leading to concerns about possible related social costs (e.g. catastrophic healthcare expenditure) and the equity of the system (ensuring universal access to health care and fair contribution to health system financing). As a consequence, as already mentioned, millions of people still face financial hardship due to medical expenses.

To be affordable, health systems should therefore focus on high-value interventions, i.e. those able to ensure high benefits compared to their costs. Such interventions include effectively governing the continuous growth of medical technologies of low value, establishing governance structures able to govern the pressure to increase consumption of unnecessary healthcare services, and addressing social determinants of health.

Adaptability: Secondly, health systems, as with all complex systems, are hard to change. However, several dynamic changes challenge the sustainability of health systems such as demographic and epidemiological changes, cultural and social changes and technological changes. Therefore health systems should be able to continuously adapt to these changes rapidly.

In Chapter 11 we have described a number of global determinants that impact population health and healthcare demand (such as changes in the eco-system, transformation of the food system, migration, the role of the internet and the market in fostering health consumerism, among others) and below we discuss how the epidemiological transition influences demand.

However, health system capacity to offer health care is also influenced by global determinants. Selective approaches (such as "vertical" global initiatives focused on single diseases or issues) prompt fragmentation, inefficiencies and inequities. Conflicts, social disruption and macroeconomic adjustment programs may further weaken fragile systems, making them unable to face public health crises (see Box 12.1).

BOX 12.1 Case study: health systems and Ebola[*]

It is as a result of weak health systems that the West African outbreak of Ebola virus disease (EVD) in 2014–2016 escalated into a full-blown epidemic, claiming

[*] Case study by Maitreyi Sahu.

more than 11,300 lives and leaving behind more than 17,000 survivors in Sierra Leone, Liberia and Guinea (World Health Organization 2016). Prior to the outbreak there was already compelling evidence of challenges in access to health services in Liberia and Sierra Leone, which both suffered from drawn-out civil wars in the 1990s and early 2000s and faced a resulting flight of health workers (Desai 2010; Kruk *et al.* 2010). Weak surveillance systems also contributed: the first cases occurred in rural Guinea in December 2013, and were not detected by the national surveillance system for another few months (Moon *et al.* 2015).

In addition, poor leadership and governance at the national and global levels played a major role in the spread of EVD. In March 2014, after cases were identified in Conakry, which houses more than one-seventh of the population of Guinea, national authorities downplayed the event in order to avoid panic and disruption of economic activity (Moon *et al.* 2015). For similar reasons, the WHO delayed in characterizing the Ebola outbreak as an international emergency until August 2014 after the outbreak was well under way in all three countries, and as a result global resources were not deployed until around the time when two US aid workers were evacuated from Liberia (Moon *et al.* 2015). The responses in Sierra Leone, Liberia and Guinea were starkly in contrast to those in nearby Nigeria, where the government declared an Ebola emergency on the same day that the first case was identified in Lagos in July 2014, immediately tracing 894 contacts of the index case (Otu *et al.* 2017) and containing the outbreak to 20 cases and eight deaths (Centers for Disease Control and Prevention).

During the outbreak, weak health systems became even weaker. For example, prior to the outbreak there was already a severe shortage of medical doctors in Sierra Leone, where in 2010 the coverage amounted to only 2.4 physicians per 100,000 population (World Health Organization 2018b). During the outbreak an unprecedented number of health workers were infected due to the high occupational risk of contracting EVD (which was approximately 21 to 32 times higher among health workers compared with non-health worker adults), and approximately two-thirds of those who were infected died (World Health Organization 2015). In Sierra Leone, this resulted in 221 health worker deaths, a staggering 21% of the country's health workforce (Raven *et al.* 2018). Across all three countries, nurses were especially hard hit: nursing staff accounted for 52% of all health worker infections, though cases were also reported among medical doctors, midwives, ambulance workers, laboratory staff, pharmacists and community health workers (World Health Organization 2015).

Sadly, Ebola also took a toll on other aspects of the health systems, including maternal and newborn care. In Sierra Leone, there was an estimated 22% decrease in coverage of antenatal care for pregnant women; this decreased utilization occurred in part because pregnant women were especially vulnerable to being denied care during the epidemic, since providers were concerned about risk of contamination from women with unknown Ebola status (Sochas *et al.* 2017). An estimated indirect mortality burden of 3600 maternal, neonatal and stillbirth deaths in 2014–2015 in Sierra Leone occurred as a result of the decrease in usage of life-saving maternal and neonatal health services (Sochas *et al.* 2017). Furthermore, some modeled estimates have suggested that the loss of doctors, nurses and midwives who were killed by Ebola could lead to an additional 4022 women dying in childbirth each year in Guinea, Liberia and Sierra Leone (Evans et al. 2015). For countries which already had some of the highest maternal death rates in the world, this was a major setback.

In the wake of the Ebola outbreak, one attribute of the health system that has been recognized as critical is "health system resilience", defined as "the capacity of health actors, institutions, and populations to prepare for and effectively respond to crises; maintain core functions when a crisis hits; and, informed by lessons learned during the crisis, reorganise if conditions require it" (Kruk et al. 2015). Utilizing this framework, it is clear that the health systems of these West African nations lacked key elements related to resilience including availability of global emergency funding which could rapidly be disbursed, a legal and policy foundation including implementation of International Health Regulations, and an adequate heath workforce including well-trained doctors, nurses, managers and community health workers (Kruk et al. 2015). Further analysis has made clear that health systems must plan for resilience long before the event of an outbreak, environmental disaster or other "health system shock".

Unfortunately, the Ebola outbreak has been the source of many missed opportunities for improvements in health systems. While short-term health system improvements were made during and in the immediate aftermath of the outbreak, including building temporary infrastructure, introducing surveillance teams and training health workers on infection control, the "slow variables of resilience" such as strengthening permanent health system infrastructure and developing human resources were largely underfunded (Ling et al. 2017). According to the government of Liberia, at the end of the outbreak there remained a US$ 700 million gap in requested versus committed funds to adequately implement Liberia's Strategic Plan for longer-term investments in health workforce and infrastructure (Government of Liberia 2015). Post-Ebola efforts to build health systems have faced challenges because the end of the outbreak coincided with a period of austerity from major donors including the governments of the United Kingdom (after the Brexit vote) and the United States (following the election of Donald Trump); additionally, funds available for global epidemics were diverted for the 2015–2016 Zika virus epidemic in the Americas.

In general, the focus on short-term improvements rather than long-term resilience has come as a result of focusing on global- and national-level priorities over local ones. A qualitative analysis of health system resilience during the outbreak in Liberia showed that global and national priorities with respect to resilience (for example surveillance and coordination) were given precedence over local-level priorities (for example improving health service delivery and breadth of health services) (Ling et al. 2017). In fact, control of the Ebola epidemic may have been impacted more by local measures rather than global ones: an analysis of situation reports in Liberia showed that the epidemic was already starting to decline prior to the introduction of global measures to control Ebola, and that the epidemic curve actually started falling when the primary measures being implemented were local ones, including deploying safe burial teams and involving local leadership to engender behavior change, rather than later on after the introduction of additional treatment-center beds (Kirsch et al. 2017). Involving local stakeholders in decision-making processes not only improves equity but can also lead to more favorable outcomes in ensuring resilience and controlling epidemics.

In August 2018, another epidemic of EVD was reported in the northern Kivu region of Democratic Republic of Congo (DRC), the second outbreak in DRC of the year, this time in a conflict-affected and difficult to access region. As of 17 September 2018, there have been 97 confirmed deaths (World Health Organization 2018a). This time, the DRC Ministry of Health, WHO and the extended international community have been faster to respond, and a vaccine developed in the 2014–2016 West African outbreak is being deployed. It remains to be seen if lessons learned from the 2014–2016 outbreak will lead to a more coordinated response and a faster end to the outbreak.

References

Centers for Disease Control and Prevention, 2014–2016. Ebola Outbreak in West Africa. Retrieved from www.cdc.gov/vhf/ebola/history/2014-2016-outbreak/index.html.

Desai, A., 2010. Sierra Leone's long recovery from the scars of war. *Bulletin of the World Health Organization*, 88(10), 725–726. doi:10.2471/BLT.10.031010.

Evans, D.K., Goldstein, M., Popova, A., 2015. Health-care worker mortality and the legacy of the Ebola epidemic. *The Lancet Global Health*, 3(8), e439–e440. doi:10.1016/s2214-109x(15)00065-0.

Government of Liberia, 2015. Investment plan for building a resilient health system in Liberia. Retrieved from https://au.int/sites/default/files/newsevents/workingdocuments/27027-wd-liberia-_investment_plan_for_building_a_resilient_health_system.pdf.

Kirsch, T.D., Moseson, H., Massaquoi, M., Nyenswah, T.G., Goodermote, R., Rodriguez-Barraquer, I., ... Peters, D.H., 2017. Impact of interventions and the incidence of ebola virus disease in Liberia – implications for future epidemics. *Health Policy and Planning*, 32(2), 205–214. doi:10.1093/heapol/czw113.

Kruk, M.E., Rockers, P.C., Williams, E.H., Varpilah, S.T., Macauley, R., Saydee, G., Galea, S., 2010. Availability of essential health services in post-conflict Liberia. *Bulletin of the World Health Organization*, 88(7), 527–534. doi:10.2471/BLT.09.071068

Kruk, M.E., Myers, M., Varpilah, S.T., Dahn, B.T., 2015. What is a resilient health system? Lessons from Ebola. *The Lancet*, 385(9980), 1910–1912. doi:10.1016/s0140-6736(15)60755-3.

Ling, E.J., Larson, E., Macauley, R J., Kodl, Y., VanDeBogert, B., Baawo, S., Kruk, M.E., 2017. Beyond the crisis: did the Ebola epidemic improve resilience of Liberia's health system? *Health Policy and Planning*, 32(suppl.3), iii40–iii47. doi:10.1093/heapol/czx109.

Moon, S., Sridhar, D., Pate, M.A., Jha, A.K., Clinton, C., Delaunay, S., ... Piot, P., 2015. Will Ebola change the game? Ten essential reforms before the next pandemic. The report of the Harvard-LSHTM Independent Panel on the Global Response to Ebola. *The Lancet*, 386(10009), 2204–2221. doi:10.1016/s0140-6736(15)00946-0.

Otu, A., Ameh, S., Osifo-Dawodu, E., Alade, E., Ekuri, S., Idris, J., 2017. An account of the Ebola virus disease outbreak in Nigeria: implications and lessons learnt. *BMC Public Health*, 18(1), 3. doi:10.1186/s12889-017-4535-x.

Raven, J., Wurie, H., Witter, S., 2018. Health workers' experiences of coping with the Ebola epidemic in Sierra Leone's health system: a qualitative study. *BMC Health Serv Res*, 18(1), 251. doi:10.1186/s12913-018-3072-3.

Sochas, L., Channon, A.A., Nam, S., 2017. Counting indirect crisis-related deaths in the context of a low-resilience health system: the case of maternal and neonatal health during the Ebola epidemic in Sierra Leone. *Health Policy and Planning*, 32(suppl.3), iii32–iii39. doi:10.1093/heapol/czx108.

World Health Organization, 2015. Health worker Ebola infections in Guinea, Liberia and Sierra Leone. Retrieved from: http://apps.who.int/iris/bitstream/handle/10665/171823/?sequence=1.

World Health Organization, 2016. Ebola data and statistics – Data from National situation reports. 11 May 2016. Retrieved from: http://apps.who.int/gho/data/view.ebola-sitrep.ebola-summary-20160511?lang=en.

World Health Organization, 2018a. Ebola situation reports: Democratic Republic of the Congo. Retrieved from: www.who.int/ebola/situation-reports/drc-2018/en/.

World Health Organization, 2018b. Global Health Observatory data. Retrieved from www.who.int/gho/health_workforce/en/.

Lack of adequate healthcare services or access pushes those who can afford it to seek services abroad. "Medical tourism" is sometimes seen as an opportunity for economic returns in the recipient countries that could benefit their national health system. However many authors agree that for those countries health tourism is a source of increased inequalities, possible cost increases and a further factor in the migration of human resources from the public to the private sector, without considering the risks (related to travel, medical-surgical intervention, the course and post-operative care) for patient-tourists (Hopkins *et al.* 2010).

Health system governance and national leadership may be hampered by global market forces and trade agreements, as well as by policies supported by international or supranational institutions. Policies and approaches defined at the global level also heavily influence the way healthcare systems are financed and organized. Finally, the generation and availability of resources (health workforce, funding, medicines, technology, etc.) are all strictly linked to global determinants. In addition, Development Assistance for Health (DAH) (see Chapter 13) plays a major role in poorer countries. All these factors must be taken into consideration when debating the sustainability of healthcare systems and their strengthening (Figure 12.3).

Acceptability: Third, to be sustainable, health systems should be accepted by all the stakeholders that contribute to them. Citizens are active components of health systems and contribute to co-create health through their behavior, lifestyle and eating and drinking habits, and eventually finance health systems either through taxation, purchasing health insurance or services paid directly out-of-pocket. The anti-vaccine movement is a good example of how lack of trust in the health system can have detrimental effects on population health. Healthcare provider behavior and efforts are also crucial to the sustainability of health systems. They need to share the mission of the health system they serve, for instance to promote appropriate use of health services and to contain costs through evidence-based prescriptions and cost-conscious behavior.

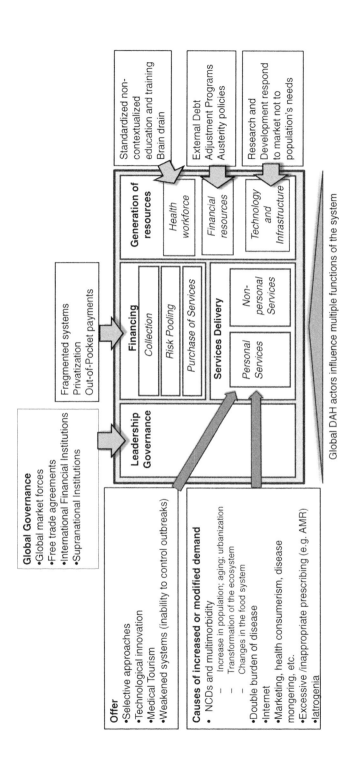

Figure 12.3 Global determinants of health system sustainability.

258 *Global policies and issues*

They also need to be happy to work for public health systems, which is often not the case in low-resource settings where health workers' salaries are low. Additionally, the industrial complex of the health sector – including pharmaceutical and biomedical companies and other health technologies manufacturers – should be engaged in the health systems serving them and respecting their objectives and not only their desire to maximize profits or reward shareholders. Regulation, inclusive governance practices and shared values are therefore important determinants of health system sustainability.

12.3.1 The epidemiological transition and the challenge of noncommunicable diseases (NCDs)

The demographic transition in many countries led to an increase in the burden of non-communicable diseases (NCDs). The steady increase in the world's population and its progressive aging are among the main causes of the increased health demand linked to NCDs. Between 2015 and 2050, the proportion of the world's population over 60 years of age will almost double, from 12% to 22%.[6]

The share of the overall burden of disease attributable to NCDs in lower-income countries has increased dramatically over the last 15 years. In 2015, NCDs accounted for over half of the total burden of disease in LMICs, and nearly one-third in low-income countries. NCDs killed 15 million people in developing countries in 2015 – 3.8 million more than in 2000 – with a corresponding increase of 28% in the burden of disease (IHME 2015).

NCDs not only require more complex healthcare services and more coordination between healthcare providers and between health and social services, but they also have a high social burden. Indeed, NCDs tend to affect people living in low-income countries at a younger age than in wealthier economies, and thus the economic impact is substantially larger. It is estimated that of all the people who die from NCDs in LMICs, 50% are under the age of 70 and 25% are younger than 60 (Nugent and Feigl 2010).[7]

Even those countries that have most successfully managed to reduce the burden of NCDs still face an absolute increase in terms of the actual impact on the health system, economy and wider society, due to the rise of the population over time and the limited capacity of the healthcare system to deal with a growing number of people diagnosed with NCDs. For instance, the fight against cancer requires a delivery system that is planned and designed to tackle and treat the conditions in due time, across different levels of care from prevention to end of life care, guaranteeing access to technologies and treatments.[8]

Although partly dependent on genetic factors, the state of health of elderly people is influenced by social, economic and environmental determinants, including the quality of food, housing conditions, family and community networks and previous experiences from early childhood. In this sense, the social determinants that affect young people today will influence the type and frequency of diseases in the coming decades. The health of the elderly is mainly characterized by geriatric syndromes, i.e. complex conditions of multimorbidity that lead to a greater demand for health care which is then not necessarily of the same quality as the traditional supply.

Aging of the population alone, however, does not explain the increased burden from NCDs. Other equally important factors include atmospheric, soil and water pollution, and social factors such as urbanization, the use of the internet and social networks, market strategies and other lifestyle factors (such as changes in diet and consumption patterns), some of which have been discussed in depth in Chapter 11.

For some chronic conditions, urban environmental factors play a major role. For example, the urban lifestyle increases the risk of diabetes by 21% (IDF 2017). In addition, in many LMICs, urban environmental factors are detrimental to a healthy lifestyle, notably the combination of increasingly sedentary jobs, the use of motorized transport to commute, and the rising popularity of fast food or street food, which is comparatively much cheaper than pursuing a heathy diet. The increase in the incidence of cancer in childhood provides further evidence of societal determinants of NCDs that go well beyond aging and are often transgenerational.

Health systems of many LMICs are largely unable to face the challenge of the growing burden of NCDs.

The WHO's 2015 Global Survey on National Capacity for the Prevention and Control of NCDs showed that while progress had certainly been made with respect to the number of low-income and lower-middle-income countries that reported having operational NCD plans or strategies, there were serious shortfalls with respect to the quality of these plans. In the WHO Africa region, less than half of the reporting countries had an operational, multisectoral, integrated NCD policy, strategy or action plan. Similarly, less than 40% of low-income countries and less than 45% of lower-middle-income countries had population-based cancer registries. Monitoring of diabetes was even less advanced: less than 20% of low-income countries had diabetes registries of any kind (WHO 2016).

SDG3 target (3.4) aims to reduce premature deaths due to NCDs by one-third by 2030 through prevention and treatment and the promotion of mental health and well-being.[9]

In order to tackle NCDs, health systems and healthcare services must rethink the magnitude, scope and modalities of their actions. Strengthening of national healthcare systems is needed. However, actions cannot happen in isolation from public policies in other sectors where the health goal should be prioritized.

Primary prevention through environmental policies, urban planning, regulation, taxation and public awareness programs could go a long way towards addressing many of these issues, with a functional health system able to promote trans-sectoral policies *for* health. The solution requires a wider approach to health and its determinants, and health system strengthening is central to respond to those global health challenges and to attain the specific goal of UHC (Topp and Sheikh 2018; Vega 2010; WHO 2014). Such an endeavor imposes new thinking and approaches, even in high-income countries.

12.4 System approaches to address contemporary global health complexity

As discussed in this book, global health is facing new challenges due to a broad array of contemporary emergent phenomena.

The financial and economic crisis that started in 2008 is changing the landscape for global health financing and further challenging national health system development, exacerbating already existing trends of fragmentation and short-term strategies. Global and national health policy-makers are experimenting with health policy and system reforms, ranging from global subsidies for essential medicines, public-private partnerships, changes to provider payment mechanisms, demand-side incentives such as conditional cash transfers, supply-side incentives such as pay-for-performance and cash-on-delivery, and new service delivery and social protection mechanisms. In this context, strengthening national health systems is fundamental to improving population health and to addressing widening health disparities, social injustice and insecurity.

260 *Global policies and issues*

In 2009, the WHO Alliance for Health Policy and Systems Research published a seminal report on System Thinking for Health Systems Strengthening (de Savigny and Adams 2009), demonstrating the need to go beyond conventional approaches to better design and assess health system interventions. The systems thinking approach is aimed at replacing the traditional linear logic of technical determinism, allowing more realistic evaluation through heuristic generalization (i.e. to achieve a clearer understanding of what is happening, what works and for whom) that can respond more appropriately to policy-makers' needs and allow them to take better account of context, system behavior and outcome effects.

Systems thinking demands a deeper understanding of the linkages, relationships, interactions and behaviors among the elements that characterize the entire system. With respect to health systems, it works to reveal the underlying characteristics and relationships of the key functions of health systems such as financing systems, human resources, information flow, service delivery and, across all these, governance and leadership. It also helps to predict and mitigate possible unintended consequences of particular actions and to exploit synergies from concerted action in the system. Yet, systems thinking approaches have been rarely applied to health systems.

Contemporary global health trends require approaches able to tackle complex challenges including a fragmented global health governance, the relevance of social determinants of health, the need for a continuum between health and social care to tackle chronic diseases and aging, the competence of health care and health professionals, and the public-private mixed nature of health systems.

12.4.1 *A fragmented global health governance*

The current global health architecture is far more complex than it once was. The increase in volume of global health financing of the last decade (Institute for Health Metrics and Evaluation 2012) has been accompanied by a proliferation of global initiatives, new actors and new modalities that have progressively rendered governance mechanisms and corresponding management structures more complex (see section 2 and Chapter 13).

Global policy making is no longer made only by national governments of rich countries and a few international organizations such as the World Health Organization (WHO). There are now multiple relevant players, including emerging donors such as foundations, financing mechanisms and transnational hybrid organizations (THO) such as the GFATM and GAVI, large global public-private health initiatives, often competing with pre-existing vertical disease control programs. In addition, newly emerging economies (NEEs) such as Brazil, Russia, India and China (the so-called BRICS), and also Mexico and South Africa, are increasingly relevant and present new opportunities and challenges for global health.

The acceleration of the globalization process requires more coordination and global regulation to manage the increase in international transfer of risks. As discussed in previous chapters, this applies not only to the spread of infectious diseases but also to lifestyles impacting health and non-health consumption. Examples of the challenges that health systems face include the increased mobility of patients and health workers, which affects national regulations, and the intensive transnational trade of health products and services both through traditional channels and via the internet.

12.4.2 Social determinants of health, demographic and epidemiological transitions

In the last decades further evidence has shown the importance of how distal social determinants of health influence societal structure and allocation of resources and power, which can in turn affect not only overall health outcomes but most importantly how health is distributed across population groups (CSDH 2008). This calls for broader approaches to protect health, for the health sector to coordinate with other sectors affecting health to guide public policy, including economic, production and environmental, housing, labor, and more generally social protection policies.

There is therefore a need for institutions that are capable of developing and implementing general public policies which improve health and coordinating multisectoral efforts. In many countries, Ministries of Health are weak and do not collaborate with other ministries, so they are not able to exercise a leadership role promoting broad approaches to support health. In addition, in modern societies the distinction between health and well-being is shrinking. This is putting more pressure on health systems to respond to citizens' increasing expectations of what the health system can provide for them.

The above-discussed demographic and epidemiological transitions, with the increase in the burden of disease accounted for by noncommunicable chronic conditions, places additional pressure on health systems. Among the implications of this change is the need for more integration between primary and secondary care, between health and social care, and between curative and preventive care. It has been shown that the achievement of a good level of integration between different care settings can lead to improvements in the quality of care and patient satisfaction as well as in the efficiency of the overall system through a reduction of the number of inappropriate and costly hospital admissions (Heard and Alexander 2013; Olden and Hoffman 2011).

In that sense, it is also essential to promote, as far as possible, the active social integration of disabled and elderly people. Extended families, communities of life and sharing of living spaces (co-housing) offer opportunities to re-evaluate intergenerational experiences of solidarity assistance, alternatives to hospitalization and institutionalization of people with reduced autonomy (Missoni 2015, 2018).

A people-centered approach to health implies a link between care provided at family or community level and the rest of the healthcare system. Approaches such as the Chronic Care Model (CCM) respond to this need, aiming precisely at ensuring the connection with community social networks (voluntary work, self-help groups, self-managed centers, etc.) and at involving the patient as an active protagonist in the care processes (Wagner et al. 2001).

The link between primary care and levels of higher complexity could also benefit from new information and communication technologies (e-health, m-health, social networks, etc.); however, unless technology and procedures are appropriate to local and national contexts and adequately regulated, they may easily increase costs and burdens on the system. In general, a systems approach to new technologies is still missing and experiences described in the literature refer almost always to pilot experiences that lack systematization (Missoni 2018). The WHO itself states that: "In order for e-health to play a full role in supporting health systems to achieve universal health coverage, a solid legal framework is needed" (WHO 2016a).

In this vein, boundaries among different levels of care have become more blurred.

Public health interventions and primary prevention are increasingly included in the realm of primary care, now taking place at different levels of healthcare systems, engaging a broader range of specialized health care and social care workforce and targeting healthy people, chronic patients and, all in all, any preventable condition causing disability.

Outpatient and ambulatory care which used to be provided at the secondary or tertiary care levels is being shifted to the primary care level; even surgery and other complex procedures can now be provided in traditional primary care centers.

To tackle chronic conditions and the aging of populations, health and social care are now being integrated at the community level, overcoming traditional boundaries between cultures, professions and indeed financing schemes to strengthen their integration.

Given the changes in the health needs, some disciplines are gaining momentum and the privileged place of their development is in primary care, to guarantee their access and integration. For instance, mental health and neurology as well as physical and functional rehabilitation or end-of-life care, a range of services which were traditionally provided by specialized professionals, are now placed at the community level and are often included in services targeted for chronic conditions.

Finally, the decreasing use of inpatient stay, with a dramatic reduction of the number of acute care beds as well as of the average length of stay, has engendered a higher degree of concentration and specialization for tertiary care services, as well as diffusion of less acute forms of inpatient stay, e.g. for intermediate care or community hospitals (Rhodes *et al.* 2014; Rittenhouse *et al.* 2009).

12.4.3 *The specialization of health care and health professionals*

Health care and health professionals are increasingly specialized. Medical education and practice is increasingly fragmented in highly specialized fields. In addition, specialized professionals are usually not inclined to participate in the multidisciplinary care teams as their specialty is not easy to integrate with other specialists. As a consequence of this compartmentalization or fragmentation, patients tend to receive the care health professionals offer, rather than the care they really need. With few exceptions, medical faculties continue to provide "information, or rather notions, detached from the context of real medicine that inevitably takes place more and more in the community, outside the hospital" (Stefanini 2014). Even the WHO in its World Health Report of 2008 denounced the "hospital-centrism" among the problems at the root of the failure to achieve the goal of health for all (WHO 2008). The doctor projected from the beginning of his studies to the examination of a "patient" in bed, "horizontal" (Missoni 2018), is formed in a context completely foreign to the social reality in which people "people are born, grow, live, work and age" (CSDH 2008). Moreover, the standardization of skills and learning objectives (specialization, high complexity, technological sophistication, etc.) is based on models that are often unsustainable even in middle-high-income countries, and elsewhere accessible only to high-income population groups, affecting the poorest countries in two major ways. On the one hand, it produces health workers who are incapable "of usefully inserting themselves into an urban or rural community, of taking care of it, of understanding its health problems and of defending its right to health" (Maccacaro 1971), with education and training that clearly contrast with local needs. On the other hand, it tends to produce a health workforce "for export". Thus, health workers and in particular doctors, unprepared and unmotivated to serve in their own communities, will seek elsewhere – first in large urban centers and then abroad – professional employment that responds to the skills and expectations prompted by their university studies, and corresponding to the globalized stereotype of the successful doctor (Missoni 2018). This "brain drain", in particular for the health workforce, is fueled by "import" agencies from high-income countries, which violate the WHO "global code of practice on the international recruitment of health personnel" (WHO 2010b).

The traditional training in public health disciplines (e.g. epidemiology) encourages us to understand determinants of health and health system behavior in linear input-output reductionist terms rather than to understand system behavior as driven by relationships among the parts of the system.

While these approaches have allowed great advances in medicine and public health, however, the expected benefits are impeded by the complexity of problems, learning failures and implementation challenges (Adam *et al.* 2012).

12.4.4 The pluralistic nature of health systems

In many countries, health systems are, in practice, pluralistic with many different public and private providers of both healthcare services and health-related goods (Lagomarsino and Nachuk 2009). This is particularly true in low-income countries, where the private sector includes many different types of service providers, from modern practitioners and certified health-care professionals to traditional healers, and from NGOs and faith-based organizations to for-profit institutions organized as individual or group practices. It also includes private providers of inputs (both physical inputs such as infrastructure, medicine and supplies as well as knowledge production inputs such as medical training institutions).

Currently, worldwide we can observe a growing share of private providers in most healthcare systems, the rise of innovative forms of contract management for commissioning services or providing therapies (i.e. shared value contracts), and the increasing search for new public-private partnership frameworks to exploit the integration of resources and competences developed as well as to outsource services for which the private market has more capacity and can operate with higher effectiveness and efficiency.

In low-income countries' health systems it is less frequent that the private sector includes financing mechanisms such as private insurance providers, community-based health insurance providers and employer-based insurance providers; however, their relevance is increasing. In many low-income countries an increased role is played by intermediate private sector actors such as NGOs or private companies, which are often used as principal recipients of the funds that are channeled into the health systems. However, national governments too often only focus on the public sector and are inexperienced in setting up or managing appropriate regulatory regimes to steer private sector behavior and performance (Sterman 2006; Lagomarsino and Nachuk 2009; Siddiqui *et al.* 2009).

Sufficient public sector capacity and the legitimacy to manage the policy-making process effectively are key to engaging the private sector in scaling up the delivery of health services (Patouillard *et al.* 2007). Because there is no single best method in this respect, the full utilization of the private sector requires a careful understanding of its potential and adequate regulatory frameworks in the specific social, economic and cultural context of each country/region (Fattore and Tediosi 2009).

How to support the development of responsive, efficient and effective health systems in LMICs remains an open issue also among global actors.

The need for systems thinking has become clearer, interest has grown in academic and research circles, and growing numbers of practical cases of its application are appearing (Adam and de Savigny 2012). However, application of these concepts at the global level is slow. Major donors are still looking for rapid impacts, and short-termism and narrow thinking still dominate global health investment decisions. An example of this is the recent experience of the Affordable Medicine Facility for malaria (AMFm), where long-term investment decisions are taken on the basis of short-term impact assessments (Tougher et al. 2012).

Both the GFATM and the GAVI have invested heavily in health system strengthening in the last decade, albeit from different approaches. However, their core investments still primarily target specific diseases or health interventions. The short-term success of disease-specific interventions has ironically revealed the inadequacies of approaches to health systems and the need to move beyond such siloed approaches which make little sense to front-line providers and policy-makers.

The need for local ownership, alignment and harmonization of donor strategies on measurable results and mutual accountability of donors and recipients has repeatedly been reaffirmed. Although sector-wide strategies have been implemented (such as IHP+) there is still a long way to go for a real common and coordinated approach among global actors of development assistance in health (DAH) (See Chapter 13).

Major advances could be achieved with more emphasis on dynamics, learning and adaptation, and on assessment of likely impacts over a longer period of time, taking into account that elements in systems are evolving continuously as are their internal and external relationships. This would help in understanding how the global changes within and outside health systems may affect population health globally, requiring more coordinated global actions for improving population health. It could also help in transforming global health governance by supporting donors to move towards more coordinated and integrated investments and modalities of partnership.

Notes

1 www.who.int/healthsystems/universal_health_coverage/en/.
2 www.who.int/sdg/targets/en/.
3 www.who.int/health_financing/strategy/dimensions/en/.
4 www.who.int/healthsystems/berlin/en/.
5 According to Frenk (2015) the creation of the Ministries of Health and the social security agencies marked the first generation of health reforms and a second generation of reforms was launched around the primary healthcare model.
6 www.who.int/en/news-room/fact- sheets/detail/ageing-and-health.
7 An important study from Barnett and colleagues (2012) based on the Scottish population, that is to say from a high-income country, proved the linkages between the early rise of morbidity and comorbidities with poverty. Out of a population of 1,751,841 individuals, 42.2% had one or more morbidities. The prevalence of multimorbidity increased substantially with age and was present in most people aged 65 years and older, but the absolute number of people with multimorbidity was higher in those younger than 65 years. Onset of multimorbidity occurred 10–15 years earlier in people living in the most deprived areas compared with the most affluent, with socioeconomic deprivation particularly associated with multimorbidity that included mental health disorders (prevalence of both physical

and mental health disorder 11% in most deprived area vs 5.9% in least deprived). Finally, the presence of a mental health disorder increased as the number of physical morbidities increased and was much greater in more deprived than in less deprived people. The work concluded with the recommendation for a complementary strategy, supporting generalist clinicians to provide comprehensive continuity of care, especially in socioeconomically deprived areas.

8 For instance, with cancer care, it has recently been demonstrated how many countries do not have the radiotherapy equipment they need to cope. In Bangladesh, for instance, where cancer accounts for 4.6% of the total burden of disease, the National Institute of Cancer Research and Hospital (NICRH) in Dhaka has only six radiotherapy machines – less than half of what it needs to accommodate current demand. And the country has only one-tenth of the number of radiotherapy centers recommended by the WHO based on its population size and burden of disease. In sub-Saharan Africa, excluding South Africa, not a single country has more than one radiotherapy machine per million people (in North America, there are ten machines per million). In the whole continent of Africa, there are 295 radiotherapy machines: excluding the 148 machines in North African countries and 82 in South Africa, that leaves 65 for the rest of the continent (Atun *et al.* 2015).

9 www.who.int/sdg/targets/en/.

References

Adam, T., de Savigny, D., 2012. Systems thinking for health systems strengthening in LMICs: seizing the opportunity. *Health Policy and Planning*, 27(Suppl. 4), 1–66.

Adam, T., *et al.*, 2012. Evaluating health systems strengthening interventions in low-income and middle-income countries: are we asking the right questions? *Health Policy Planning*, 27(Suppl. 4), iv9–19.

Barnett, K., *et al.*, 2012. Epidemiology of multimorbidity and implications for health care, research, and medical education: a cross-sectional study. *The Lancet*, 380, 37–43.

Boerma, T., *et al.*, 2014. Monitoring Progress towards universal health coverage at country and global levels. *PloS Medicine*, 11, e1001731. doi:10.1371/journal.pmed.1001731.

CSDH, 2008. *Closing the gap in a generation: health equity through action on the social determinants of health*. Final Report of the Commission on Social Determinants of Health. Geneva: World Health Organization.

De Savigny, D., Adams, T., 2009. *System Thinking for Health Systems Strengthening*. Geneva: World Health Organization, Alliance for Health Policy and Systems Research.

Fattore, G., Tediosi, F., 2009. Attaining universal health coverage: the role of governance and management. In Missoni, E. (Ed.), *Attaining Universal Health Coverage. A Research Initiative to Support Evidence-Based Advocacy and Policy-Making*. Milan: Egea, 31–51.

Franklin, P., 2017. *Sustainable Development Goal on Health (SDG3): The opportunity to make EU health a priority*. EPC Discussion Paper.

Frenk, J., 2015. Leading the way towards universal health coverage: a call to action. *The Lancet*, 385(9975), 1352–1358.

Global Burden of Disease Health Financing Collaborator Network, 2018. Trends in future health financing and coverage: future health spending and universal health coverage in 188 countries, 2016–40. *The Lancet*, 391(10132), 1783–1798.

Haider, M., Nibb, K., 2017. *Universal health coverage and environmental health: an investigation in decreasing communicable and chronic disease by including environmental health in UHC*. In Comite, U. (Ed.), *Advancement in Health Management*. Intechopen.com. 129–146. Available from: http://doi.org/10.5772/intechopen.69922.

Hearld, L.R., Alexander J.A., 2013. Patient-centered care and emergency department utilization: a path analysis of the mediating effects of care coordination and delays in care. *Medical Care Research and Review*, 69, 560–580.

Hopkins, L., Labonté, R., Runnels, V., Packer, C., 2010. Medical tourism today: what is the state of existing knowledge? *Journal of Public Health Policy*, 31(2), 185–198.

IDF, 2017. *Diabetes Atlas – Eight Edition 2017*. Brussels: International Diabetes Federation.

IHME, 2012. *Financing Global Health 2012: The End of the Golden Age?* Seattle, WA: Institute for Health Metrics and Evaluation.

IHME, 2015. Global Burden of Disease Study 2015 (GBD 2015), GBD Results Tool. Institute for Health Metrics and Evaluation. Available from: http://ghdx.healthdata.org/gbd-results-tool.

IHME, 2018. *Financing Global Health 2017: Funding Universal Health Coverage and the Unfinished HIV/AIDS Agenda*. Seattle, WA: Institute for Health Metrics and Evaluation. Available from: www.healthdata.org/sites/default/files/files/policy_report/FGH/2018/IHME_FGH_2017_fullreport_online.pdf.

Kieny, M.P., Evans, D.B., 2013. Universal health coverage. *Eastern Mediterranean Health Journal*, 19(4), 305–306.

Kieny, M.P., *et al.*, 2017. Strengthening health systems for universal health coverage and sustainable development. *Bulletin of the World Health Organization*, 95(7), 537–539.

Lagomarsino, G., Nachuk, S., 2009. *Public Stewardship in Mixed Health Systems*. Washington DC: Results for Development Institute.

Maccacaro, GA., 1971. Una facoltà di medicina capovolta. Intervista. *Tempo Medico*, November.

Missoni, E., 2015. Degrowth and health: local action should be linked to global policies and governance for health. *Sustainability Science*. doi:10.1007/s11625-015-0300-1.

Missoni, E. 2018. Determinanti globali della salute e (in)sostenibilità dell'obiettivo di copertura sanitaria universal. *Welfare e Ergonomia*, in press.

Nugent, RA., Feigl, RB., 2010. Where have all the donors gone? Scarce donor funding for non-communicable diseases. *CGD Working Paper 228*, Center for Global Development. Available from: www.cgdev.org/content/publications/detail/1424546.

OECD, 2016. Universal health coverage and health outcomes. Available from: www.oecd.org/els/health-systems/Universal-Health-Coverage-and-Health-Outcomes-OECD-G7-Health-Ministerial-2016.pdf.

OECD/DAC, 2005. *Paris Declaration on Aid effectiveness*. High-Level Forum, Paris, February 28–March 2.

Olden, P., Hoffman, K.E., 2011. Hospitals' health promotion services in their communities: Findings from a literature review. *Health Care Management Review*, 36, 104–113.

Obrist, B., *et al.*, 2007. Access to health care in contexts of livelihood insecurity: a framework for analysis and action. *PloS Medicine*, 4, e308. doi:10.1371/journal.pmed.0040308.

Patouillard, E., *et al.*, 2007. Can working with the private for-profit sector improve utilization of quality health services by the poor? A systematic review of the literature. *International Journal for Equity in Health*, 6, 17.

Rhodes, K., *et al.*, 2014. Primary care access for new patients on the eve of health care reform. *JAMA Internal Medicine*, 174(6), 861–869.

Rittenhouse, D, Shortell, S., Fisher, E., 2009. Primary care and accountable care – two essential elements of delivery-system reform. *New England Journal of Medicine,* 361(24), 2301–2304.

Siddiqui, S.T., *et al.*, 2009. Framework for assessing governance of the health system in developing countries: gateway to good governance. *Health Policy*, 90, 13–25.

Stefanini, A., 2014. "Capovolgere" la facoltà di medicina? L'eredità di Giulio A. Maccacaro. *Salute Internazionale*, 22 April. Available from: www.saluteinternazionale.info/2014/04/capovolgere-la-facolta-di-medicina-leredita-di-giulio-a-maccacaro/#biblio.

Sterman, J.D., 2006. Learning from evidence in a complex world. *American Journal of Public Health*, 96, 505–514.

Tediosi F., *et al.*, 2016. BRICS countries and the global movement for universal health coverage. *Health Policy and Planing*, 31(6), 717–728.

Tougher S., *et al.*, for the ACTwatch Group, 2012. Effect of the Affordable Medicines Facility – malaria (AMFm) on the availability, price, and market share of quality-assured artemisinin-based combination therapies in seven countries: a before-and-after analysis of outlet survey data. *The Lancet*, 380, 1916–1926.

Topp, S.M., Sheikh, K., 2018. Are we asking all the right questions about quality of care in low and middle income countries? *International Journal of Health Policy Management*, 7(10), 971–972. Available from http://ijhpm.com/article_3502_ce28ca05043391e0a0ff251aad89fe87.pdf.

UN, 2012. Resolution adopted by the General Assembly on 12 December 2012 67/81. Global health and foreign policy. Available from: www.un.org/en/ga/search/view_doc.asp?symbol=A/RES/67/81.

Vega, F.J., 2010. Universal health coverage with equity: what we know, don't know and need to know. Available from: http://healthsystemsresearch.org/hsr2010/images/stories/9coverage_with_equity.pdf.

Wagner, E.H., *et al.*, 2001. Improving chronic illness care: translating evidence into action. *Health Affairs*, 20, 64–78.

WHO, 2000. *World Health Report 2000*. Geneva: World Health Organization.

WHO, 2005. WHA58.33. Sustainable health financing, universal coverage and social health insurance. Available from: http://apps.who.int/iris/bitstream/10665/20383/1/WHA58_33-en.pdf?ua=1&ua=1&ua=1.

WHO, 2007. *Everybody's Business – Strengthening Health Systems to Improve Health Outcomes – WHO's Framework For Action*. Geneva: World Health Organization.

WHO, 2008. *World Health Report 2008. Primary Health Care, Now More Than Ever*. Geneva: World Health Organization.

WHO, 2009. *Systems Thinking for Health Systems Strengthening*. World Health Organization, Geneva.

WHO, 2010. *Key Components of a Well Functioning Health System*. Geneva: World Health Organization. Available from: www.who.int/entity/healthsystems/EN_HSSkeycomponents.pdf?ua=1.

WHO, 2010a. *Health systems Financing: The Path to Universal Coverage*. Geneva: World Health Organization.

WHO, 2010b. The WHO global code of practice on the international recruitment of health personnel. www.who.int/hrh/migration/code/code_en.pdf.

WHO, 2011. WHA58.33 Sustainable health financing, universal coverage and social health insurance. Available from: http://apps.who.int/iris/bitstream/handle/10665/20383/WHA58_33-en.pdf?sequence=1.

WHO, 2014. *Making Fair Choices on the Path to Universal Health Coverage. Final Report of the WHO Consultative Group on Equity and Universal Health Coverage*. Geneva: World Health Organization.

WHO, 2016. Assessing national capacity for the prevention and control of noncommunicable diseases: report of the 2015 global survey. Available from: http://apps.who.int/iris/handle/10665/246223.

WHO, 2016a. *Global Diffusion of eHealth: Making Universal Health Coverage Achievable. Report of the Third Global Survey on eHealth*. Geneva: World Health Organization.

Wickramasinghe, N., *et al.* 2008. *Encyclopedia of Healthcare Information Systems*, Vol. 3. Medical Information Science Reference.

World Bank, 2017. *Tracking universal health coverage: 2017 global monitoring report*. Washington DC: World Bank Group.

Unless otherwise indicated, all websites were accessed on 9 August 2018.

13 Global health financing and Development Assistance for Health

13.1 Introduction

Independently from the debate about the definition of development and the best way to measure progress in development (see Chapters 2 and 4), international cooperation with less advanced and poorer countries has been an important component of foreign policies of most advanced, although diversely defined and organized, OECD countries. Specifically, nations which form the Development Assistance Committee (DAC) have shared the idea of "Development Assistance" or "Development Aid" as an instrument to promote the economic growth of "developing" countries and their integration in the market economy, "with recipients in a hierarchical relationship of dependence on donors" (Moon and Omole 2017).

At least at the beginning, OECD policies were intended to oppose analogous international cooperation policies of the Soviet Union aiming to affiliate countries that were becoming independent to the socialist family, in the name of socialist internationalism (Missoni 2017). Although the development debate in the UN was more inclusive, investment and technical cooperation programs of the main multilateral development actors, such as the UN Funds and Programs, the World Bank and other specialized agencies of the UN, were mainly influenced by Western (i.e. market economy) countries, which have always been their largest contributors.

With the dissolution of the Soviet Union and the socialist block, in the early 1990s the "development agenda" became a globally shared agenda, and a sequence of Summits eventually led to the adoption of the Millennium Development Goals in 2000 and of the Agenda 2030 with its 17 Sustainable Development Goals in 2015 (see Chapters 2 and 4).

Over the same period an alternative conceptual framing of DAH emerged,

> including 'cooperation' which implies a more equal relationship based on the principle of mutual benefit; 'national security', based on the argument that infectious diseases or other health threats arising in a foreign country may spread back to the donors' country unless managed at the source; 'global public goods', which emphasizes the responsibility of all states to contribute to the shared benefit of health; 'health diplomacy', which can include the use of DAH to achieve a donor's other foreign policy goals; 'investment', eyeing future commercial relationships to be built between a donor and recipient country; 'restitution', which emphasizes obligations to remedy past and/or ongoing wrongs; 'global solidarity', based on the notion of the emergence of a global society bound together by relationships of interdependence.
>
> (Moon and Omole 2017)

The number and typology of actors also changed substantially. Emerging economies joined the donor's club, starting their own development cooperation programs, often in a horizontal "South-South" fashion or collaborating with traditional donors in "triangular" cooperation. Some of those countries also joined the OECD-DAC group (e.g. South Korea) or are now aiming to become members (e.g. Turkey, Chile, Mexico); others take a clear distance from it (e.g. China)[1] or aim at newly creating, or consolidating,[2] more horizontal approaches with their partners (e.g. Brazil, India, Venezuela, Cuba, Argentina, South Africa, Egypt, Malesia, Thailand) (Rowlands 2010). Besides new donor countries, new actors – both non-profit and for-profit – emerged in the private sector or grew in their capacity to influence the agenda. Finally, global public-private partnerships and new financial mechanisms leveraging financial markets to support development strategies increasingly contributed to modify the development assistance architecture (see Section 2).

Indeed, development cooperation – not exclusively in the health sector – is among the "transnational health determinants and solutions" impacting health and health systems at national and local level, and is thus an important component of what we have defined as Global Health (see Chapter 1).

In this chapter we specifically analyze Development Assistance in Health (DAH) and other mechanisms of global health financing, in terms of both financial flows and ways of operating. DAH includes both Official Development Assistance (ODA), i.e. aid from governmental sources,[3] and financial and technical assistance from non-state actors (NSA).

An important challenge to any quantitative evaluation of health aid is the lack of agreement on what exactly counts as health aid. For quantitative analysis, we refer mainly to the Institute for Health Metrics and Evaluation (IHME) yearly reports. Accordingly, we refer to DAH as all financial and in-kind contributions from global sources and channels with the primary purpose of maintaining or improving health in low-middle-income countries (according to the World Bank classification), and specifically for the health sector, and not for all sectors that influence health, thus excluding assistance to "allied sectors like water and sanitation as well as humanitarian aid" (IHME 2009: 15; IHME 2018).

In addition, due to lack of information and reporting, aid flows analyzed by IHME do not include health aid from non-OECD countries such as Brazil, China, India and South Africa, nor data on South-South cooperation. Only data related to DAH from the United Arab Emirates are currently captured by the IHME database (IHME 2018; Bendavid *et al.* 2018).

DAH flows from sources to implementers are very complex. In a simplified way, three levels can be identified: (a) sources of funding, (b) channels that transfer funds and (c) implementing organizations that use the funds to finance health programs (Figure 13.1).

Sources include aid budgets of national (and subnational) governments, which are also fed by debt repayments from previous development assistance loans, and private sources including citizens, philanthropic organizations and companies making corporate donations.

Multiple organizations such as the EU, multilateral institutions and global public-private partnerships (GPPPs) act as channels of assistance that receive funds from multiple public and private sources and pass them onto implementing institutions in recipient countries. In many cases, sources of funding also act as channels of their own

270 *Global policies and issues*

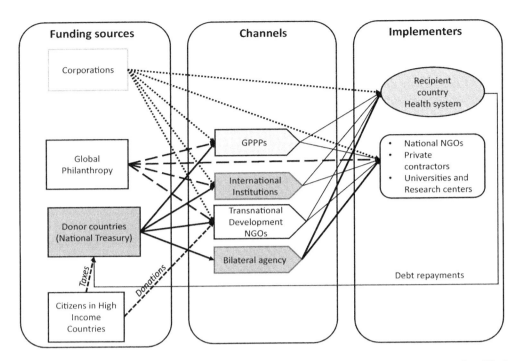

Figure 13.1 DAH sources, channels, implementing organizations and flows (a simplified representation).

funding and sometimes even implement part of those resources directly in recipient countries. This is the case for most donor countries (bilateral donors) whose funds are channeled through their development cooperation agencies, and often implemented in recipient countries through direct technical assistance (consultants, local contracts, etc.).

However, implementing actors in recipient countries are mostly national and local institutions (e.g. health authorities, municipalities, etc.), as well as other public (e.g. universities, research and training centers, etc.) and private organizations (e.g. NGOs and grassroots organizations, local consultancies, etc.) that execute health programs.

Globally, though essential for many countries, DAH represents only a tiny part of total health spending. In most recipient countries, DAH accounts for only a small part of the total health spending, which consists of the sum of government health spending, prepaid private health spending, out-of-pocket health spending and DAH (IHME 2018).

Between 1996 and 2015, total health spending grew considerably worldwide, at an annualized rate of 3.1%, with growth being largest in upper-middle-income countries (5.4% per capita) and lower-middle-income countries (4.2% per capita), reaching US$ 9.7 trillion in 2015. The largest part of the spending occurred in high-income countries (50% of the total spending in only six countries), whereas only 0.7% of it was spent in low-income countries. Of worldwide health spending, 59.7% was financed through public sources, 22.3% was spent out-of-pocket, 17.6% was financed through private insurance and 0.5% was financed through DAH, which in 2017 amounted to $37.4 billion (Dieleman *et al.* 2018; IHME 2018).

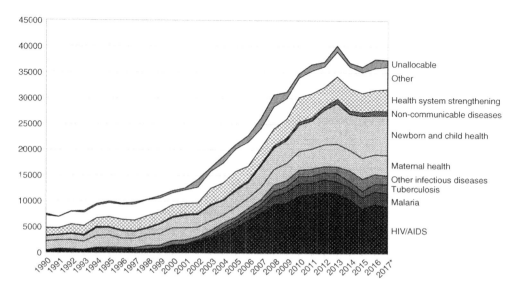

Figure 13.2 Development Assistance for Health 1990–2017 (US$ millions).
Source: authors' elaboration on IHME (2018) data.

Between 1990 and 2017, development assistance for health increased by 394.7%. In 2017, one-quarter of the estimated $37.4 billion of development assistance being disbursed for health was targeted for HIV/AIDS (Dieleman *et al.* 2018) (Figure 13.2).

Low-income countries rely heavily on DAH. In at least 15 low-income countries DAH represents more than 30% of total health expenditure, and in four countries it represents more than 50%. Middle-income countries which are highly dependent on DAH are mostly small states (WHO 2017).

To provide financing for global health in addition to traditional DAH, following the International Conference on Financing for Development in Monterrey, Mexico, in 2002, a Taskforce on Innovative International Financing for Health Systems was established. Global Innovative Financing *Instruments* (GIFIs) – i.e. financing schemes that generate and mobilize funds, normally based on market mechanisms – have contributed to increasing the availability of resources for health-related products (medicines and vaccines) that have been pooled or channeled by GPPPs (see Chapter 9). Some of these schemes have also been referred to as innovative financing *mechanisms* (such as the Global Fund to Fight AIDS, Tuberculosis and Malaria [GFATM] and GAVI) for the novelty they have introduced in pooling and using resources beyond traditional ODA (Atun *et al.* 2017).

BOX 13.1 Sources of DAH data

Development Assistance for Health (DAH):
  Financial and in-kind resources that are transferred through major health development agencies (such as UNICEF, the United Kingdom's Department for International Development, or the Bill & Melinda Gates Foundation) to low- and

middle-income countries with the primary purpose of maintaining or improving health.

Analyzing DAH is challenging due to the lack of a systematic system for tracking it.

OECD-DAC: The main source of data is the OECD-DAC database. It is compiled from information provided by each donor, guided by a set of consistent reporting objectives. It consists of two only databases. One database lists aggregate commitments and disbursements figures. The other contains details regarding projects for all OECD-DAC donors. www.oecd.org/dac/stats/.

AidData: Some information on non-OECD countries DAH is available from the AidData database PLAID (Project Level Aid). www.aiddata.org/.

Institute for Health Metrics and Evaluation (IHME) Development Assistance for Health Database 1990–2017: The IHME maintains a database on DAH and regularly publishes a Financing Global Health report. The DAH Database includes "estimates for 1990–2017, which are based on project databases, financial statements, annual reports, IRS 990s, and correspondence with agencies. The DAH Database enables comprehensive analysis of trends in international disbursements of grants and loans for health projects in low- and middle-income countries from key agencies. The data are disaggregated by source of funds, channel of funding, country and geographic region, health focus areas, and program areas". http://ghdx.healthdata.org/record/development-assistance-health-database-1990-2017.

13.2 Development Assistance for Health and global financing instruments

In this section we describe the main global health actors; some of them are important financial sources of DAH, others act mainly as channels of those resources. In addition, most of them are at least in part also implementers.

ODA from high-income countries is still the most important source of DAH. There are two main measures of ODA: ODA as a percentage of GNI, and absolute ODA, normally reported in millions of US$ at fixed prices. The 'weight' of a donor on the global DAH scene is mainly related to the absolute amounts of money spent on DAH. This measure, however, gives no information about the quality and specifically the effectiveness of the aid in terms of its contribution to health outcomes. The effectiveness of DAH is difficult to measure, and is related to how the aid is channeled and implemented.

The resources for ODA, i.e. the donor country "aid budget", are provided by national (and subnational) treasuries and collected through taxes, royalties on natural resources, lotteries, etc., but also reflows (payment of debt service) from previous loans conceded to recipient countries. Debt forgiveness is also recorded as ODA but does not correspond to new financial flows; however, in some cases, debt is not forgiven right away but renegotiated into the indebted country's commitment to invest the owed amounts in local development programs (e.g. poverty reduction programs, health programs, etc.).

ODA can be transferred to partner countries along the *bilateral* channel, and be either directly (e.g. through general budget support [GBS] or sector-wide approach programs [SWAps]) or indirectly (through governmental or non-governmental agents) spent in the recipient country. It can also be transferred using the *multilateral* channel, through financial contributions – both "core" and "non-core" – to supranational (e.g.

the European Union) and international institutions (see Chapter 6) and GPPPs (see Chapter 9).

ODA provided through the bilateral channel is negotiated bilaterally between the donor and the recipient country and may use multiple development assistance instruments, such as technical cooperation,[4] projects, programs, humanitarian interventions, and the above-mentioned actions on debt, and may involve a great variety of implementers in both the donor and the recipient country (public entities, NGOs, universities, companies, etc.). Financing may be through *grants* or *loans*. In order to be recorded as ODA, loans must be concessional in character with "a grant element of at least 25 per cent".[5]

Multilateral aid is negotiated between the recipient country and the international institution. In addition, *multi-bilateral* ODA refers to voluntary contributions provided by donor countries to a multilateral institution earmarked by the donor for specific purposes normally agreed upon with the recipient country (World Bank 2008).

Other sources of DAH include global philanthropies, corporate donations, funds raised from the general public by NGOs and other charitable actors in development. These resources also may be directly or indirectly (financing local implementers) spent in recipient countries, or channeled through international institutions, GPPPs, transnational non-state actors (NSAs) (see Chapter 8) and others.

National and local implementers of DAH in recipient countries include the national and local health authorities, and a great variety of other public and private organizations. The increasing number and diversity of channels and implementers has led to a highly crowded aid scene, at both the global and country level, with challenges that we discuss below.

The latest IHME report on Global Health Financing trends (IHME 2018) shows the dramatic increase in DAH over the last three decades and the changing relevance of sources and of institutions channeling DAH. The data indicate some important trends that are worth highlighting.

Regarding the sources of DAH:

> In 2017, the US, UK, and Germany provided $12.4, $3.3, and $2.0 billion, respectively, to development assistance for health. These figures represented 0.06%, 0.10%, and 0.05% of these countries' GDP, respectively. Other nations, though contributing smaller dollar figures, stood out as providing substantial assistance as a fraction of GDP. The UK and Luxembourg devoted the highest fractions of their GDP to DAH, dedicating 0.103% and 0.102%, respectively. By this metric, the US was the sixth most generous contributor. […]. Since 2010, Germany, France, South Korea, and the UK have contributed an increasing amount of DAH as a share of GDP. Countries decreasing DAH as a share of GDP since 2010 include Australia, Canada, Norway, and the US.
>
> (IHME 2018)

Regarding channels that transfer funds:

> While bilateral development agencies disburse a majority of DAH (34.0% between 1990 and 2017), a great deal of DAH was also disbursed by multilateral development agencies. The World Bank and WHO disbursed $1.6 and $2.3 billion, respectively, and the public-private partnerships, the Global Fund to Fight AIDS, Tuberculosis and Malaria and Gavi The Vaccine Alliance, disbursed $4.6 and $1.5

billion, respectively. Notable growth in the last decade is seen in the Global Fund and Gavi, up 32.8% since 2010, and NGOs and private foundations, up 10.5% since 2010. The very high growth rate from 2000 to 2010 for DAH, especially for financing from Gavi and the Global Fund, is associated with the MDGs and the founding of these two partnership programs.

(IHME 2018)

Regarding the geographical distribution of DAH and health focus areas:

> Across regions, sub-Saharan African countries were the recipients of 32.9% of 2016 DAH funds, while 5.0% flowed to South Asia. [...]
> Across health focus areas targeted in 2017 the distribution of DAH was: 31.0% to maternal, newborn, and child health, 24.2% to HIV/AIDS, 11.3% to health systems strengthening/SWAps, 7.1% to malaria, 4.6% to tuberculosis, 4.5% to other infectious diseases, 2.2% to non-communicable diseases, and 11.6% to other health focus areas.

(IHME 2018)

13.2.1 Global Innovative Financing Instruments (GIFIs)

In a recent analysis Atun *et al.* (2017) identified ten GIFIs in the health sector responding to criteria such as funding from new sources and not from traditional donor financing: the Advanced Market Commitments Pilot for Pneumococcal Disease (AMC), the Affordable Medicines Facility for Malaria (AMFm), the Airline Solidarity Levy (Airline Levy), the Children's Investment Fund Management which financed the Children's Investment Fund Foundation (CIFF), Debt2Health, the GAVI Matching Fund, the International Finance Facility for Immunisation (IFFIm), the Japan International Cooperation Agency ODA Loan Conversion Program for Polio (ODA Loan Conversion), Product(RED) and the World Bank Investment Partnership for Polio International Development Assistance Buy-Back Program (IDA Buy-Back).

All the ten GIFIs operate along one or more stages of the value chain, i.e resource mobilization, pooling, channeling, allocation and implementation. The sources of revenue vary by instrument. For example, Product(RED) and the Airline Levy generate revenue through direct contributions via retail sales; IFFIm, AMC and AMFm mobilize resources from the market, but finally associated costs are covered with contributions from governments and charitable foundations; for IDA Buy-Back and ODA Loan Conversion, the source of revenue is the portion of the loan or credit converted and available for pooling or channeling. The Children's Investment Fund Management, which manages hedge funds, is the revenue source for CIFF (see Table 13.1). Financing from IFIs is primarily channeled to GPPPs such as GAVI, the Global Fund and UNITAID, and thus primarily supports vertical programs to control communicable diseases (vaccination programs, HIV/AIDS, tuberculosis, malaria, pneumococcal disease) and only marginally funds health system strengthening.

Nevertheless, academic reviews suggest that innovative financing mechanisms such as front-loading of aid and international transactions taxes may provide an important opportunity to generate additional funds to address the rising burden of noncommunicable diseases (Meghani and Basu 2015).

Table 13.1 Global Innovative Financing Instruments (GIFIs)

Instrument	Focus area	Strategy and channel
International Finance Facility for Immunization (IFFIm) (established 2006)	Vaccines for preventable diseases; health system strengthening	Long-term donor pledges are converted to bond instruments, which are issued based per funding demand. Funds are pooled and channeled via GAVI.
Advance Market Commitments Pneumococcal Pilot (AMC) (established 2009)	Vaccines for pneumococcal disease	Long-term purchase commitments are used to encourage vaccine manufacturers to invest in needed vaccines. Payments are pre-negotiated and are subsidized by donors and recipients. GAVI serves as an intermediary by connecting donors, suppliers and recipients. The World Bank serves as the custodian for all donor payments, which are made either per a schedule or on demand. UNICEF serves as procurement intermediary for vaccines. Funds are released by the World Bank to UNICEF per GAVI's directive. WHO oversees procurement, acting as a prequalification authority.
Product(RED)™ (established 2006)	HIV/AIDS, Tuberculosis and Malaria	Product(RED)™ is marketed and licensed as a health-specific philanthropic brand. Partner companies adopt the brand on select products and a percentage of profits gained through the sale of those products ismobilized to health-specific programs. Product(RED)™ is hosted and managed by UNITAID. However, funds are pooled/channeled via the Global Fund.
Debt2Health (established 2007)	HIV/AIDS, Tuberculosis and malaria	A creditor forgoes a portion of a debt on the condition that the beneficiary invests an agreed counterpart amount on national health programs. The investment is made by contributing to the Global Fund, per a schedule established as a part of the debt swap agreement. The Global Fund mobilizes the funds for country-specific programs. The debt swap agreement is executed between the creditor and the beneficiary. All counter payments are made to the World Bank and are disbursed to the Global Fund for country-specific channeling.
The World Bank Investment Partnership for Polio-IDA Buy-Back Program (IDA Buy-Back) (established 2003)	Oral polio vaccines	A donor commits to pay (buy-down) principal and/or interest of an IDA credit. The buy-down is contingent on the recipient achieving predefined performance targets within implemented programs. Required funds are held in trust until program performance levels are met and principal and/or interest has been bought by the donor. The buy-down relationship exists strictly between the donor and the recipient/debtor. Funds are channeled via the Global Polio Eradication Initiative

(*continued*)

Table 13.1 (Cont.)

Instrument	Focus area	Strategy and channel
GAVI Matching Fund (established 2011)	HIV/AIDS, tuberculosis and malaria	Private sector corporate donors make funding contributions to GAVI. GAVI works with the donors to engage their customers, employees and other business partners. The cumulative funds generated by each donor are matched by the UK government (for UK partners) and by the Bill & Melinda Gates Foundation (for American partners). GAVI manages donor and partner engagement, fund generation, and subsequent pooling/channeling.
Airline Solidarity Levy (established 2006)	HIV/AIDS, tuberculosis and malaria	Participating countries implement a tax (levy) on airline tickets for flights originating from local destinations. Resulting proceeds are donated to UNITAID either as a companion to budgetary contributions or as an independent contribution. Funds are pooled and disbursed via the Global Fund to programs implemented by UNITAID partners.
Affordable Medicines Facility for Malaria (AMFm) (established 2009)	Malaria artemisinin-based combination therapies (ACTs)	Prices of ACTs are negotiated so that public/private first-line buyers pay the same reduced price. A further portion of this reduced price is paid by the host, the Global Fund. The price reduction is passed on to patients, thereby ensuring that the price of ACTs is lower or equal to competing monotherapies. Organization AMFm is hosted and managed by the Global Fund. As host, the Global Fund negotiates prices with drug manufactures for select ACTs. The Global Fund also finances the buyer co-payment by involving other donors such as UNITAID, the UK Department of International Development (DFID) etc. UNITAID also assists with market forecasting and procurement.
Japan International Cooperation Agency ODA Loan Conversion program for Polio (ODA Loan Conversion) (established 2011)	Oral polio vaccines	Loans falling under official development assistance (ODA) are repaid (bought back) based on program performance. If performance targets are met, then the loan is repaid by a donor, thereby converting the loan to a grant. The Japan International Cooperation Agency (JICA) provides the loan under ODA. The performance criteria for the recipient (debtor) are established by the donor, The Bill & Melinda Gates Foundation. If met, the loan is repaid by the donor. The loan agreement is traditional and exists between the creditor and debtor. The repayment agreement is tri-party with performance agreements between the donor and the debtor and repayment agreements between the donor and the creditor.
The Children's Investment Fund Foundation (CIFF) (established 2007	Children's health, education, nutrition, climate change and environment	Revenue is generated via income from the Children's Investment Fund Management, which manages the London-based hedge fund, Children's Investment Fund. All funds are channeled by CIFF.

Source: adapted from Atun et al. 2017.

Global health financing 277

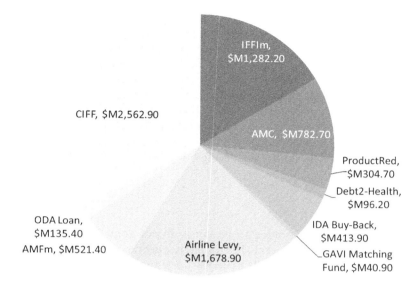

Figure 13.3 Global Innovative Financing Instruments (GIFIs): cumulative revenue by instrument (2002–2015).

Despite the hype about GIFIs, altogether the absolute amounts and the proportion of global health funding from innovative financing have been modest compared with donor assistance from traditional sources (see Figure 13.3). Besides the risk of creating excessive expectations about the yield and sustainability of innovative financing, there are risks associated with high start-up costs and high volatility in the contributions from non-bilateral donors (Atun *et al.* 2012, 2017).

13.3 DAH modalities and health systems

DAH may be implemented along different modalities. These vary in terms of duration (short- to long-term), scope (selective and focused on single issues of geographical areas or country- and sector-wide) and alignment to recipient countries' national strategies and administrative procedures. The way in which DAH is delivered has an impact on the recipient country's health system.

> A system is a set of integrated components working together to achieve a given objective. […] Thinking systemically means considering the whole and the possible effects on all components of actions targeting only one or few of them. Thinking systemically is exactly what many donors and many organizations do not do when they intervene in the health systems of poor countries.
>
> (Murru and Tediosi 2009)

13.3.1 Project aid

A project is defined by a specific purpose and a series of activities aimed at the delivery of a limited number of outputs, within a defined time period and with a defined budget, to contribute to the resolution of a specific problem (European Commission 2004; Fernandes Antunes *et al.* 2008).[6]

Generally donors are highly involved in the whole project cycle, from identification, through programing, financing, implementation, monitoring and evaluation. Projects are thus seen to be donor-driven and, especially in the health sector and other service-related projects, their long-term financial sustainability may be affected once donor financing has concluded. The project approach evidently comes with limited local ownership of projects and has contributed to the current fragmentation of DAH. When several projects on related issues are funded by different donors, each with their own management and reporting arrangements, the high transaction costs for the recipients may undermine local capacity and accountability. Fungibility is another issue related to the project approach (see 13.4.1).

13.3.2 Program assistance

The OECD/DAC defines program assistance as aid consisting of contributions made available to a recipient country for general development purposes (i.e. balance of payment support, general budget support and commodity assistance, not linked to specific project activities). According to the OECD definition, program aid is channeled directly to partner governments, uses local accounting systems and is not linked to specific project activities (OECD 1991). Program aid aims to improve the level of resources available to an economy or to a specific sector (OECD 1991), though sector-wide approach (SWAp) programs (see below) have often used multiple financing modalities.

Program assistance includes different planning, financing and implementation modalities.

Direct budget support

Direct budget support (DBS) refers to financial assistance for macro-level policies and to government budgets with funding channeled through the national treasury. The funds are managed by the recipient government, using its existing budget and financial management systems.

Although in some cases DBS can maximize ownership and coherence with national policies whilst minimizing transaction costs (European Commission 2004), it can also be subject to conditionalities imposed by the donor, thus undermining ownership in the recipient country. This has been the case of Structural Adjustment Programs (SAPs) agreed upon by Bretton Woods Institutions, which require macroeconomic reforms (see Chapter 4).

DBS targets result delivery over a longer-term horizon than project aid does. Over the past decade, it has been accompanied by a focus on the importance of good governance to generate capacity for sustainable development. In contrast to project aid, it concentrates on outcomes rather than outputs, and emphasizes the importance of ownership of policies and programs by recipient countries (Fernandes Antunes *et al.* 2008).

However, DBS is only appropriate as a mechanism of assistance to the public sector. Unlike the project modality, it cannot be used for direct support to the private sector or NGOs (European Commission 2004).

Two main categories of DBS can be identified: General Budget Support (GBS) and Sector Budget Support (SBS).

The major characteristic of *General Budget Support* is "the absence of earmarking of funds to particular sectors or activities" (Fernandes Antunes *et al.* 2008). The donors can influence to some extent the sector allocation process through policy dialogue. However, recipient countries allocate funds between sectors according to national planning and decision-making processes and procedures. GBS maximizes ownership and coherence with national policies, whilst minimizing transaction costs. Yet it is the ministries of finance and/or planning offices which have the most influence on the process through their role in the formulation of the general budget and GBS program negotiations, and these offices tend not to be concerned with social and health issues. Thus, it is important that ministries of health take an early role in negotiations of GBS programs and that any reforms which often come as part of GBS programs are appropriate to the specificities of the health sector (European Commission 2004; Fernandez Antunes *et al.* 2008).

Sector Budget Support provides additional funding to a specific sector (e.g. the health sector), supporting a stated sector policy and agreed spending framework. Financial contributions may either be sector ear-marked and channeled through the national treasury, or they can be directly transferred to the relevant ministry with an overall allocation to the sector. These funds often contribute to Common Pooled Funds (or "common basket funds") which fund all or part of the Sector Program or target specific budget items.

The earmarking of funds in SBS ensures that they are not retained in the central banks as currency reserves or used for other purposes, such as debt repayments. Ministries of health tend to appreciate this type of funding because it allows them to respond to identified needs; however, ministries of finance and planning offices sometimes react by reducing domestic financial commitment to health (see below *fungibility*) and may see SBS as in contrast with macroeconomic stabilization (Fernandes Antunes *et al.* 2008).

Sector-wide approach

Sector-wide approach programs (SWAps) aim to reduce fragmentation of development assistance typical of project aid (Table 13.2) by engaging all donors active in a defined sector in a structured manner through joint planning, financing, implementation and monitoring arrangements.

SWAps in health were developed in the early 1990s in response to fragmentation introduced by donor-sponsored projects and prescriptive macroeconomic adjustment lending. SWAps were intended to produce a shift from donor-driven policies to policies fully owned by recipient countries which responded to their needs and were in line with their national strategies. In addition, by design, the SWAp promotes transparency in resource allocation and accountability for donors and country governments (Peters *et al.* 2013).

SWAps may use various financing and implementing mechanisms. These can be summarized in three modalities: ear-marked SBS channeled through the national budget "Treasury" (Channel 1); SBS with donors contributing directly to the sector budget, where funds are managed through special accounts outside the regular government system, including pooled funding arrangements (Channel 2); and donors' direct financing of operations through projects, financing of specific budget items such as capital equipment, or technical assistance (Channel 3). In this third channel, expenditures are undertaken directly by the donor's agency or by non-governmental organizations

280 *Global policies and issues*

Table 13.2 Comparing project assistance and sector-wide approach

Sector-wide approach	Project approach
View on entire sector	Focus on projects to support narrowly defined objectives
System approach; promotes reduction of fragmentation	Favors "vertical" and piecemeal initiatives
Partnerships with mutual trust accountability	Recipient accountable to donor
Collective policy dialogue between donors and partner country	Bilateral negotiations and agreements
Procedures aligned to local system	Parallel implementation arrangements
Long-term support toward health system strengthening	Short-term disbursement, success based on project outputs
Process-oriented approach through learning by doing	Standardized approach
Promotes respect of Aid effectiveness principles	Principles of Aid effectiveness are scarcely followed

Source: adapted from OECD, 2006.

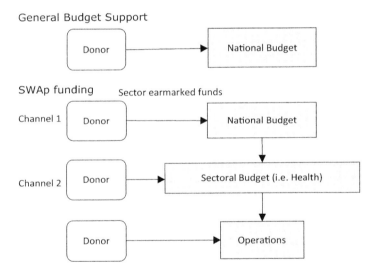

Figure 13.4 Program assistance financing.

(NGOs) on its behalf; a government may receive assets or services in kind but does not handle the funds itself (Handley 2009) (Figure 13.4).

The introduction of SWAps represented an increasing focus on health system strengthening by both the World Bank[7] and the World Health Organization (WHO) and an approach consistent with aid effectiveness principles. However, in practice implementation presented considerable challenges. Some challenges were linked to factors related to their implementation mechanism. Tensions implicit in donor-partner asymmetry became evident, coordination mechanisms required on occasion additional technical assistance to address local institutional weakness and pooling of finances did not become the main route of financing, with projects (along Channel 3) remaining the dominant mode of aid delivery. Finally, most donors participating in SWAps would maintain parallel project aid; few, if any, SWAps engaged all donors; and although supportive of SWAps, a number of donors were constrained by their own administrative rules from providing direct financing, participating in pooled funding or using the partner country's national systems for procurement or monitoring (Hill et al. 2012).

Another challenge was related to the significant change in the global architecture of DAH at the beginning of the new Millennium. Global health initiatives, such as the Roll Back Malaria Partnership, Stop TB Partnership, GAVI, the Global Fund to Fight AIDS, TB and Malaria, and the President's Emergency Plan for AIDS Relief (PEPFAR) all focused on priority diseases and had their own governance arrangements, thus contributing to fragmentation (Peters et al. 2013).

The International Health Partnership (IHP) was launched with the purpose of overcoming the increasing fragmentation challenge in DAH and reframing the discourse on coordination in the health sector according to the global Aid Effectiveness Agenda.

13.3.3 From International Health Partnership to UHC2030

The IHP initiative launched in September 2007 by the British government was later implemented as IHP+ (i.e. IHP and Related Initiatives). The "+" symbol signified the bringing together of a range of other similar initiatives aiming to accelerate the achievement of the health-related MDGs in line with the Paris Declaration.[8] IHP+ opposed the emphasis on selective (i.e. vertical) approaches, focusing instead on horizontal health system strengthening and on the coordination of global health actors at all levels in order to provide solutions to issues such as fragmented DAH, weakened ministries of health and dysfunctional health systems.

In 2016, IHP+ was transformed into UHC2030 to respond to the health-related Sustainable Development Goals, and expanded its scope to include the goal of universal health coverage (UHC). While the new partnership would continue the work on improving effective development cooperation in countries receiving external assistance, it would also broaden the scope to focus on health system strengthening and domestic spending in all countries.

The initiative grew from 26 partners in 2007 to 66 partners in 2016, including governments, international organizations, civil society organizations and global philanthropies. Although encouraged to join as partners, to date the business sector, academia and media are not yet among the signatories of the UHC2030 Global Compact.

As with IHP+, UHC2030 links global and national coordination processes to promote and support investment in a single national health plan and monitoring framework for better coordination of health aid. Similarly to the UHC2030 Global Compact, national compacts also commit recipients and donors to this goal.

The UHC2030 presents itself as "a multi-stakeholder platform to promote collaborative working in countries and globally on health systems strengthening" and is configured as a GPPP initiative (see Chapter 9). It has a Steering Committee of 20 members who represent the different constituencies of the partnership, and a Core Team which is co-hosted by the WHO and the World Bank, which serve as the joint secretariat for the partnership (Moon and Omole 2017; UHC2030 2018).

282 *Global policies and issues*

Positive changes in practices among IHP+ signatories have been reported together with progress in strengthening national planning processes, mutual accountability, and donor alignment with national budgets. However, also documented is a lack of progress in the use of recipients' financial management and procurement systems, reporting and information systems (Moon and Omole 2017).

13.4 Main issues and challenges

Over the last two decades DAH has grown faster than development assistance overall, leading to significant results especially in focus areas that were identified as priorities, such as those related to the Millennium Development Goals (MDGs).

The global aid architecture and particularly that of DAH underwent important changes, shifting from a scheme of near-complete reliance on bilateral and multilateral ODA to an overcrowded and highly fragmented system of very diverse actors (see Chapter 5). Although ODA remains the largest source of DAH, accounting for over 70% of the total, the Bill & Melinda Gates Foundation, with funding of about US$3.3 billion in 2017, is the single largest contributor to global DAH after the USA and the UK. Indeed, despite a proliferation of initiatives in global health, much of the financing for global cooperation comes from a few powerful donors, with the USA, the UK and the Gates Foundation keeping the lion's share (Clinton and Sridhar 2017). Enormous amounts of funds are channeled through GPPPs, whereby the highest amount of resources is channeled through NGOs (IHME 2018).

13.4.1 DAH resources

Notwithstanding the increased amount of global resources for DAH, financial resources dedicated to health still fall short of needs in terms of both support to countries and financing of global public goods and leadership (Moon and Omole 2017; Schäferhoff *et al.* 2015).

In addition, disbursement of DAH is irregular and unpredictable. The share of external assistance in health spending varies from year to year within countries.

Volatility and uncertainty of financing particularly affect funding of recurring costs in the health sector such as salaries, drugs and transport, and can undermine longer-term investment in health system strengthening and countries' efficient use of resources. Some estimates show that volatility reduces the value of aid to recipients by 15–20% (WHO 2017).

Fungibility of external funds, particularly in low-income countries, is often a consequence of external conditioning. Fungibility refers to displacement of domestic financing for health as a response to external financing: development assistance is spent in the health sector, but the recipient government re-allocates its own resources to fund other priorities, resulting in a decrease of domestic resources devoted to health (WHO 2017). This often happens due to debatable macroeconomic reasons, generally inspired by IFIs' prescriptions compelling governments to fix spending ceilings for single sectors. When main donors' DAH is aligned only to a minimum extent with national priorities and the national strategic sectoral plan, while a large proportion of spending is on overheads, unrequested Technical Assistance (TA), unnecessary activities or "tied" to donors' expensive goods and services (see below), the consequences of reduced national public spending in the health sector in order to keep expenditure below allowed ceilings can be detrimental (Murru and Tediosi 2009). In addition, once levels of DAH are reduced (e.g. due to erratic aid disbursement), governments typically do not increase spending on health again (Dieleman and Hanlon 2014).

Critiques have also been raised regarding fungibility between various priorities within health spending (such as between HIV and NCDs) (Moon and Omole 2017).

It has also been noted that often the proportion that is transferred to or spent in developing countries is unclear and/or inadequate. "Phantom aid" refers to the proportion of aid that remains in the donor country, for example, through administrative costs or grants to donor-linked NGOs (Moon and Omole 2017). Debt relief is also recorded as grant, in amount equal to the nominal amount of the cancelled repayments and interest due, and in arrears. Some also consider it "phantom aid" (Moon and Omole 2017) or "non-genuine" aid (CONCORD 2017), due to the fact that there is no fresh transfer of resources to the recipient country. In the case of cancellation of unpayable debts, and in a number of other situations,[9] being recorded as aid may be inappropriate (CONCORD 2017); however, in other cases, debt relief can free resources that the recipient can use for development purposes (e.g. poverty alleviation programs).

OECD-DAC also allows for reporting in-country refugee costs as ODA. Specifically, admitted spending items include living costs for the first 12 months of the refugees' stay, temporary subsistence costs, and some costs for resettlement. Clearly, as civil society organizations (CSOs) have been pointing out

> although it is vital to support refugees in Europe, counting donor refugee costs as ODA is misleading: this type of spending has little to do with development aid and does not link directly with the core purpose of ODA, which is to alleviate poverty in developing countries.
>
> (CONCORD 2017)

Another long-standing concern about aid resources is related to the macroeconomic argument that rapid inflow of large amounts of foreign exchange in a country could lead to a loss of competitiveness either by raising inflation or by appreciating the exchange rate. As a consequence, the recipient country's exports, productivity and economic growth may slow down. This phenomenon is known as the "Dutch disease" after the macroeconomic impact of natural gas discoveries in the Netherlands in the 1960s, which caused appreciation of the exchange rate and a crisis of the manufacturing sector. Since then, the concept of "Dutch disease" has been used to refer to other types of foreign exchange inflows, including rapid increases in external development assistance. However, the impact of inflows from DAH, if any, depends on an array of country-specific factors. It has been demonstrated that it is possible to effectively mitigate the risk of "Dutch disease" following an increase in DAH (Cavagnero et al. 2008).

Countries that are recipients of DAH may face challenges in efficiently using the resources received. A well-known problem is the fiscal impact of aid. In many areas, including the health sector, aid is used to invest in capital goods such as building new health facilities or infrastructure to reach them. Typically these investments require additional domestic resources to make them functional and to maintain them. These are not only financial resources that recipient countries must allocate, but also human resources and management capacity. Several low-income countries have limited management capacity and often limited trained human resources to efficiently absorb DAH.

It is therefore crucial to plan DAH in the broader context of National Development Plans that takes into account fiscal and health sector constraints. Ideally DAH should be aligned with National Health Plans that include the financial and human resources required to effectively benefit from external funding.

13.4.2 Fragmentation

As mentioned above, the number of actors in development assistance has increased enormously. Indeed, "the number of international organizations, funds and programs is now higher than the number of developing countries they were created to assist" (World Bank 2008: 14). Wide consensus exists on aid effectiveness principles formally adopted with the Paris Declaration on Aid Effectiveness in 2005: recipient countries set their own objectives and strategies (Ownership); donors align behind these objectives and use local systems (Alignment); donors coordinate, simplify procedures and share information to avoid duplication (Harmonization); recipient countries and donors shift focus to development results and results get measured (Results); and donors and partners are reciprocally accountable for development results (Mutual accountability) (OECD 2005). Nevertheless, a diverse and uncoordinated aid community not aligned to the beneficiary country's system imposes an additional strain on already weak implementation capacities in low-income countries.

> Managing aid flows from many different donors is a huge challenge for recipient countries, since different donors usually insist on using their own unique processes for initiating, implementing, and monitoring projects. Recipients can be overwhelmed by requirements for multiple project audits, environmental assessments, procurement reports, financial statements, and project updates.
>
> (Radelet 2006, cited in World Bank 2008)

The health sector is the one with the highest number of "development actors" and the highest level of proliferation of such actors. In addition, in recipient countries not all health-related activities are under the responsibility of the Ministry of Health or equivalent health authority. Instead many aspects are managed by other ministries. For example, the Ministry of Education may be the official authority for health workers' training; salary and disciplinary matters can fall under the responsibility of the Ministry of Public Services; other ministries may autonomously manage their healthcare systems (e.g. the Ministry of Defense and the Ministry of Interior); and social insurance may be a competence of the Labor or Social Welfare Ministry. "At least 100 identifiable organizations operate in the heath sector, but financial flows and initiatives are in the thousands" (Murru and Tediosi 2009).

Among donors' specific requirements there is often an obligation for the recipient country to spend the financial resources provided by the donor to buy goods and services in the donor country itself, sometimes at costs higher than those that could be obtained on the free market, or of lower quality or technically inappropriate (e.g. with different standards, creating dependence for the donor country for maintenance and spare parts). Thus, in open contrast with the principles of ownership and alignment, aid is often "tied" to the donors' market. OECD reports that tied aid can increase the costs of a development project by as much as 15 to 30%. Untying aid, i.e. removing the legal and regulatory barriers to open competition for ODA-funded procurement, gives the recipient country the freedom to procure goods and services on the global market (OECD 2018). Analysis of OECD/DAC donor countries' compliance with the DAC Recommendation on Untying ODA at least to the Least Developed Countries (LDCs) and non-LDC Highly Indebted Poor Countries shows that almost all (99%) of the aid that should be untied remains tied, and concerns "project type interventions", mostly in the areas of health (22%) (OECD 2018a).

In response to effectiveness principles and in an attempt to increase coordination amongst themselves and with the recipient countries, a number of donors have moved toward program aid and budget support (see 13.3). In search of system-wide coherence, since the mid-1990s the United Nations system has engaged in reforms aimed at increasing inter-agency coordination at global as well as country levels. A "Delivery as One"[10] (DaO) strategy was launched in 2006 and was progressively implemented in an increasing number of countries. The expected benefits of the DaO model included better alignment of the UN system organizations' programs with national priorities and multilateral funding tied to them, increased attention to cross-cutting issues, reduction of transaction costs, and easier interaction between the UN system as a whole and countries' governments (Missoni and Alesani 2013).

Since 2011 the European Union (EU) has adopted EU Joint Programming for EU members, a major flagship initiative to strengthen the coherence, transparency, predictability and visibility of EU external assistance. Implementing Joint Programming at the country level has led to more effective division of labor and reduced aid fragmentation (EC 2018).

Indeed, the implementation of aid effectiveness principles lags far behind, and even donors that have engaged in horizontal, well-aligned systemic approaches such as General Budget Support and program aid, in parallel still finance and/or implement project aid and both bilateral and multilateral vertical initiatives, including support to GPPPs such as the GFATM and GAVI.

13.4.3 Verticalization

The mushrooming of development assistance actors has been particularly evident in the health sector, which has also suffered a high degree of "verticalization". Indeed, the vast majority of these actors earmark their DAH for communicable diseases, and often only on the "big three" diseases: HIV/AIDS, tuberculosis (TB) and malaria. Another major focus area has been maternal and child health, including vaccinations.

These specific focus areas have also explicitly been pursued by donors to help countries reach the MDGs on child mortality (MDG 4), maternal health (MDG 5) and HIV/AIDS, TB, and other major diseases (MDG 6) (Bendavid et al. 2017).

"Verticalization" of ODA also characterizes some bilateral assistance programs. The US government's PEPFAR has been driving the increase in DAH focused on HIV/AIDS.

Questionably, noncommunicable diseases received the least funding of categories tracked by IHME (2018). Indeed, allocation criteria remain a highly debated issue in terms of both focus and geographical area.

According to Bendavid et al. (2018), "Health aid resources cannot fully subsidize the health sector of even the poorest countries, and decisions for prioritizing disease areas and programs are unavoidable". Although one can agree on the obvious need for prioritization, the selective focus on specific diseases, often with tight earmarking of donors' resources, has led to the verticalization and fragmentation of DAH and to donors losing sight of the complexity of health systems. In this sense, the key issue is not with identifying which criterion to use for choosing disease priorities for health aid (such as disease burden, cost-effectiveness of interventions, or diseases afflicting "the most ill", i.e. persons with lower healthy life expectancy) (Bendavid et al. 2018), but rather with identifying and addressing the dysfunctions of the health system that limit universal access to prevention and care, and thereby prioritizing people most in need (i.e. not their diseases). In other words, DAH should principally aim to strengthen health systems, taking into account complexity and contextualizing approaches, and following a systemic approach to health and health care,. *What* is implemented is as important as *how* it is done, and the extent to which DAH is "embedded" in the health system should be part of the assessment of success (Cleary et al. 2018).

The 2030 Agenda mandates an integrated approach to the 17 SDGs, thus implying that DAH should be coordinated with interventions in other sectors and, according to ownership and alignment principles, be further integrated with country development plans. Besides, noncommunicable diseases (NCDs) now account for 71% of the global burden of disease, and 85% of these "premature" deaths occur in low- and middle-income countries (WHO 2018). NCDs pose a much higher burden on the health system than acute infectious diseases, with the risk of making the goal of Universal Health Coverage (SDG3, target 3.8) unsustainable. Thus, investment for health, i.e. a health in all policies approach with clear intersectoral strategies, will require an indispensable shift toward a social determinants approach, including for DAH (Missoni 2018).

If UHC is deemed to be the cornerstone of the SDG3, then sector-wide support is the most effective and direct way toward the goal (Buffardi 2018).

An increasing part of DAH is spent on transnational health issues, including epidemics and antimicrobial resistance. Yet the share of DAH that should be allocated globally to control these kinds of threats remains an open question (Schäferhoff et al. 2015; Bendavid et al. 2018). In any case, in the absence of well-functioning health systems at the country level, global investments may prove ineffective.

13.4.4 Geographical allocation

Allocation criteria should guide decisions about which countries are eligible for assistance, how much assistance each country will be offered, levels of co-financing required of recipients, and other necessary conditions for receiving funding. These criteria may consider countries' needs, effectiveness of delivered aid and a number of cross-cutting issues (Ottersen et al. 2017).

The gross national income (GNI) per capita criterion has been traditionally used to determine countries in need. In fact, to be recorded as ODA, financial and technical assistance must be allocated to "developing" countries, a category including all low- and middle-income countries based on GNI per capita as published by the World Bank (OECD 2018b). Obviously international cooperation (including technical and scientific cooperation in health) has always gone beyond assistance eligible to be recorded as ODA, but even considering only ODA, most donor countries have not defined the geographical priorities of their bilateral development cooperation purely on GNI per capita. Indeed, political and economic foreign policy criteria have always played a role in the definition of ODA geographical priorities (Ottersen et al. 2017).

GNI does not, however, represent countries' needs or capacity to make the best use of external support and "agreement is growing that GNI per capita is an inadequate basis for deciding which countries are eligible for health aid and how much each country should receive" (Bendavid *et al.* 2018).

As discussed in Chapter 2, GNI by itself is not an indicator of the life conditions, including health status, of the majority of a country's population. GNI per capita typically masks within-country inequalities and fails to capture context-specific aspects critical to making aid effective (Haakenstad *et al.* 2018). In addition, with the ongoing economic transition, due to the growth of their GNI many formerly low-income countries (LICs) have moved to middle-income status, but in many cases inequalities in income and health persist or have actually increased. Today over 75% of the world's poor and almost 70% of the world's disease burden are in middle-income countries (Ottersen *et al.* 2017), which may be regarded as too rich to qualify for aid (Schäferhoff *et al.* 2015).

Bendavid *et al.* (2018) summarize the debate about the use of GNI as a criterion for resource allocation as follows: some question "whether GNI per capita thresholds should be used at all to determine eligibility for health aid", others suggest "maintaining GNI per capita as a criterion, but supplementing it with criteria directly linked to health needs in the country", and finally some believe donors should "go beyond countries and average measures such as GNI per capita and focus more on the subnational allocation of health aid".

The question remains open about what other criteria should be used, as well as whether or not these criteria should be combined with GNI per capita; however, few would argue that GNI per capita correlates with need for DAH or countries' autonomous capacity to provide health services or to deal with domestic challenges, which is another criterion that may be used to determine the recipient country's need for assistance (Ottersen *et al.* 2017).

Alternative indicators of need include the Human Development Index (HDI), life expectancy at birth, under-five mortality rate (U5MR) and burden of disease.

Effectiveness criteria aim to allocate aid where it will be most effective, an approach which is also related to expected impact, country performance and absorptive capacity. Past performance is for example one of the criteria adopted by the GFATM to determine eligibility for grant renewal (Ottersen *et al.* 2017).

A number of adopted criteria have limited association with need or effectiveness, or are to a certain extent crosscutting to both. These include criteria such as population size, aid from other donors and country effort.

Finally, allocation criteria may involve some form of conditionality, such as co-financing requirements or targeting to specific population groups (e.g. discriminated ethnic groups, refugees, etc.) (Ottersen *et al.* 2017).

As mentioned above, an increasing amount of DAH is spent at the global level, but at least part of that effort is not reported through the Development Statistics databases of the OECD/DAC. In the attempt to provide a more comprehensive picture of donor support for health, Schäferhoff *et al.* (2015) have extended the analysis of official DAH to include additional public spending for pharmaceutical R&D for neglected diseases that is not reported as ODA, characterizing this as "ODA+", and arguing that this "expanded thinking" may have the potential to reshape how policy-makers approach their support for global health. After classifying international ODA+ into three global functions (Supplying global public goods,[11] Management of cross-border externalities[12] and Exercising leadership and stewardship[13]) and a fourth function related to providing support for country-specific purposes,[14] Schäferhoff et al. (2015) analyzed the spending of eight major donors and concluded that 21% of ODA+ spending went to financing global functions (14% to supplying global public goods, 4% to management of cross-border externalities and 3% to exercising leadership and stewardship) and 79% went to country-specific DAH. They concluded that "funding for global functions should be strengthened", and emphasized that donors spent remarkably little on leadership and stewardship, among other important areas, contributing to a situation where "WHO remains a central actor for delivery of this role, but its core budget continues to shrink" (Schäferhoff et al. 2015).

Notes

1 China's engagement in global health is rapidly expanding financing of projects and providing technical assistance in other countries; it has been a leading player in promoting and supporting inter-BRICS country initiatives in health. Partnerships between China and other low- and middle-income countries have led to new, lower-cost product pipelines for new drugs, vaccines and diagnostics. However, to date China's contribution to multilateral initiatives has been minimal, and limited transparency around its health- and development-related activities does not allow one to properly track and measure the impact of China's official health financing activities in Africa (Grépin et al. 2014).
2 For example, Cuba has for over five decades provided direct assistance to staff public health systems and support to training of human resources for health over the past five decades. Havana's Latin American Medical School has graduated 25,000 international students since 2005, primarily from and for poor communities in developing countries; the school also provided full scholarships to over 200 US students (MEDICC 2015).
3 According to OECD: Official Development Assistance is defined as: "those flows to countries and territories on the DAC List of ODA Recipients and to multilateral institutions which are:
  (1) *provided by official agencies*, including state and local governments, or by their executive agencies; and
  (2) each transaction of which:
      (a) is administered with the promotion of the *economic development and welfare of developing countries* as its main objective; and
      (b) is *concessional in character* and conveys a grant element of at least 25 per cent (calculated at a rate of discount of 10 per cent).
  Military equipment or services are not reportable as ODA. www.oecd.org/dac/stats/officialdevelopmentassistancedefinitionandcoverage.htm.
4 Includes both (a) grants to nationals of aid-recipient countries receiving education or training at home or abroad and (b) payments to consultants, advisers and similar personnel as well as teachers and administrators serving in recipient countries (including the cost of associated equipment). See: www.oecd.org/dac/dac-glossary.htm#TC.
5 The formula used to calculate the grant element includes three parameters: Maturity (i.e. duration the date at which the final repayment of a loan is due), grace period (i.e. interval to first repayment of capital) and interest rate. According to the OECD reporting guidelines, the grant element "measures the concessionality of a loan, expressed as the percentage by which the present value of the expected stream of repayments falls short of the repayments that would have been generated at a given reference rate of interest". Under the current system (since 1969) the reference interest rate is 10%. However, interest rates have been much lower than the 10% reference rate for many years. This has implied that the required grant element could be easily met, and even official loans extended at market rates could easily qualify

as ODA. This limit is being corrected. With effect from 2019 reporting on 2018 flows, loan concessionality will be assessed based on differentiated discount rates taking into account factors such as time preference, inflation and risk (Scott 2017).
6 In the context of the project cycle management (PCM) a project is defined in terms of a hierarchy of objectives (inputs, activities, results, purpose and overall objective) plus a set of defined assumptions and a framework for monitoring and evaluating project achievements (indicators and sources of verification) (European Commission 2004).
7 With the purpose of reducing fragmentation of development assistance, in the 1990s the World Bank introduced Sectoral Investment Programs (SIPs). SIPs contained the key elements of what would later be called the sector-wide approach, or SWAp (Hill *et al.* 2012).
8 Currently the UHC2030 partnership includes the following "related initiatives": health system specific initiatives: Alliance for Health Policy and Systems Research, P4H Network for health financing and social health protection, Global Health Workforce Network, Global Service Delivery Network, Health Data Collaborative, Health Systems Global, Health Systems Governance Collaborative, Inter-agency Pharmaceutical Coordination Group, Inter-agency Supply Chain Coordination Group, Joint Learning Network for UHC, Primary Health Care Performance Initiative, Universal Health Coverage Partnership. Other related initiatives: Global Health Security Agenda, Non Communicable Diseases Global Coordination Mechanism, Partnership for Maternal, Newborn and Child Health, Global Health Cluster, The Elders, UHC Coalition. www.uhc2030.org/about-us/related-initiatives/.
9 Among the reasons indicated for considering debt cancellation as "non-genuine" aid there are: "in debt cancellation donors can count both the principal and future interest; and since many of the debts are long-term, counting future interest can inflate the figure significantly; the relationship between the debt and development objectives is often unclear. Research conducted by Eurodad shows that 85% of the bilateral debts cancelled between 2005 and 2009 were debts resulting from export credit guarantees. The mandate of export credit agencies is to support national (donor-country) companies by encouraging international exports – not to support development" (CONCORD 2017).
10 One program; one leader and team; one budgetary framework and one office.
11 Including: Research and development for health tools; Development and harmonization of international health regulations; Knowledge generation and sharing; Intellectual property sharing; Market-shaping activities.
12 Including: Outbreak preparedness and response; Responses to antimicrobial resistance; Responses to marketing of unhealthful products; Control of cross-border disease movement.
13 Including: Health advocacy and priority setting (convening of policy-makers for negotiation and consensus building for strategy and policy) and Promotion of aid effectiveness and accountability.
14 Including: Providing support to low-income, lower-middle-income and upper-middle-income countries for country-specific purposes; Achieving convergence – i.e. for control of infectious diseases and to provide reproductive, maternal, newborn and child health interventions and services; Controlling noncommunicable diseases and injuries; Health system strengthening.

References

Atun, R., *et al.*, 2012. Innovative financing for health: what is truly innovative? *The Lancet*, 380(9858), 2044–2049.
Atun, R., Silva, S., Knaul, F.M., 2017. Innovative financing instruments for global health 2002–15: a systematic analysis. *The Lancet*, 5, e720–e726.
Bendavid, E., *et al.*, 2017. Development Assistance for Health. In Jamison, D.T., *et al.* (Eds.), *Disease Control Priorities: Improving Health and Reducing Poverty. Disease Control Priorities* (3rd edn.), Vol. 9. Washington DC: World Bank, 299–313.

Buffardi, A.L., 2018. Sector-wide or disease-specific? Implications of trends in development assistance for health for the SDG era. *Health Policy and Planning*, 33(3), 381–391.

Cavagnero, E., et al., 2008. Development assistance for health: should policy-makers worry about its macroeconomic impact? *Bulletin of the World Health Organization*, 86, 864–870.

Cleary, S., et al., 2018. The everyday practice of supporting health system development: learning from how an externally-led intervention was implemented in Mozambique. *Health Policy and Planning*, 33(7), 801–810.

Clinton, C., Sridhar, D., 2017. Who pays for cooperation in global health? A comparative analysis of WHO, the World Bank, the Global Fund to Fight HIV/AIDS, Tuberculosis and Malaria, and Gavi, the Vaccine Alliance. *The Lancet*, 390(10091), 324–332.

CONCORD, 2017. *CONCORD Aidwatch 2017. EU aid uncovered how to reach the target on time*. Brussels: CONCORD Europe. Available from: https://library.concordeurope.org/record/1891/files/DEEEP-REPORT-2017–022.pdf.

Dieleman, J.L., Hanlon, M., 2014. Measuring the displacement and replacement of government health expenditure. *Health Economics*, 23(2), 129–140.

Dieleman, J.L., et al., 2018. Spending on health and HIV/AIDS: domestic health spending and development assistance in 188 countries, 1995–2015. *The Lancet*, 391(10132), 1799–1829.

European Commission, 2004. *Aid Delivery Methods. Volume 1. Project Cycle Management Guidelines*. Brussels: European Commission.

European Commission, 2018. The EU approach to development effectiveness. Available from: https://ec.europa.eu/europeaid/policies/eu-approach-aid-effectiveness_en.

Fernandes Antunes, A., Carrin, G., Evans, D.B., 2008. *General budget support in developing countries: Ensuring the health sector's interest*. Geneva: World Health Organization.

Grépin, K.A., et al., 2014. China's role as a global health donor in Africa: what can we learn from studying under reported resource flows? *Globalization and Health*, 10(1), 273.

Haakenstad, A., Templin, T., Lim, S., Bump, J.B., Dieleman, J., 2018. The financing gaps framework: using need, potential spending and expected spending to allocate development assistance for health. *Health Policy and Planning*, 33(suppl.1), i47–i55.

Handley, G., 2009. *Sector Budget Support in Practice Literature Review*. London: Overseas Development Institute and Mokoro.

Hill, P. S., et al., 2012. Development cooperation for health: reviewing a dynamic concept in a complex global aid environment. *Globalization and Health*, 8(1), 5.

IHME, 2009. *Financing Global Health 2009: Tracking Development Assistance for Health*. Seattle, WA: Institute for Health Metrics and Evaluation.

IHME, 2018. *Financing Global Health 2017: Funding Universal Health Coverage and the Unfinished HIV/AIDS Agenda*. Seattle, WA: Institute for Health Metrics and Evaluation. Available from: www.healthdata.org/policy-report/financing-global-health-2017.

MEDICC, 2015. Global Health Cooperation: International Relations' New Frontier. *MEDICC Review*, 17(3), 3.

Meghani, A., Basu, S., 2015. A review of innovative international financing mechanisms to address noncommunicable diseases. *Health Affairs*, 34(9), 1546–1553.

Missoni, E., 2017. L'architettura e la governance dello sviluppo e dell'aiuto alla ricerca di nuovi assetti. [The architecture and governance of development and aid in search of new settings.] In Ianni, V. (Ed.), *Lo sviluppo nel XXI secolo. Concezioni, processi, sfide*. Rome: Carocci editore, 151–162.

Missoni, E. 2018. Global health determinants and the (un)sustainability of the Universal Health Coverage goal. *Welfare & Ergonomia*.

Missoni, E., Alesani, D., 2013. *Management of International Institutions and NGOs. Frameworks, Practices and Challenges*. Abingdon: Routledge.

Moon, S., Omole, O., 2017. Development assistance for health: critiques, proposals and prospects for change. *Health Economics, Policy and Law*, 12(2), 207–221.

Murru, M., Tediosi, F., 2009. Official Development Assistance and health cooperation. In *Global Health and Development Assistance. Rights, Ideologies and Deceit. 3rd Report of the Italian Global Health Watch*. Pisa: ETS, 41–60.

OECD, 1991. *Development Assistance Manual. DAC Principles for Effective Aid*. Paris: Organization for Economic Co-operation and Development.

OECD, 2005. *Paris Declaration on Aid Effectiveness*. High-Level Forum, Paris, 28 February–2 March.

OECD, 2006. *Harmonising Donor practices for Effective Aid Delivery. DAC Guidelines and reference Series*. Vol. 2. Paris: Organization for Economic Co-operation and Development.

OECD, 2018. Untied aid. Available from: www.oecd.org/dac/financing-sustainable-development/development-finance-standards/untied-aid.htm.

OECD, 2018a. *2018 Report on the DAC Untying Recommendation. DCD/DAC(2018)12/REV2*. Paris: Organization for Economic Co-operation and Development, 13 June. Available from: www.oecd.org/dac/financing-sustainable-development/development-finance-standards/DCD-DAC(2018)12-REV2.en.pdf.

OECD, 2018b. DAC List of ODA Recipients. Available from: www.oecd.org/development/financing-sustainable-development/development-finance-standards/daclist.htm .

Ottersen, T., et al., 2017. Development assistance for health: what criteria do multi- and bilateral funders use? *Health Economics, Policy and Law*, 12(2), 223–244.

Peters, D. H., Paina, L., Schleimann, F., 2013. Sector-wide approaches (SWAps) in health: what have we learned? *Health Policy and Planning*, 28(8), 884–890.

Rowlands, D., 2010. 'Emerging Donors' and the International Development Assistance Architecture. In *NORRAG, A brave New World of 'Emerging', 'Non-DAC' Donors and their Differences from Traditional Donors*, NN44 Policy Brief, September. Geneva: NORRAG, 29–31.

Schäferhoff, M., et al., 2015. How much donor financing for health is channeled to global versus country-specific aid functions? *The Lancet*, 386(10011), 2436–2441.

Scott, S., 2017. *Working Paper No. 339: The grant element method of measuring the concessionality of loans and debt relief. OECD DEV/DOC/WKP(2017)5*. Paris: Organisation for Economic Co-operation and Development.

UHC2030, 2018. UHC2030 is the global movement to build stronger health systems for universal health coverage. Available from: www.uhc2030.org/.

WHO, 2017. *New Perspectives on Global Health Spending for Universal Health Coverage*. Geneva: World Health Organization.

WHO, 2018. Noncommunicable diseases. 1 June. Available from: www.who.int/news-room/factsheets/detail/noncommunicable-diseases.

World Bank, 2008. *Aid Architecture. An Overview of the Main Trends in Official Development Assistance Flows*. Washington DC: The World Bank Group.

Unless otherwise indicated, all websites were accessed on 9 August 2018.

14 Career opportunities in global health

14.1 Global health trends and education

As described in other chapters of the book, the growth in global health relevance and funding has been accompanied by the proliferation of global initiatives and new actors that have increased the complexity of the health-related global governance and management structure. In fact, the mushrooming of new private actors (including corporate, philanthropic and civil society organizations) and a vast array of global alliances and public-private partnerships, together with the growing role of emerging countries, has brought about considerable changes in global governance.

In the last decades, with the acceleration of the globalization process, the interdependency among national health systems and the interconnectedness between health and the multifaceted aspects of development have dramatically increased. A wide range of social, economic, political and environmental determinants are of planetary relevance and transnationally influence population health: medical technologies are developed and traded globally by transnational companies, medical and health-related knowledge is shared by a global community of professionals, and both patients and the healthcare workforce have fluid national borders.

A report titled "The Dramatic Expansion of University Engagement in Global Health", published by the Center for Strategic & International Studies (CSIS), includes evidence of the increasing importance of global health and development education. This aspect is well explained in a paragraph of the report that reads:

> The looming threats of another SARS-like outbreak, a pandemic of avian influenza, or the global spread of multi-drug resistant tuberculosis (for example) create a domestic public health imperative for investing in global health. This national interest in 'self-protection' is closely tied to the investment in global health as a strategic foreign policy imperative for both political and economic reasons. It has been suggested that investment in global health is a concrete way in which the United States can exercise its 'soft power' to reach out to those living in poverty, save lives, and repair the U.S. image abroad.
>
> (Merson and Chapman Page 2009)

In the same report the rapid growth of global health education is clearly stated:

> Global health is experiencing an unprecedented and palpable surge of attention and growth on universities' campuses across the United States. Curricula, programs, centers, departments, and institutes of global health are being established [...].

There are at least three root causes or drivers of the growth of global health on American campuses:

(1) significant changes in American higher education that places greater emphasis on and resources for internationalization, in response to students' greater awareness of the world starting at an early age and facilitated by the global media;
(2) heightened public visibility of the global health agenda, as a matter of US foreign policy, and as part of a larger movement for greater global equity;
(3) expansion of resource flows: US government, foundations and corporate and private philanthropy have generated new opportunities for universities, and potential career paths for students.

The majority of college graduates now enter the workforce with some kind of global experience on their resume. The reality of globalization brings greater international connectedness, including ease of communication through innovations in information technology, which has created more opportunities to work overseas.

(Merson and Chapman Page 2009)

The number of courses that are dedicated to global health and contribute to a "Master in Global Health" degree has mushroomed over the past decade, both in the large universities in the USA and in Europe. Most top academic institutions are now offering PhD programs in global health-related fields (e.g. Harvard University, Johns Hopkins University, University of London, University of Geneva). Nevertheless, the international offer of graduate programs is highly dominated by programs taught in medical or public health schools. These programs, which often fail to combine health sciences with economic, social and management sciences, also tend to target medical and health sciences students. Due to the complex characteristics of the global health arena and the multidisciplinary nature of the field, post-graduate employment and continued research in the field inevitably necessitate a more comprehensive, interdisciplinary skill set which covers scientific, political, social and economic disciplines. It is only with this interdisciplinary mindset that it is possible to effectively perform analyses, engage in policy-making and manage activities both among the various sectors as well as between highly intertwined, yet separate, actors, including the public sector, the private sector and civil society (Missoni and Tediosi 2013).

The subject attracts new generations of students and scholars and the offer of courses in this new area is booming. However, there is still wide discrepancy in the content among global health courses offered around the world and sometimes the denomination global health is arguably used to refurbish pre-existing courses in "international health", "tropical medicine" and others in a mere response to marketing needs (Koplan *et al.* 2009). This presents an interesting conundrum because, as pointed out by Bozorgmehr (2010), "social innovations are unlikely to evolve if 'Global Health' becomes or remains a cosmetic re-labeling of old patterns, objects, and interests".

A group of leading global health experts of four academic institutions in Switzerland have even conceptualized the term Academic Global Health (AGH) to analyze the increasing importance of transforming global health education, research and practice (Wernli *et al.* 2016). They state that the primary goal of AGH is to foster transformative knowledge, which implies both new models of thinking and new types of research. At the operational level, this translates into a process of mutual learning for change and health improvement, through sharing and comparing across systems and cultures, using both qualitative and quantitative methods, validating new evidence internally and externally, and making interdisciplinary and international collaborations a prerequisite. [...]

In education, the main challenge is to extend the topics and methods taught both in the curricula of global health in medicine, public health, and engineering, and in other programs granting global health degrees, while maintaining sufficient coherence and disciplinary depth. Mixing students from diverse backgrounds is paramount to foster collaboration across disciplines and to develop the reflexive and synthesizing mind in a competence-based education.

(Wernli *et al.* 2016)

They conclude by emphasizing that in order for academic institutions to keep their social relevance, they

should develop new intellectual spaces to pursue the production of knowledge across disciplines while drawing on the achievements of two centuries of disciplinary organization of science.

(Wernli *et al.* 2016)

Thus, education in global health should aim to provide skills beyond "health" studies and supplementary to those acquired through training in specific disciplines, and its outcome should produce professionals who, whatever their specific field of training may be (e.g. medicine, economics, sociology, natural sciences, engineering, etc.), understand how their professional work on local levels can feed into or be linked with global action (Bozorgmeher *et al.* 2011) in a truly "g-local" approach.

We have included the term equity in our definition of global health (see Chapter 1). Equity has a moral and an ethical dimension and implies the overcoming of inequities. In order to describe a certain situation as inequitable and identify the strategies and tools to correct it, the cause has to be examined and judged to be unfair in the context of what is going on in the rest of society.

The inclusion of equity in the definition also has methodological implications. In our view, global health studies should engage students ethically, and the teaching of technical skills should also promote a reflection on the values and social mission of future health and for health professionals. In other words, global health teaching should also imply an ethical commitment to educate future professionals in social justice and their non-neutral role in correcting global processes at the root of human suffering and inequities in health (Missoni and Martino 2011).

14.2 "Hands-on" training: internships and first steps in the "career"

An important link between education in global health management and policy and the professional career in that domain is an initial period of experience and training "on the job". Most postgraduate programs described in the previous paragraphs include a short period of internship in fulfillment of the requirements of the degree.

Formalized and educationally focused unpaid work embedded into degree programmes that are well supervised and have clear learning outcomes is generally considered by educators, students and prospective employers to provide much-needed exposure to professional practice and valuable learning opportunities.
(Grant-Smith and McDonald 2018)

Beside the educational importance of such experience, the inclusion of an internship period is an important element of the marketing of postgraduate courses, as ranking of schools is also based on rate of placement after obtaining the degree, and increasingly a student placement or internship represents the first international experience for professionals engaging in global health.

Thus, due to the proliferation of courses in "global health" which include a period of internship, and despite internships being in most cases non-paid,[1] access to such an experience has become highly competitive.

Search for the placement may be a cause of anxiety and frustration for students, especially when training institutions leave the search for the "position" entirely to the autonomous initiative of the student. The training institution's formal network may not be sufficient to ensure the required placement; faculty members may provide additional support through their informal personal networks. There is also a growing market of private "brokers" that offer services to identify and negotiate placements in domestic or international internships, and typically charge significant fees (Grant-Smith and McDonald 2018). In any case affordability of unpaid work represents an open equity issue, as students from less well-off circumstances will clearly face more difficulties to settle, especially in expensive capital cities where international institutions' headquarters are based. "Access to unpaid work experience opportunities are identified in the literature as being highly classed, raced, gendered, ageist and subject to geographical inequalities" (Grant-Smith and McDonald 2018). In addition, interns often feel to be tasked with institutional work without adequate supervision, while bearing responsibilities which go beyond those legitimately entrusted to non-paid trainees.

This book deals with management and policy in global health, thus we do not discuss experiential educational offerings that involve health workers (medical doctors and nurses) in developing countries, i.e. internships, also described as "global health" fieldwork or international medical electives. Nevertheless, it is important to stress that these educational experiences, as well as volunteering in medical field missions, entail important ethical issues. "Ethical blunders are frequent when students and faculty act in service before they have sufficient education and understanding of complex global health contexts." Some of these medical electives "allow students to provide healthcare services usually reserved for licensed healthcare workers [...]. Such efforts done in the name of 'global health' are a shame, disregarding basic tenets of health equity and evidence-based medicine" (Neil Arya and Evert 2017). To a lesser extent, field experiences in the area of management also face similar ethical challenges and one should not underestimate the need for interdisciplinary training (socio-cultural, anthropological, political, etc.) in preparation for the internship period. Some of these aspects are further discussed below (see 14.4).

For early-career professionals who have just completed studies as well as for mid-career professionals who wish to transition into a global health-related field, the first step is again often volunteering, whether they want to work with an international institution or NGO, a bilateral development agency, or any other of the actors that we described in previous chapters and that are summarized in Table 14.1. In this case the professional is involved in an elective form (i.e. the experience is not required as part of a formal educational program) of unpaid work which results in the delivery of pro bono productive work. "Although there may be benefits for the participant in terms of enhanced employability, the work is structured around the delivery of productive work for an 'employer'" (Grant-Smith and McDonald 2018). Indeed, many global health organizations value previous international experience in job candidates, whether the experience was paid or unpaid.

14.3 Working in global health

The growing relevance of global health and the resulting changes in higher education systems are coupled with a growing demand for professionals who combine a thorough understanding of health-related challenges, with multidisciplinary analytical, policy-making, economic and management skills, as well as the capability to interact with diverse stakeholders at all levels.

The global job market is in fact offering unprecedented opportunities for graduates with these skills in both the private and the public sector, as well as in the emerging area of public-private endeavors. International institutions, pharmaceutical, biotech, and medical devices companies, central and local governments, public authorities and intergovernmental organizations, transnational development NGO, civil society organizations and networks, transnational commercial health providers and insurance companies are generally the favored organizations among graduates with competencies related to global health. The need for research in global health is also growing and is increasingly using innovative approaches that link health to political economy, social and management sciences and international law.

The health sector is one of the largest single industries, with a total annual revenue in excess of US$ 7.3 trillion (in 2015),[2] equivalent to one-tenth of the global GDP and employing in excess of 59 million staff (WHO 2006). The relevance of the health sector has been constantly expanding; health expenditure has been increasing over the past decades, in both absolute and relative (compared to the GDP growth) terms. Professionals trained in global health are needed by national bodies such as the Ministry of Health, Ministry of Finance, public health agencies, Ministry of Foreign Affairs, national and regional development cooperation agencies, Ministry of Trade, Ministry of Education and finally also ministries and departments concerned with environmental issues, industrial and technological research and development. Training in global health is obviously fundamental for those who will occupy a position in international institutions, NGOs and public-private partnerships, and not solely in those institutions or departments related directly to the health sector.

Possible career opportunities for graduates in Global Health Management and Policy include working in innovative professional contexts in health-related national and international organizations requiring strategic, managerial and economics skills.

Indeed, there is an increasing emphasis on global governance for health (Frenk and Moon 2013); ensuring that health becomes a priority in all global policies may push international organizations in other sectors (such as economy, trade, environment, agriculture and many others) to recruit officers with a good understanding of health issues and the capacity to design policies for health. A broad international perspective is also needed by professionals in multinational pharmaceutical, biotechnology and medical devices companies, which in recent decades have ranked highest in terms of earnings and growth among instituttions which work at the global level.

Both healthcare providers and insurance companies are increasing their international interdependencies because the big players operate in the global market, especially in emerging countries. On both the public and the private side, health and social care providers are increasing their average size, through processes of mergers and acquisition, by asking for more skilled management with clear strategic skills and familiarity with international best practices. The medical research market is a global arena for funding, working and publishing; international consulting in global health has also been expanding (World Health Profession Alliance 2007).

Health and the health sector are peculiar in many respects; from the economics of ill health and health systems, to services management and policy-making, these fields require specific competences. This explains the poor performance of professionals with a "generalist" background in dealing with health-related issues (whether within or outside the "health sector"). This problem is seen in a wide range of jobs from economists working in Ministries of Finance, to managers of healthcare organizations, global health initiatives and foundations, to academics, to local, national and global politicians. Higher-education programs should, therefore, reflect these peculiarities, and try to capture the interest of future professionals who may not work for their entire career in direct contact with health services.

International consulting in global health "is increasingly becoming big business" (WHPA 2007). Devex International Development, which is meant to be the largest provider of business intelligence and recruitment services to the development community, provides an example of the demand for experts in global health. Out of the 4995 job openings, a search with the key words "Health" returned 1170 jobs.[3]

According to WHPA (2007), access to the positions on the global health market often requires a doctoral degree or a master of public health (MPH), health administration (MHA), global health or health economics, and "even candidates with a medical doctorate or nursing degree may need a master's that covers management, policy, social or economic topics in this multidisciplinary field" (WHPA 2007).

A recent study on career opportunities in global health reviewed online job postings that included 178 employment opportunities from 26 websites (Eichbaum *et al.* 2015). The findings showed, among other qualifications, the importance of advanced academic credentials and of public health training and program management skills. Sixty-seven percent of the positions were in non-governmental organizations (NGOs) in both developed countries and LMICs. When combined with multinational organizations such as the WHO and the World Bank, the two employer types accounted for 89% (158/178) of the total. Only 14% of the positions involved clinical disciplines, primarily medicine. Fifty percent of job posts requested applicants to have the kind of knowledge and skills normally acquired in schools of public health offering courses relevant to global health; 51% of the listed opportunities required at least a Master's degree level of qualification or doctoral degree (23%); 84% of the positions were program-related, and included roles in planning, program direction, finance, management and other supportive functions.

A non-comprehensive list of areas and institutions increasingly offering opportunities to graduates with a global health and development education is included in Table 14.1.

Table 14.1 List of areas and institutions interested in global health recruitment[a]

Type of institution	Description
UN system and other intergovernmental (public) organizations	These organizations (see Chapter 6) – whether dealing only or mainly with health issues such as the World Health Organization, the United Nations Fund for Population Activities (UNFPA) or UNAIDS, or with a multi-sectoral mandate such as the World Bank or the International Labor Organization (ILO) – often search for graduates with a specialization in global health. It is often considered an asset to be specialized in one sector.
Governmental development agencies and national health authorities	All governments of high-income countries have established semi-autonomous agencies to implement their development cooperation strategies (see Chapter 7). These agencies employ a substantial number of people specialized in each of the sectors they work in. The share of the total budget for development cooperations accounted for by the health sector increased constantly over the last decades. Agencies such as USAID (USA), the DFID (UK), AUSAID (Australia) and GIZ (Germany) have huge health sector programs. Over time, they have also supported a number of consultancy companies that have dramatically expanded their personnel needs in the health sector. Also national health authorities and other governmental agencies in both rich and poor countries need professionals with specific competency in global health in offices related to international relations and the negotiation of global health policies, regulations and agreements affecting their national policies and economy (i.e. national delegations to WHO, FAO, WTO, etc.).
International NGOs	Many international NGOs engaged in global health are now large and complex organizations (see Chapter 8). They often require specialized professionals for both the managerial and the technical positions. To give an example, PATH, an international non-profit specialized in global health, started in 1977 with a modest grant from the Ford Foundation and since then its revenue has increased from less than $20 million to more than $280 million. It has various offices around the world.
Foundations and private philanthropic organizations, advocacy groups	Some major foundations also invest a large amount of their resources in global health. The most prominent example is the Bill & Melinda Gates Foundation, which has made the global health program its main priority (see Chapter 8).
Global health initiatives	The increase in global financing for health development has been accompanied by the proliferation of global health initiatives and independent public-private partnership organizations (see Chapter 9). Organizations such as the Global Fund to Fight AIDS, Tuberculosis and Malaria and the GAVI Alliance continuously search for specialized graduates. Innovative financial mechanisms for financing global health also require personnel with new competencies acquired through global health coursework which are based on economic and managerial skills.
Corporations producing health-related commodities – pharmaceuticals, vaccines and other bio-medical technologies	Pharmaceutical companies and the emerging biotechnology companies offer opportunities for graduates specialized in global health. Besides the core business function, more and more, the corporate sector is going beyond traditional corporate social responsibility and looking into creating social values, making global health part of its core business (see Chapter 8).

Table 14.1 (Cont.)

Type of institution	Description
Management and economics consulting firms and media	Several major management consultancy companies have specialized groups working in global health. In addition, there are several international consultancies that only focus on global health and compete to obtain mandates from major global health donors.
Health insurance companies	Several private insurance companies are global players interested in managing their health insurance business at the global level. The management of these organizations will increasingly include experts able to monitor the global health market both to expand the business in low- and middle-income countries and to monitor global trends affecting the performance of the health insurance business.
International health and social care providers	There are an increasing number of healthcare companies which operate in an international environment, both in the traditional developed world (e.g. France, German, Swedish multinational healthcare providers) and in the emerging countries, which are asking for increasing health and social protection, after a period of time very much focused only on economic and industrial development.
Research and development	Besides strategic and managerial functions, some of the above-mentioned actors also offer career opportunities to those who prefer to have a strong research content in their profession. In that view, universities and other public and private research centers may offer academic careers in the areas of global health, development economics and social health sciences. The increasing opportunities in applied research are shown by the growing community working in health system research. In 2012, this community formed a new membership society named Health System Global. The mission of Health System Global is to "Convene researchers, policy-makers and implementers from around the world to develop the field of health systems research and unleash their collective capacity to create, share and apply knowledge to strengthen health systems".[b] The Global Symposium organized every two years attracts around 1500–2000 academics and practitioners each time.

a The Duke Global health institute website provides a useful list of areas in which it is possible to develop a career in global health. See: https://globalhealth.duke.edu/careers (accessed 9 August 2018).
b www.healthsystemsglobal.org/vision/ (accessed 9 August 2018).

Source: authors' experience and search.

14.4 The ethical global health professional

The decision to undertake a career in global health management and policy can be due to a variety of motivations and may be influenced by background studies and previous experiences. In our experience, students choosing a postgraduate course specifically dealing with global health management, economics and policy, open to any previous field of studies or experience, have included professionals with backgrounds in health sciences, basic sciences, economics and business, pharmacy, law, humanities and other less represented disciplines. Students were mainly "shifters", i.e. professionals with some previous experience in unrelated fields who felt the need to shift to activities related to health in an international environment (whether in the private or public sector) (Missoni et al. 2013).

Such a shift, or more in general the desire to engage in health internationally, can be a response to very diverse personal motivations. These may include desire for a broader perspective on public health, genuine humanitarianism, idealism, employment and professional opportunities, sense of mission and the challenge of a different setting in which new skills can be mastered. However, "excessive idealism, overconfidence (in your tools, role, abilities, or approach), and ignorance about the realities of international health can pose insurmountable impediments and grave damage on local populations" (Birn et al. 2009: 701).

Whether working at the global headquarters of an organization or in the field, i.e. in a country office or at community level as part of a development program/project, professionals engaged in health-related management and policy must be aware of the global social, economic, political and environmental determinants of health and how these interact with national systems. Especially for those engaging in development aid

> it is essential to become historically, culturally, and politically aware – that is, to appreciate the relationship among local conditions and national and international policies and forces, as well as the profoundly political underpinning of most international health aid.
>
> (Birn et al. 2009: 706)

However, beyond knowledge transfer and the acquisition of technical skills ("how to do"), the learning process in, but especially *for* global health, needs to include the "how to be" in a globalized world with health and equity as common goods and fundamental human rights (Tediosi and Missoni 2013).

Current and future generations of professionals, managers and policy-makers involved in various ways in global health will have to deal with increasingly challenging issues inherent to the acceleration of the globalization process, which directly or indirectly affect population health. In this sense, we believe that the professional engaged in global health, whether working in the public sector, with an NGO or in the complex and competitive environment of a transnational company, should respond to the highest ethical standards, and constantly ask her/himself about the impact of her/his behavior, managerial attitudes and decisions in terms of the common good, and specifically how their decisions will influence the health of the people.

The communal approach to ethics, which better applies to management and policy-making, indeed

> focusses on the common good and on the ways in which actions or policies promote or prohibit social justice or ways in which they bring harm or benefits to the entire community [...].
> Ethics concerns conscious and free actions and behaviors that try to differentiate between good and bad in search of the good.
>
> (Missoni and Lupu 2014)

All aspects of global health are full of ethical dilemmas. These are often related to asymmetries in power and resources within and between countries; regulations which affect access to drugs; marketing strategies which prompt unhealthy consumption;

trade of harmful products; professionals' right to migrate against the consequence of brain-drain; restrictive migration policies and humanitarian assistance; donor-driven programs contrasting with locally perceived priorities; funding needs and donor-imposed constraints; investment choices and public health outcomes; and many others (Birn *et al.* 2009).

Ideally, global health professionals, even more than any other international or transnational workers, should adopt "ethics as an attitude for life, a responsible life, open to the problems of our world, with commitment to bringing about change toward the common good" (Missoni and Lupu 2014). It may be hard to reconcile this vision with a position in an organization that may have different interests or whose practice may have lost connection with its stated values and objectives.

It is the daily behavior, the actions and decisions of its members at every level of the hierarchy, that allow an organization to be consistent with the mission, the high human values and the ethical principles, which are formally and publicly stated in the theoretical frames and belong to the public discourse of most international institutions, NGOs, philanthropies and other organizations with public health among their goals. The ethical culture of the organization is the result of the commitment to the constant search for the "good", and specifically "health for all", of each and every one of the individuals in the organization personnel, managers and leaders (Missoni and Lupu 2014). Thus, the higher the position in the management of the organization, the higher is the responsibility to be consistent and to ensure consistency with ethical principles, or to change the organization from within to that end. "The ethics of leaders is the most tangible and vital component of the ethics of an organization" (Missoni and Lupu 2014: 396).

The opportunities to contribute to improving global health may often be a key motivation to engage in global health. As Birn *et al.* (2009) put it

> Individuals working within mainline international health agencies can also play a major role in reforming international health endeavors to be true to their stated mission, rooted in local agenda-setting, and sensitive to the international political economy context. For example, the struggle against unaccountable private sector influences through PPPs at the WHO has been spearheaded by WHO employees themselves, supported by international activists and researchers.
>
> (Birn *et al.* 2009)

For a manager in an organization whose policies may have an indirect impact on public health (e.g. the World Trade Organization), or for whom the health sector is only the market for goods and services it offers (e.g. the pharma industry) or may otherwise have an impact on public health (e.g. the food industry), the ethical dilemma may become difficult to face. In such a context there may or may not be space for negotiation to positively influence the policies and strategies of the organization (for example developing areas of "true" corporate social responsibility, or even promoting new sustainable business models; see Chapter 8). In any case, the ethical professionals will have to identify and manage such a space and maneuver between *loyalty* to the organization, *voicing* their dissatisfaction in an attempt to negotiate and activate a process for the restoration or initiation of an ethical orientation for the organization, and, if unsuccessful, a definitive *exit*. This option may also represent an ethical option. "Exit may in fact mean 'Resign under protest' and, in general, to denounce the organization from without instead of working for change from within" (Missoni and Lupu 2014 cited Hirschman 1970). The alternative may be to risk "to become Prisoners of the Organization, instead of being Servants of the Spirit" (Brown 1947).

An ethical perspective may offer inspiration and guidance to the global health professional in taking difficult decisions and assuming responsibility for his or her choices.

Notes

1 In May 2018, the 71st World Health Assembly passed a resolution requesting the Director-General to take the necessary steps to implement an organization-wide internship program (WHO 2018). A few months later the international press were informed that WHO was to offer paid internships for the first time to boost access for those applying from developing countries. www.bbc.com/news/world-45605768 (accessed 26 September 2018).
2 www.who.int/health_financing/data-statistics/en/.
3 www.devex.com/jobs/ (search performed on 27 July 2018).

References

Birn, A.E., Pillay, Y., Holtz, T.H., 2009. *Textbook of International Health. Global Health in a Dynamic World.* New York: Oxford University Press.
Bozorgmehr, K., Saint, V.A., Tinnemann, P., 2011. The 'global health' education framework: a conceptual guide for monitoring, evaluation and practice. *Global Health.* 7(1), 8.
Bozorgmehr, K., 2010. Rethinking the 'global' in global health: a dialectic approach. *Global Health*, 6, 19.
Brown, W.P., 1947. Imprisoned ideas. *The Spectator*, 19 September. Available from: https://fee.org/articles/imprisoned-ideas/.
Eichbaum, Q., et al., 2015. Career opportunities in global health: a snapshot of the current employment landscape. *Journal of Global Health*, 5(1), 010302.
Frenk, J., Moon, S., 2013. Governance challenges in global health. New England Journal of Medicine, 368(10), 936–942.
Grant-Smith, D., McDonald, P., 2018. Ubiquitous yet ambiguous: an integrative review of unpaid work. *International Journal of Management Reviews*, 20, 559–578.
Hirschman, A.O., 1970. Exit, voice and loyalty. In *Responses to Decline in Firms, Organizations and States.* Cambridge, MA: Harvard University Press.
Koplan, J.P., et al., 2009. Towards a common definition of global health. *The Lancet*, 373, 1993–1995.
Merson, M.H., Chapman Page, K., 2009. *The Dramatic Expansion of University Engagement in Global Health. Implications for U.S. Policy.* A Report of the CSIS Global Health Policy Center. Washington DC: Center for Strategic and international Studies. Available from: https://csis-prod.s3.amazonaws.com/s3fs-public/legacy_files/files/media/csis/pubs/090420_merson_dramaticexpansion.pdf.
Missoni, E., Lupu, G., 2014. Ethics and international organizations. In Missoni, E., Alesani, D. (Eds.), *Management of International Institutions and NGOs. Frameworks, Practices and Challenges.* Abingdon: Routledge, 391–405.
Missoni, E., Martino, A., 2011. L'insegnamento della salute globale. In Cattaneo, A. (Ed.), *Salute Globale. InFormAzione per cambiare. 4° Rapporto dell'Osservatorio Italiano sulla Salute Globale.* Pisa: Edizioni ETS, 21–34.
Missoni, E., Tediosi, F., 2013. The need for policy-making and management training of future health-relevant professionals. In Missoni, E., Tediosi, F. (Eds.), *Education in Global Health policy and Management.* Milan: Egea, 11–17.

Missoni, E., Tediosi, F., Pacileo, G., Procacci, C., 2013. Teaching global health and development in a school of management and economics. In Missoni, E., Tediosi, F. (Eds.), *Education in Global Health policy and Management.* Milan: Egea, 97–112.

Neil Arya, A., Evert, J., 2017. Introduction. In Neil Arya, A., Evert, J. (Eds.), *Global Health Experiential Education: From Theory to Practice.* Abingdon: Routledge.

Tediosi, F., Missoni, E., 2013. Conclusions. In Missoni, E., Tediosi, F. (Eds.), *Education in Global Health policy and Management.* Milan: Egea, 161–164.

Wernli, D., *et al.*, 2016. Moving global health forward in academic institutions. *Journal of Global Health*, 6(1), 010409.

WHO, 2006. *Working Together for Health: World Health Report 2006.* Geneva: World Health Organization.

WHO, 2018. *Reform of the global internship programme.* Seventy-First World Health Assembly. A71/B/CONF./1. Geneva: World Health Organization.

WHPA, 2007. A core Competency Framework for International Health Consultants, World Health Profession Alliance. Available from: www.whpa.org/pub2007_IHC.pdf.

Unless otherwise indicated, all websites were accessed on 9 August 2018.

Index

abuse 53, 98, 117; drug 68, 183 219; human rights 56, 162; sexual 217
Academic Global Health (AGH) 293
access to health: care 56, 162, 214, 252; information 231–232; products 226, 228; services 34, 51, 132, **218**, 221, 233, 253
adaptability 208, 252
Advance Market Commitment (AMC) 63, 171, 176n13, 274–**275**, *277*
advocacy 28n1, 90, 103, 111, 150–153, 289n13; groups 48, **298**
affordability 219, 251, 295
Affordable Medicine Facility for malaria (AMFm) 264, 266, 274, **276**, *277*; *see also* malaria
African Regional Office of WHO (AFRO) 93
African Union Commission 133
Aga Khan Foundation 156
agenda 18; 2030 for sustainable development 20, 66–67, 163, 183, 196, 268; Accra 63; aid effectiveness 65, 281; G8 56, **59**, 61, 130–131, 135; global 17, 55, 64, 97, 99, 112, 130, 134, 149; global health 39, 134, 293; international development 13; political 79, 129, 169. 181; world 17, **97**
Agreement on the Application of Sanitary and Phytosanitary Measures (SPS) 115–116, 207
AIDS Indicator Surveys 35
Alma Ata 47, 64, 133; Declaration 33, 46–47, 53, 94, 100, 170, 249; spirit of 52
American Regional Office of WHO (AMRO) 93
Annan, K. 55, 59, 161
antimicrobial resistance 119, 134, 136, 200, *257*, 286, 289n12
apps 229, 232; *see also* eHealth
Arusha Declaration 14
Atlantic Charter 84

balkanization 170
Ban Ki-Moon 65
basic needs approach 14–15, 45, 88

Bellagio 47, 162
Bellamy, C. 167
Berkley, S. 201
Beyond debt relief 58
Big Data 232–234
Big Food 144, 203
Big Pharma 61, 143, 223
big three diseases 285
Bill & Melinda Gates Foundation 37, 52, 57, 63, 150, 162, 170–171, 174, 176n7, 271, 276, 298; funding from 157; non-state actor 65, 80, 100–102, 153, 156; history and structure 154; contribution to global DAH 282
biomedicalization 190
Board of Governors 106–108; *see also* International Monetary Fund
bovine spongiform encephalopathy 198, 201
breast-milk substitutes 48, 91, 94, 144, 151, 160
Bretton Woods 70n6, 105, 107; agreements 105; financing system 49; institutions 22, 49, 52, 142, 278; International Conference 113; organizations 106; origins 105
BRICS 65, 79, 81, 128–129, 136, 137n3, 288n1; *see also* emerging economies
Brundtland, G.H. 54, 95–98, 169
budget support: direct 278; general 53, 272, 278–179, *280*, 285; sector 278–279
burden of diseases 38, 42n9, 196
Buruli ulcer 221
Bush, G.W. 60, 98

Candau, M.G. 89, 94
capability approach 16
capitalism 21, 189
Carnegie Endowment for International Peace 153
centralist approach 48; *see also* disease specific approach
Chief Executive Board for Coordination (CEB) 86
chikungunya virus 194, 199

Index   305

Children's Investment Fund Foundation (CIFF) 274, **276**, *277*
Chirac, J. 63
Chisholm Brock, G. 89
cholera 91, 194, 198
Chronic Care Model (CCM) 261
Churchill, W. 84
civil society 40, 57, 59, 62, 64, 66, 79, 86, 97, 102, 112–113, 146, 173, 293; activists 61; actors in 131; expression of 142, 145; groups 141, 149, 152, 161; international 150; initiative 150; market and 140, 164; partnerships 163; sectors 104, 181, 185
Civil Society Organizations (CSOs) 65, 98, 103, 119, 130, 150–153, 158n3, 161, 171, 281, 283, 296; alliance with 62, 184; meaning of 145–146; private sector and 57, 162, 292; representative of 58, 65; *see also* third sector
climate change 23, 190, 195–196, 209–210, 213; agreement 182; combat 67; effects of 194; global 192; and health 197; impacts *195*; risks of 193; targets 79
cluster approach 86
Codex Alimentarius 116, 207, 236n14
Commission on Ending Childhood Obesity 100
Committee for Food Security 209
Commission on Intellectual Property Rights, Innovation and Public Health 223, 226
Commission on Macroeconomics and Health 55, 96, 183
Commission on Social Determinants of Health 26, 62–64, 98, 100, 183, 220
Common Pooled Funds 279; *see also* sector budget support
communicable diseases 23, 68, 85, 137, 195, 214, 228; control 274; DAH for 285; treatment of 112; *see also* infectious diseases
Comprehensive Economic Trade Agreement 62, 120
Conference of Sixteen 12
cooperation 13, 17, 48, 58, 90, 103, 105, 131, 136n2, 145, **218**, 296; agreements 107; forms of 77; global 282; development 60, 65–66, 160–161, 251, 270, 281, **298**; international health 52; inter-sectoral 54; multi-sectorial 196; policies 12, 80; programs 136, 268–269; public-private 137; social 11; technical 268, 273; trilateral 119
Corporate Social Responsibility 142, 144, 156–157, 168, **298**, 301
corporate donation 143, 269, 273
country-specific approach 110
cross-sectoral approach 220

Cuba 220, 269, 288n2
cyber-bullying 230

Declaration on the TRIPS agreement 119
Declaration on Health Environment and Climate Change 196
Debt2Health 174, *175*, 176n23, 274–**275**
de-growth 19
Demographic and Health Survey 34, 38–39
dengue 162, 194, 199, 221; *see also* infectious diseases; communicable diseases
determinants of health *25*, 135, 183, 246, 249, 263; environmental 62, 79, 102, 300; epidemiological transitions 261; key 64; political 69, 104; social 26, 47, 78, 182, 190, **218**, 220, 252, 260; system sustainability *257*, 258
development: agenda 13, 17–18, 53, 66, 108, 251, 268; aid 12, 53, 56, 162, 174; goals 53, 66, 85, 88, 160–161; human 16, 18–19, 20; social 17, 29, 66, 108; sustainable 16, 18–19, 67–68, 84, 104, 108, 134–135, 175n4, 278
Development Assistance Committee (DAC) 12, 17, 66, 161, 268, 288n3
Development Assistance in Health (DAH) 57, 63, 67, 112, 127, 147, 156, 180, 256, 268–269, 274, 283–285, 287; agenda 183; country specific 288; database 272; fragmentation 278, 281, 286; global actors *257*, 264; global resources for 282; modalities 277; sources of *270*, 271, 273, 282
Development Cooperation Forum (DCF) 66, 70n18
development-partnership approach 65
diabetes 204, 259; *see also* non-communicable diseases
Disability Adjusted Life Years (DALYs) 38, 193–194
disease specific approach 45, 48, 95, 132–133, 180
Doctors without Borders (MSF) 149, 152
Dodgson, R. 80, *81*, 127, 180
Doha: Declaration 61, 68, 117, 119, 224, **225**, 229; Development Agenda 122n28; Ministerial Conference 117
Duke, J.B. 210
Dutch disease 283

Eastern Mediterranean Regional Office of WHO (EMRO) 93
Ebola 55, 85, 111, 198; case study 252; crisis 99, 199; epidemic 70n12, 85, 101, 133–134, 151, 201, 253–254; post 254; virus 23, 135
eHealth 191, 229, 230–235, 237n34, 237n37
eLearning 232–233
electronic health record 232
Elmau Summit 134

emerging economy 65, 79, 115, 225, 260, 269
environmental health 190–191, 196, 235n6; *see also* climate change
equality *see* equity
equity 17, 33, 38, 46, 53–54, 96, 122n23, 218, 246, 249, 251–252, 254, 294; in access health 247; social 26; global 196, 293; in global health 27, 151; health 64, 295, 300
Essential Drugs Program 48, 94
European Central Bank 106, 219 *see also* Troika
European Commission 70n16, 120, 129, *175*, 219, 278–279, 289n6
European Recovery Program 12
European Regional Office of WHO (EURO) 93
European Union (EU) 56, 83, 106, 115, 135, *175*, 205, 207, 219, 226, 236n14, 237, 285
evergreening 223
evidence–based medicine 182, 295
Executive Boards 87

Farrar, J. 201
female genital mutilation 217
five no approach 137
Flu: avian 23, 55, 132, 182, 198, 292; Spanish 198; swine 23, 55, 99, 101, 192, 198
food: safety 116, 119–120, 204–207, **206**, 236n14, 236n15; security 67, 133, 204–205, **206**, 208–209, 235n12, 236n16; sovereignty 204, 208; system 191, 202, 208–210, 252, *257*
Food and Agriculture Organization (FAO) 78, 89, 109, 116, 160, 204, 236n14, 236n16, **298**
Ford Foundation 47, 156, **298**
Forum on China-Africa Cooperation 136n2
Fourth Ministerial Conference 61
Framework Convention on Tobacco Control (FCTC) 45, 62, 91, 96–98, 144, 151, 180, 211–212
Framework of Engagement with Non-State Actors (FENSA) 103, 140, 144, 149–150, 156
Free Trade Agreement of the Americas 226
fungibility 278–279, 282–283

G7 58, 129, 133–136, *175*
G8 55–58, 60–61, 63–65, 78, *81*, 128–135; Genoa Summit 59, 163, 172
G20 64, 79, 128–129, 135–136
GAVI Alliance 170, 201, 273, **298**
Gender Inequality Index 28n4
General Agreement on Trade in Services (GATS) 61, 114–115, 118, 211, 237n36
General Agreement on Trade and Tariffs (GATT) 22, 113–115, 211
generic top-level domain 234

Geneva Conventions 147–148
Genoa Trust Fund for Healthcare 59
Ghebreyesus, A.T. 93, 104
global: environment 27, 58 197, 235; faith 18; partnership 56, 65, 68, 163–164, 175n4, 180; policy 24, 55, 79, 143, 151, 161, 181, 189, 208, 235, 260
Global Action Network 163, *165*
Global Alliance for Vaccines and Immunizations (GAVI) 54, 57, 63, 70n16, *81*, 111, 132, 143, 156, 162–163, 166, 169, 175n2, 176n10, 176n12, 176n14–16, 260, 264, 271, 274, **275**, **276**, *277*, 281, 285; board 171; model 164; partners 172
Global Alliance for TB Drug Development 162
Global Burden of Disease 210, 250, 286
Global Compact 161, 281
Global Conference on Air Pollution and Health 197
Global Financing Facility (GFF) 111, 134
Global Fund to fight HIV/AIDS Tuberculosis and Malaria 55, 57–59, *81*, 111, 135, 156, 163, 172–174, 176n19, 23, 271, 273–274, **275**, **276**; creation of 113, 132; global health initiatives 281, **298**; global partners 143; launch of 64
global governance for health 62, 77, 79, 175, 180–183, 197, 296
Global Health Diplomacy 79
Global Health and Foreign Policy 85
Global Health Governance 79, *81*, 83, 102–104, 121n11, 151, 153, 163, 182, 200, 264; actors of 150, 172; challenges 38, 180, 183; concept of 78; fragmented 260; map 80, 127; mechanism 184; system 128
global health education 292–293; *see also* Academic Global Health
Global Health Observatory (GHO) 36
global health security 92, 182; agenda 133, 289n8; approach 201
Global Health Watch 46, 62, 95, 97, 101, 104, 143, 152; Italian 20, 51, 170
Global Innovative Funding Instruments (GIFIs) 167, 271, 274, **275**, *277*
Global Observatory for eHealth 231, 235
Global Partnership for Effective Development Cooperation (GPEDC) 65–66
Global Public-Private Partnerships (GPPPs) 54, 57, 59, 65, *81*, 95–96, 156, 160, 162–163, *165*, 168, 175n1, 251, *270*, 271, 273, 282, 285; classification 70n13; initiative 281; model 60, 170; organizations 164, 166–167, 169, 172
Global Strategy on Diet, Physical Activity and Health 99, 121n12, 144
Global Strategy and Plan of Action on Public Health 119, 228

Global Urban Ambient Air Pollution
  Database 191
globalization 17, 23, 51, 134, 175n2, 185,
  202, 209, 220, 229; characteristic of 140;
  contemporary; definition 21–22; economic
  161; and health 24–25, *26*, 78, 81, 217;
  neoliberal 181, 189–191; process 69, 77, 150,
  198, 293, 300
governance; architecture 165, 182; challenges
  180–181, 231; component 103; global social
  149; and human rights 69; issues 18, 58,
  135; models 142; reform 102; scenario 185;
  structure 164, 174, 252; system 128, 168,
  234; the term 77
Great Acceleration 27
Great Depression 105
gross domestic product (GDP) 12–13, 16,
  57, 60, 136n1, 220; fractions of 273;
  global 21, 296; growth 19–20, 55, 252;
  per capita 127
gross national income (GNI) 127, 286–287
growth: economic 12–13, 16–19, 20, 54–55, 65,
  67, 109, 131, 189, 200, 251, 268, 283; zero
  nominal 48; zero real 48
Guterrez, A.M. 84

H1N1 *see* swine flu
H5N1 *see* avian flu
Harare Conference 53
hard law 79, 184
Health 4.0 229, 231–133
Health Data Collaborative 37, 289n8
health expenses 251–252
Health for All 45–47, 53, 94, 98, 180, 249,
  262, 301
Health Impact Assessment 181, 185n1
health indicators 20, 33–34, 36–7, 39, 41,
  130, 218
Healthy Life Expectancy (HLE) 20, 286
health policy 34, 41, 98, 119–20, 119, 153,
  259, 289n8; global 33, 152, 181, 249;
  international 78
health system' building blocks 247, *248*
High-level Political Forum 66, 86
HIV/AIDS 36, 55, **59**, 110, 130, 173–174, 198,
  221, 224, *271*, 274, **275**–276, 285; cause of
  162; control of 57, 101, 112; data on 113;
  emergence of 182; epidemic 55, 67–68, 85;
  fight against 56, 113, 132; treatment 98, 131,
  223, 151, 167
horizontal approach 269
hospital-centrism 262
Human Development Index (HDI) 16–17,
  28, 287
human rights 16, 24, 69, 79, 89, 127, 130, 161,
  190, 233; based development approach 17;
  for all children 88; fundamental 300; and
health 64; respect of 11, 84; violations 23,
  162, 219
hunger 56, 67, 154, 203–205, 208

immunization 48, 88, 131, 162, 171–172, 199
Import Risk Analysis (IRA) 207, 236n15
industry-wide approach 97
inequality 17, 20, 67, 109, 150, 155, 190, 198,
  200, 204; health 46, 196
infectious diseases 57, 59, 91, 130, 132, 193,
  199, 200, 214, 268, *271*, 274, 286, 289n14;
  centered action on 183; combat 55; control
  of 56, 94; outbreaks of 23, 182, 200–201;
  spread of 136, 191, 194, 197–198, 260;
  treatment of 131
influenza *see* flu
Innovation for Uptake, Scale and Equity in
  Immunization (INFUSE) 172
Institute of Health Metrics and Evaluation
  (IHME) 37–39, 269–270, *271*, 272–273, 285
integrated approach 52, 54, 57, 64, 98, 133,
  163, 286
international aid 12, 15, 51, 65
International AIDS Vaccine Initiative (IAVI)
  54, 162, 221
International Bank for Reconstruction and
  Development (IBRD) 11, 105, 107, 109
International Conference on Financing for
  Development 134
International Conference on Nutrition 209
International Conference on Population and
  Development 88
International Cooperation 11, 44, 61, 84, 132,
  268, 286
International Court of Justice (ICJ) 84, 86
International Development Association (IDA)
  107–109, **275**, *277*
International Federation of Pharmaceutical
  Manufacturers and Associations (IFPMA)
  149–150
International Finance Corporation (IFC) 107,
  111, 122n21
International Financing Facility for
  Immunizations (IFFIm) 63, 167, 171,
  176n11, 274, **275**, *277*
International Health Conference 24, 89, 94
International Health Governance 77–78
International Health Partnership 63, 70n15,
  70n16, 264, 281–282
International Health Regulations (IHR) 45,
  99, 101–102, 121, 133, 136, 151, 180, 182,
  200–201, 254, 289n11; definition 91–92
International Labor Organization (ILO)
  48, 78, *81*, 88–89, 108, 112, 164–165,
  176n6, **298**
International Lender of Last Resort
  (ILLR) 50

308　*Index*

International Monetary Fund (IMF) 15, 22, 28, 49, 50, 53, 56, *81*, 95, 112, 122n20, 122n25, 132, 160 219; beginning of 105; members of 107; structure and functions 106
International Monetary and Financial Committee (IMFC) 106–107
International Partnership against AIDS in Africa 54
international organizations 37, 47, 58, 63–64, 83, 90, 93, 95, 106–107, 121n5, 131, 144, 147, 157, 227, 260, 281, 284, 296
International Organization for Migration (IOM) 195, 213, *214*, 217, 236n20
International Sanitary Conference 78
International Telecommunications Union 233, 237n38, 237n40
International Tobacco Control Treaty 211
International Trade Organization 105, 113
internet health 229; *see also* eHealth
intersectoral approach 44, 46, 110
iron deficiency 205

Kanasnakis (Canada) 132
Key Indicators Surveys 35
Keynesian economism 182
Kyoto Protocol 197

Lancet Commission on Climate Change 193
League of Nations 11, 78, 83, 89 176n6
Least Developed Countries 62, 69, **225**, 285
Lee Wong, J. 62, 98–99, 121n12
Lee's flagship initiative 98
legislation based approach 79
Lehman Brothers 22
List of Essential Medicines 223
Local Health Systems 52–53, 199
low-middle income countries (LMICs) 34–35, 38, 40–41, 172, 175, 192, 210, 249, 252, 259, 269, 270, 286, 288n1, **299**
Lyon summit 130

McNamara, R. 15, 108–109
macroeconomic: approach 28; outcome 106; policies 48, 50, 55, 105, 108–109, 112, 136; process 191, 217; reforms 278
Mahler, H. 45–48, 52, 54, 94–95
malaria 33, 42n3, 55–56, 85, 88, 110, 173–174, 196, 210, 221, 224, *271*, 274, **275**, **276**, 285; control of 57, 131, 137n2; drugs 132, 167; epidemics 68; eradication 45, 48, 194; report 36; treatment of 63, 157n1
Malaria Indicator Surveys 35
Malaria Medicine Initiative 54
malnutrition 55, 109, 193, 196, 204–205, 219
market-based approach 208
Marmot, M. 98

Marshall Plan 11–12
maternal health 17, 36, 56, 85, 98, 216, *271*, 285
MDG summit 65
Mectizan Donation Program 142
medical expenses 251–252
medical tourism 118, 256, *257*
Medicus Mundi 150
mental health 90, **195**, 216–217, **218**, 219, 236n27, 262; disorders 215, 264n7; and well-being 68, 208, 259
mHealth 229, 231; *see also* eHealth
microplastic 192–193
Middle-Income Countries 20, 65, 110, 119, 127, 211, 249, 271–272, 287
migration 26, 38, 79, 194, 213, 217, 236n25, 263n30, 252, 256; direct drivers 195; health 214, 216, **218**, 236n23; human 191, 213; phases of *215–216*; policies 301
Millennium Declaration 17, 162
Millennium Development Goals (MDGs) 17, 33, 56–57, 67, 97, 108, 133, 173, 268, 274; health related 39, 63–64, 102, 183, 281–282, 285; achievement of 65–66, 109;
Modernization Theory 13
Monterrey International Conference 60, 271
mortality: maternal 33, 39, 57, 67–68, 253; rate 33, 55, 219; child 36, 39, 56–57, 65–66, 68, 112, 130, 133, 219, 253, 285, 287
Multilateral Investment Guarantee Agency (MIGA) 107, 122n21
Multiple Indicator Cluster Surveys 34–35, 38
multi-stakeholder approach 77, 161
Muskoka 64; Declaration 65; Initiative 133

Nabarro, D. 96
Nakajima, H. 95
National Evaluation Platform 41
National Treatment 115, 211
neglected disease 132, 171, 192, 201, 221, 287; tropical 68, 134, 235n3
neoliberalism 95, 189
New International Economic Order (NIEO) 14–15, 160
New Partnership for Africa's Development 132
New York Declaration for Refugees and Migrants 217
Nixon, R. 49
noncommunicable diseases (NCDs) 103, 183, 285–286, *257*; burden of 55, 65, 250, 258, 274; challenges of 102, 259; climate change on **195**, 197; control of 85, 100, 209, 289n14; reduce 68, 208
non-governmental organizations (NGOs) 23, 59, 78, *81*, 90, 93, 97, 101, 110, 113, 121n4, 131, 140, 147, 150–153, 158n4, 160–161,

166, 171, 173–174, 175n1, 207, 228, 251, 263, *270*, 273–274, 278–280, 282, 296–297, **298**, 300–301; business-interest 149, 158n3; definition 141, 146; public-interest 149, 158n3
non-targeted approach 110
North American Free Trade Agreement (NAFTA) 226
North-South approach 65, 67
nutrition 67, 87–89, 90n3, 110–112, 117, 131, 204, **206**, 208, 210, 220, 236n16, **276**; climate change on **195**; deficits 55; initiatives 133; policy 209; programs 109; transition 190, 204
Nyerere, J.K 14

obesity 235n10, 11; childhood 100, 203–204; epidemic 209
OECD/DAC 53, 57, 155, 269, 278, 285, 287
Office for the Coordination of Humanitarian Affairs (OCHA) 86
Official Development Aid (ODA) 14, 50, 52–53, 57, 60, 160, 271–273, **276**, *277*, 282–287, 288n3, 288n5; for health 55; verticalization of 285
Official Development Assistance in Health (ODAH) 127
Okinawa summit 56
OMOV principle 106
one health 134–136
Organization for Economic Cooperation and Development (OECD) 12, 17, 56, 65–66, 161–162, 212, 268, 284, 288
Oslo Ministerial Declaration 80
Ottawa: Declaration 94; Charter 53, 68
out-of-pocket expenditure 250, 252
Oxfam 151–152

Pan American Health Organization (PAHO) 53, 93, 121n9
Pan American Sanitary Conferences 121
Paris agreement 134, 197, 235n8
Paris Declaration on Aid Effectiveness 63, 65, 133, 281, 284
Pearson Commission 60, 160
people centered approach 153, 261
People's Health Movement (PHM) 150–151
petrodollars *49, 105*
phantom aid 283
Pharmaceuticalization 190
philantro-capitalism 156
Philip Morris 97, 211–212
Plan of Action on Nutrition 209
polio 132, 176n9, **275**
Political Declaration 85, 100, 209
pollution 13, 23, 62; air 191, 196, 197, 235n2; water 68, 258

poverty 14, 17–18, 53–54, 111, 131, 150, 154, 195, 198–199, 214, 219, 228, 236n31, 250–251, 264n7, 283, 292; eradication 57, 67, 108–109; reduction strategies 56, 162, 189, 272
Poverty Reduction Strategy Papers (PRSP) 53
Primary Health Care (PHC) 33, 45–46, 48, 53, 63, 94, 98, 100, 132–133, 202, 249, 289n8; selective 47
privatization 50, 69, 109, 120, 190, 200, 217, 248, *257*; health service 51, 143
program: aid 53, 278, 285; disease eradication 45, 95; disease oriented 48
project: aid 53, 277–279, 281, 285; approach 278, **280**
public health 62, 68, 87, 90, 99, 104, 110, 115, 120n3, 136n2, 144–145, 162, 167–168, 181, 182, 190, 192, 197, 199, 202, 207, 213, 219, 225–229, 232, 248–249, 251–252, 292, 301; advocates 54, 97; challenges 116–117, 119, 214; emergency 61, 101, 134, 199, 224; global 102, 201, 230, 234; international 78, 131, 140; interventions 183, 200, 202, **218**, 262; policy 98, 100, 153, 169, 236n19; practices 91, 231; problem 194; risk 92; schools 263, 293–294, 296–297; system 258, 288n2
Public Health Emergency of International Concern (PHEIC) 92, 101, 199, 201

qualitative growth 19
quality of care 38, **218**, 235, 261
quality data 39, 41

Reagan, R. 15
Realpolitik 79
Red Cross: International Committee of the Red Cross 147–148; International Conference of 147, 164–165; International Federation of the Red Cross and the Red Crescent Societies 147–148
refugees 23, 213–215, 217, 283, 287; health of **218;** *see also* migration
Regular Budget Funding 94
report: A better World for All 56, 162; Brundtland 18; CIPIH 226–227; CMH 55; Commission on Social Determinants of Health 63; Human Development Report 16; Intergovernmental Panel on Climate Change 193; Investing in Health 38, 51; UNAIDS Global AIDS monitoring 36; World Development Report 38, 109; World Health 62–64, 98, 100, 246, 249, 262; World Health Statistics Annual 36; World Malaria 36, 42n3
result-based management approach 103
return on investments 168

Index

Rockefeller Foundation 47, 94, 153, 156–157, 158n8, 162, 249
Roll Back Malaria 54, 130, 170, 176n19, 281
Rome Declaration 209–210
Roosvelt, F.D. 84, 105

San Francisco Conference 121n9
San Juan summit 129
SARS *see* severe acute respiratory syndrome
Save the Children 151
Sea Island summit 132
Seattle Conference 115
Sectorial Investment Programs 53, 289n7
sector-wide approach programs (SWAps) 53, 272, 278–279, *280*, 289n7
selective approach 51, 60, 63, 132, 170, 200, 252, *257*; *see also* vertical approach
Service Provision Assessment 35
severe acute respiratory syndrome 23, 55, 132, 182, 200–201, 292
sexually transmitted diseases 198; *see also* infectious diseases
sherpas 130
Sixth World Health Promotion Conference 62
smallpox 45, 91, 176n7
socialist internationalism 268
soft law 79, 184
South-East Asia Regional Office of WHO (SEARO) 93
state of health 24, 58, 258
Stop TB 166, 170; initiatives 54; partnership 143, 176n19, 281
Structural Adjustment Programs (SAPs) 15, 50–51, 105, 108, 248, 278
sustainable: agriculture 66, 208; economic growth 67, 251; health system 54, 96, 110, 251, 256
Sustainable Development Goals (SDGs) 18, 33, 35, 66–67, 183, 196, *216*, 217, **218**, 249, 251, 268, 281, 286; definition of 18; health related 37, 134
syphilis 45; *see also* infectious diseases; *see also* sexually transmitted diseases

TB *see* tuberculosis
Task Force on the Prevention and Control of Noncommunicable Diseases 85
Task Force on Tobacco Control 85
Technical Barriers to Trade 114–115, 211
telehealth 229, 231
Thatcher, M. 31
third sector 140, 145–146
tobacco 111, 119, 142, 213, 217, 236n17, 236n18, 236n19; control 151, 183, 212; epidemic 191, 210; industry 97–98, 144 211
Toyako Framework for Action 133

Toyako summit 64
trachoma 142; *see also* infectious diseases; *see also* sexually transmitted diseases
Trade Policy Review Body 114
Transatlantic Trade and Investment Partnership (TTIP) 62, 115, 226
Transnational companies 52, 59, 61, *81*, 141, 161, 210–211, 225–226, 251, 292
Transnational Hybrid Organizations (THOs) 164, **165**, 175n1, 260
trans-national non-state actors 77, 140, 149–150, 160, 164, 273
Transnational Relations 77
Troika 106, 219
Trump, D. 120, 190, 197, 254
tuberculosis 55, 68, 110, 130–133, 167, 173–74, *271*, 274, **275**, **276**, 285; global report 36; mortality 131, 210, 219; multi drug resistance 200, 224, 292; TB alliance 162; treatment 63, 221
typhus 91, 197, 221; *see also* infectious diseases

UN Climate Conference: COP21 134, 210; COP22 196
UN Economic and Social Council (ECOSOC) 66, 70n18, 84–86, 88, 112, 146–149
UN Secretary-General 55, 59, 65, 84–87, 113
UN Security Council 55, 70n12, 84–85, 120n4, 201
UN Trusteeship Council 84, 86, 120n4
UNAIDS 36, 42n4, 59, 63, 67, 70n16, 78, *81*, 87–88, 130, 173, **298**; origins 112; structure and function 113
UNITAID 63, 113, 143, 167, *175*, 176n19, 274, **275**, **276**
United Nations Centre on Transnational Corporations (UNCTC) 160
United Nations Charter 84, 88, 146
United Nations Conference on Sustainable Development (Rio+20) 18, 66
United Nations Conference on Trade and Development (UNCTAD) 14, 233
United Nation Department of Economic and Social Affairs (UNDESA) 86
United Nations Development Group (UNDG) 86–87
United Nations Development Programme (UNDP) 16–17, 19, 22, *81*, 88, 109, 112, 146
United Nations Educational Scientific and Cultural Organization (UNESCO) 48, 112, 233
United Nations Environment Program (UNEP) 15, 196
United Nations Framework Convention on Climate Change (UNFCCC) 196, 197

United Nations Fund for Children (UNICEF) 35, 47–48, 60, 63, 70n3, 16, 78, *81*, 87–88, 94, 112, 144, 160, 167, 170–171, 271, **275**

United Nations General Assembly (UNGA) 15, 63, 84–85, 87, 100, 121n6, 162, 209, 249

United Nations High Commissioner for Refugees 88

United Nations International Conference (UNHCR) 84, 87, 112, 213

United Nations Mission for Ebola Emergency Response (UNMEER) 201

United Nations Monetary and Financial Conference 105

United Nations Population Division (UNPD) 33

United Nations Population Fund (UNFPA) 63, 70n16, 78, *81*, 87–88, 112, **298**

Universal Declaration of Human Rights 24, 44

Universal Health Coverage (UHC) 34, 68, 70n15, 85, 102, 111–112, 134–136, 183, **218**, **231**, 32, 248–251, 259, 261, 264n1, 281, 289n8

Uruguay Round 113, 211

USAID 47, 94, 249, **298**

vaccine 63, 101, 110, 130–132, 154, 156, 163, 169, 171–172, 176n9, 183, 190, 199, 200–201, 221, 227, 247, 271, **275**, 288n1, **298**; anti- 256; for all 68, 249; HIV 162; *see also* immunization

vector-borne disease 193, 194, 198–199

Verona Initiative 54

vertical; approach 180, 183, 281; initiatives 54, 95–96, 101, 135, 285; programs 47, 95, 170, 199, 274

verticalization 285–286

Virchow, R. 197

vitamin A deficiency 205

Washington: Consensus 15, 28n2, 50; Declaration 84

water-borne diseases 68, 192–193

welfare 17, 50, 69, 90, 117, 155, 222, 288

Wellcome Trust 156, 158n8, 201

Western Pacific Regional Office of WHO (WPRO) 93

WHO Global Outbreak Alert and Response Network 132

WHO Health Systems Framework 247

World Bank 15, 22, 28n2, 38, 47, 51–53, 58, 63, 79n16, *81*, 88, 89, 94–96, 105–106, 122n22, 132, 134, 146, 155, 157, 166, 171–173, 236n38, 268, 273, **275**, 280–281, 286, 289n7, 297, **298**; activity of 50; Advisory Board 108; group 11, 107–108, 112; health policies 109

World Economic Forum (WEF) 63, 133, 137n6, 161–162, 174

World Food Program (WFP) 78, 87–88, 112, 143

World Health Assembly (WHA) 46, 90–5, 99, 100, 102–103, 121n8, 121n9, 153, 196, 209, 211, 215, 217, 223, 226–228, 230, 233–234, 249, 302n1

World Health Organization (WHO) 24, 26, 36, 44, 70n16, 86, 88, 97, 131, 140, 189, 191, 260, 280, **298**; health system approach 246; origins 78, 89, 94

World Health Statistics 36

World Intellectual Property Organization (WIPO) 119

World Meteorological Organization (WMO) 194, 197

World Organization for Animal Health (OIE) 236n15

World Telecommunications Standardization Assembly 233

World Trade Organization (WTO) 52, 61–62, *81*, 113–119, 122n29, 152, 205, 207, 211–212, 222–224, **225**, 229, **298**, 301; Ministerial Conference 114–115

years lived with disability (YLDs) 38

years of life lost (YLLs) 38

zika virus 199, 254; *see also* infectious diseases

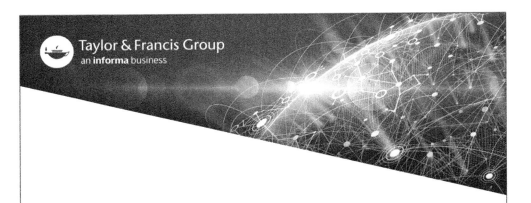